SURVIVING AND THRIVING
ON THE LAND

SURVIVING
AND THRIVING
ON THE LAND

How to use your time and energy
to run a successful smallholding

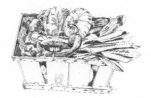

Rebecca Laughton

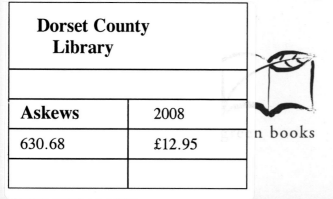

n books

First published in 2008
by Green Books Ltd
Foxhole, Dartington
Totnes, Devon TQ9 6EB

Text printed on 100% post-consumer waste paper.
The colour plates and covers are on 75% recycled materials.

Printed by TJ International Ltd, Padstow, Cornwall, UK

ISBN 978 1 900322 28 7

Contents

Dedication

I dedicate this book to all those who are working to create a greener, more socially equitable future. May your wisdom, vision and generosity endure.

I would also like to dedicate it to the memory of Samson, the Shire horse at Tinker's Bubble, who died in March 2008 aged 21, after 13 years of service and companionship. His strength, character and gentle nature made him a central part of the community, and fired my enthusiasm for the potential of draught-horses to contribute to sustainable agriculture.

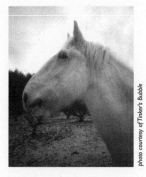

photo courtesy of Tinker's Bubble

Acknowledgements

Many, many people have helped and inspired me during the journey of writing this book. Their help has come both in obvious and in more subtle ways, and I am indebted to each and every one, whether or not they are mentioned here. I would specifically like to thank the following people, without whom writing this book would have been impossible.

Firstly, thanks must go to all the smallholders and community members, who generously shared with me their time, knowledge and experiences, to provide the interview material upon which this book is based. Often they also hosted me, for a meal or several days, sometimes I worked alongside them, and all have been willing for me to ask searching questions in my quest to learn about how they manage their own energy, whilst working the land. I count myself as fortunate in having made many new friends in the process of this research, and deepening friendships as a result of the conversations provoked by the interviews.

Whilst writing, I have been able to enjoy the almost perfect balance of head and hand work, through living and working at Tamarisk Farm, in Dorset. Daily contact with the soil, plants in the market garden, and animals on the farm, has kept me in touch with the realities of working the land, providing further valuable inspiration and time to think about ideas before returning to the computer. Thank you to Josephine and Arthur Pearse, and to Ellen and Adam Simon, for giving me this opportunity. Thanks also to my fellow WWOOFers at Tamarisk, whose good humour and support have carried me through this project.

The following friends and family members have offered constructive comments and proofreading services: Nigel Buchan, Wilf Richards, Simon Fairlie, Peter Wright, Jonathan Rouse, Adam and Ellen Simon, Josephine Pearse, Clare and Anthony Laughton. Other friends and colleagues provided specific practical help and encouragement along the way. They include Kristin Olsen, who hosted me for a month in Edinburgh and encouraged me to explore the possibility of writing a book about human energy; Diana Jansen, for her enthusiasm about my initial ideas; John Coleman, who helped me to find a publisher; Barbara Beyer, Mark and Catherine Beaumont and Simon Fairlie, who lent me books and journals; Tim Crabtree, who shared his knowledge of Community Land Trusts; Carolyn Spencer and Avril Taylor, who have helped me understand the importance of prioritising personal needs as a first step in balancing the human energy equation; and Rob McCall, who has offered encouragement and support during the final stages of writing.

In recent months I have benefited from the experience and advice of my editor, Amanda Cuthbert, and the rest of the team at Green Books. I would like to thank them for their support and patience when the pressing needs of the market garden have competed with writing time.

I am also grateful to Andrew Leppard for embracing the job of illustrating *Surviving and Thriving on the Land* so wholeheartedly, and for his patience during the creative process.

I would like to thank my parents, Anthony and Clare Laughton, for keeping faith in me despite my choosing to follow an unorthodox path in my life.

I think I would have been less likely to start on this adventure of low-impact, land-based living, had it not been for Ben Law, who first showed me that it is possible. Without his courage, imagination and ground-breaking example I might well have chosen a more conventional route towards sustainable agriculture.

Above all, my appreciation and heartfelt thanks go to both past and present members of the community at Tinker's Bubble. My four and a half years there changed my life in countless ways, and provided the most significant inspiration of all, to start investigating how to balance low-impact living, earning a land-based livelihood and being part of a community. Each and every individual that makes up the community has taught me valuable lessons, and the joy and strength I feel from belonging to such a group are immeasurable. I am deeply grateful that they have trusted me to write this book, and encouraged me each step of the way.

Introduction

Living lightly on the land can be both a deeply satisfying and a pleasurable experience, and extremely hard work. Unfortunately, in traversing the narrow tightrope between these two extremes, many people and projects topple over into exhaustion, illness or stress-induced conflict, and the potential benefits of their activities are lost as they give up. Yet as the imperative to cut fossil-fuel use increases, both to reduce greenhouse gas emissions and conserve our dwindling oil supplies, the matter of deriving an ecologically sustainable livelihood from the land may turn from one of choice into one of survival. If a project is failing, it may no longer be as easy as it is now to get another job and buy food, fuel and other necessities. This book starts from the premise that meeting one's needs for shelter, food, fuel, water and livelihood directly from the land, using minimal fossil-fuel-powered machinery and off-farm inputs, is a practical and powerful way of solving the pressing problems which are afflicting Planet Earth.

For four and a half years I lived at Tinker's Bubble, a small community which endeavours to manage 40 acres of forest, grassland, vegetable gardens and orchards without the use of fossil-fuel-powered machines. Trees are felled using hand tools, extracted with a shire horse, Samson, and planked-up using a saw bench powered by a wood-fuelled steam engine. Hay is cut with scythes, turned by a horse-drawn tedder (hay turner) and gathered in on a cart, and gardens are cultivated mainly with hand tools, but occasionally a horse-drawn plough or harrow. Houses and communal buildings are built by residents using timber grown on site mixed with a variety of recycled materials, bought-in straw bales and subsoil. Space and water are heated by stoves fuelled with hand-cut firewood, electricity is generated by wind and solar power, and communal meals are cooked over an open fire or a wood-fuelled Rayburn. It would be inaccurate to claim that the community is fossil-fuel-free, since paraffin is used in hurricane lamps when the electricity fails, two shared cars are run off-site, some food is bought in, and much of the equipment used is made from oil (polytunnel plastic, plastic mulch, solar panels etc). However, the policy of not using fossil-fuel-powered combustion engines has given me a deep insight into the issues, pleasures and sheer hard work of life without abundant oil.

Above all, the experience of living at the community has made me aware that for a project to be sustainable it is not enough for it to be ecologically benign and economically viable. If the people who make the project happen are not happy, healthy and willing, its long-term future is likely to be uncertain.

The effects of human-induced climate change are showing themselves already. Melting ice caps and permafrost in the Arctic and Alaska, and extreme weather conditions such as droughts, floods and hurricanes are causing devastation worldwide, and are making the urgency to dramatically reduce our CO_2 emissions greater than ever. Significant steps that can be taken to cut CO_2 emissions include production of our food, wood-fuel and building materials and energy provision from renewables such as wood, wind, sun and small-scale hydroelectricity generators. However, widespread adoption of these practices will not occur unless the people who are choosing to live in this way are leading healthy and fulfilled lives. And without the widespread adoption of energy-efficient living, the rest of us may as well not bother because climate change will happen anyway.

It was with these ideas in mind that I set off on my bicycle in 2005 for a seven-month sabbatical to visit organic farms and communities in the UK and France. I was particularly interested in learning more about how working horses could be used in growing vegetables, and had heard that in France this is more common than in the UK. At this stage my aims were purely personal, to find out how other people were managing to derive a livelihood from the land, whilst living sustainably both in ecological and human energy terms. It was, and still is, my intention to set up a project to supply organic fruit, vegetables and eggs to local people, whilst living in a way that will make other people want to emulate my environmentally low-impact lifestyle. I created a set of 12 questions to ask people at each of the projects I visited, to find out how they felt their land-based livelihoods and lifestyles were affecting them (see Appendix 1).

Starting in April 2005 I cycled through France, staying at four different organic farms and communities during four months. As I talked to people about their experiences, asked my questions and had countless hours to think whilst weeding long rows of vegetables and pedalling my way across country, my ideas developed and this book was conceived. I returned to England and continued my journey, also visiting projects in Wales and Scotland. As the days grew shorter, my deadline for returning home grew closer, and the list of interesting places to visit grew longer, I started travelling by train as well as bicycle! On my way I attended a two-week Permaculture Design Course at Ragman's Lane Farm in Gloucestershire. Throughout my travels I was encouraged by others to write about how people maintain their health, energy and enthusiasm whilst working on the land. I was amazed to find, when I started searching for literature, that very little has hitherto been written about it.

Since beginning my journey I have visited 28 farms, smallholdings and communities, and interviewed over seventy people who are involved in land-based activities, either commercially or for subsistence. My interpretation of these case studies is based on over ten years of working on farms and market gardens, and academic study of sustainable agriculture, as well as a broad knowledge of local food production and marketing gained whilst working for Somerset Food Links. The case studies I refer to include farms and communities that have been working well for a long time, as well as ones that are struggling or have even had to stop due to shortages of human energy. Others are in their infancy, still full of optimism and the energy of youth, yet in a position to benefit from the experience of more established projects. Only time will tell which of these have found a successful formula for survival.

Whilst most of the smallholdings, farms and communities described are named, a few requested that their identities and locations were not revealed. In these cases, therefore, I have changed the names of the smallholdings or communities, and the individuals involved. I would like to request on behalf of the projects I have described, that readers have respect for the privacy and time of the people running them. While some run courses or host visitors through exchange schemes such as WWOOF (World Wide Opportunities on Organic Farms), too many offers of help or requests for information can become overwhelming. Every year more land-based projects are becoming established, and I would encourage anyone seeking experience of smallholdings or communities to look beyond the ones described in this book to those listed by WWOOF or in directories such as *Diggers and Dreamers* (see Appendix 2).

The scope for this book is enormous, and I am aware that I am only skating over the surface of subjects that demand much more thorough examination. My main objective is to pass on the experiences that people I met on my travels were kind enough to share with me. By highlighting some of their choices relating to energy use and quality of life, I hope to help those who are embarking on land-based initiatives improve their chances of designing a truly sustainable project. However, I also hope that my findings will stimulate further discussion and that perhaps others will develop these ideas to greater depth. I, meanwhile, will be returning to the field to grow vegetables, plant fruit trees, and apply the lessons I am attempting to convey in these pages to my own life!

Chapter One

The Human Energy Equation

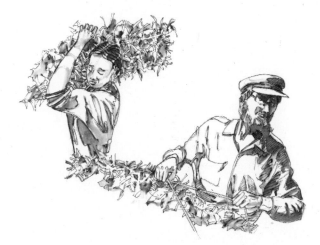

A new generation of small-scale, land-based initiatives is establishing itself throughout the United Kingdom. These include smallholdings, organic farms, land-based communities, forestry initiatives, permaculture projects and community-supported agriculture schemes. The people starting these initiatives are usually driven by a desire to address some of the pressing environmental problems of the twenty-first century, such as climate change, biodiversity loss and soil erosion. Often those wishing to work on the land see their domestic arrangements as part of an integrated endeavour to minimise their personal environmental impact. Alongside organic farming or forestry, they choose to build energy-efficient homes from local or recycled materials; harvest rainwater from their roofs; generate electricity using wind generators, solar panels or hydroelectric turbines and use firewood for cooking and heating their homes. Some smallholders wish to meet the growing demand for food which has been produced locally to high environmental standards. Others are motivated by the belief that their quality of life will improve if their own basic needs are met directly by living and working on the land. Their food will be fresher and taste better, their water cleaner, their environment more pleasant, they will be able to work from home and spend more time with their families, and they will have the freedom to choose how to use their time.

The price of bucolic bliss

Such an idyllic rural existence is entirely achievable, but it comes at a price – hard work. To generate a livelihood from the land in modern Britain, whilst minimising your environmental impact, is demanding. Firstly, for the aspiring self-sufficient or commercial smallholder, finding an affordable property is a challenge. Buying a bare land holding, let alone a house with enough land to grow your own vegetables and keep a few chickens, is an expensive business, unless you have large reserves of capital or a well-paid job. Secondly, despite the recent increase in demand for local and organic food, it is still hard for farmers to charge prices that realistically value their time as well as covering the cost of production. The establishment of a successful agricultural enterprise requires skill and efficiency, imaginative marketing skills and the willingness to work extremely long hours for very low pay. Thirdly, government bureaucracy and manifold regulations – including DEFRA paperwork, organic certification, planning laws and environmental health legislation – result in time-consuming and sometimes expensive extra work. Without some forethought and care, the rural idyll can turn into a slog through a never-ending list of chores or a stressful succession of bureaucratic battles with various authorities.

At best, these clouds in the blue sky of bucolic bliss are frustrating and tedious. At worst they can lead to exhaustion-related ill health or injury, marital breakdown and sometimes, tragically, suicide. It can be hard to maintain motivation and harmony with your nearest and dearest when the work is relentless, financial viability uncertain, and security on the land or in your home tenuous. I know smallholders who have had to give up their dreams due to work-induced back problems, or the energy-sapping inconvenience of not being allowed by the planning authorities to live on their land. Others have come to grief when long working hours regularly disrupt family life, or stress and over-tiredness cause couples to get irritable with one another. Sometimes running a smallholding is more a matter of surviving than thriving.

Yet such discomforts and disasters are not inevitable. Organic farmers, market gardeners and self-sufficient smallholders have been enjoying the benefits of a land-based lifestyle for years. Some are running successful businesses selling fresh, high quality food to local individuals, shops and restaurants. Others are content to produce vegetables, eggs, cheese or meat solely for their own consumption, alongside other income-generating professions. There are those who operate alone or with their partner and family, and those who choose to live and work in a community, sharing responsibility for land and its produce. Sometimes life is tough for them, but they survive and on the whole they are happy and fulfilled.

I have written this book to help aspiring and existing, but struggling, smallholders find a way to thrive, rather than merely survive. My aim in visiting the smallholdings, farms and communities featured in this book, was to learn how I could maximise the chances of maintaining my own health, enthusiasm and energy while establishing an organic market garden. On the way I have discovered that there are many ingredients in the recipe for land-based projects which successfully meet the needs of the humans running them. I have used the term 'Human Energy' as a shorthand way of referring to the precious entity that enables people to maintain their physical and mental health, and remain motivated, happy and harmonious with their family and fellow workers, despite hard physical work, long hours and stressful times, when every job is demanding to be done immediately. Like a natural resource, such as fish or wild herbs, human energy requires careful stewardship in order to prosper and multiply.

What is 'Human Energy'?

The word energy has a variety of meanings, depending on the context in which it is being used. It is defined in the Oxford English Dictionary firstly as, "force, vigour (of speech, action, person etc); active operation, individual powers in use; latent ability".[1] Secondly, there is a scientific definition, "the ability of matter or radiation to do work" before the dictionary goes on to define the different types of energy – kinetic, potential and mass energy. We are interested in how to maintain the ability of humans to work on smallholdings – an occupation which requires considerable vigour, force and active operation!

Whilst physical energy is a vital ingredient in the ability to run a smallholding, equally important for the farmer are mental and emotional energy. Without these, quality of life is diminished and the length of time the smallholder will continue is likely to be curtailed. Scientifically speaking, human energy comes from the chemical energy contained in food, but the definition of human energy used in the context of this book is broader and includes:

- Physical energy – Energy required to perform work and play; physical health.

- Mental energy – Ability to engage mentally in the project, juggling several tasks, such as gardening, animal husbandry, marketing and childcare. Decision-making and problem-solving both require mental energy.

- Emotional energy – Feeling happy, or at least content; support from those around you; being appreciated for the role you play.

- Spiritual energy – Feeling of fulfilling one's role on Earth, vocation; opportunities to be creative; integrating spiritual values into daily life.

Physical energy

This is the energy used when humans work, and is the result of respiration; the 'burning' at cellular level of the chemical energy contained in food. Respiration is a combustion reaction, akin to burning wood or oil, which produces carbon dioxide and water as by-products of heat, light and the ability to perform work. Hence, food can be seen as the 'fuel' which enables muscles to contract and provides physical human energy – the ability to run, dig, lift or do anything else that requires exertion.

A balanced diet, composed of carbohydrates, proteins and lipids, or fats, should provide a healthy human being with sufficient energy to undertake some degree of physical work, depending on one's level of fitness. Most of the energy liberated in aerobic respiration comes from the oxidation of hydrogen to water. The energy density of different food types depends, therefore, on the number of hydrogen atoms in the food substrate molecule. Lipids, or fats, have more hydrogen atoms per molecule than carbohydrates, and so lipids have a greater energy value per unit mass, or energy density, than carbohydrates or proteins, as shown in table 1.1 below.[2] In practical terms this is evident when hard physical work increases our desire to eat thick slabs of butter or cheese. The high energy density of lipids is reflected by the traditional diets of land-based labourers, which often contained significant amounts of fatty foods such as bacon, suet, lard and cheese, whenever they were available. Although proteins have a higher energy density than carbohydrates, they tend to be used for growth and repair of cells rather than as an energy provider, except in the absence of carbohydrates and lipids.

Respiratory Substrate	Energy Density (kJ g-1)
Carbohydrate	15.8
Lipid	39.4
Protein	17.00

Table 1.1 – Typical energy values of different food types.

Refined sugar in cakes, biscuits, drinks and cereals can give an instant energy boost because it can quickly be broken down into glucose and transported to cells via the bloodstream. It is the complex carbohydrates (rice, millet and root vegetables) that provide sustained and stable energy levels, as sugars are released more slowly. Over-consumption of highly processed sugary foods and cereals has led to increased incidence of diet-related illnesses, such as diabetes. Other conditions, such as food intolerances related to gluten, are more controversial. The symptoms of gluten intolerance include fatigue or tiredness, and many people who have cut out gluten from their diets claim to have significantly more energy and motivation. However, many health professionals and organisations are sceptical about whether the prevalence of gluten intolerance is on the increase, and caution against exclusion diets which they believe can lead to poorer nutrition.

Closely related to physical energy is injury. Back pain, slipped discs, repetitive strain injury, broken bones, sprained joints and other injuries can temporarily, and sometimes permanently, impair our ability to do physical work. Such problems can have a severe impact on the viability of businesses, especially when they put someone out of action at a critical time like hay-making or lambing. Their cause may be something other than land-based work, but the physical nature of farming exposes people to the risk of injury, especially when they are unaccustomed to manual labour. Injuries are sometimes caused by over-exertion or loss of concentration, due to fatigue. In other cases, wear and tear on joints as a result of age and prolonged strain is the main culprit. It is possible to reduce the risk of injury by learning techniques, such as how to lift heavy weights, and by adopting a mindful attitude to the way we use our bodies. Likewise, the thoughtful design of systems to avoid excess carrying of, for example, bales or manure, combined with the appropriate choice of equipment, can ease strain on joints and muscles. Investment of time and attention in such skills and details of design is invaluable, since an injury which could have been avoided can return to haunt you over years and may eventually put an end to dreams of a land-based lifestyle.

Mental energy

By mental energy, I mean the energy that is required to think clearly and solve problems. In some ways it is easier to describe the absence of mental energy. All readers will at some time or another have experienced the very specific kind of exhaustion which comes from mental over-exertion. It is the feeling you get when you've worked at a computer for hours, or endured a long and intense meeting. It is a very different fatigue from that experienced after physical exertion, which can be quite pleasant as long as you have got the time to rest and enjoy it. Compared with the mildly aching muscles and sense of having stretched yourself that comes from a day's gardening, hay-making or a long walk, mental tiredness results in people feeling less alert, indecisive and downright lethargic. From time to time, such a feeling of fatigue is perfectly normal. However, when it becomes a chronic condition that impairs people's ability to make decisions, plan each day's activities or engage mentally in their work, mental exhaustion can reduce quality of life. It can even lead to illnesses such as depression, anxiety or chronic fatigue syndrome.

Smallholders need mental energy as much as physical energy. An alert mind and an ability to make decisions and solve problems are needed to plan crop rotations, care for animals, maintain infrastructure and equipment, and make a smallholding work financially. Management of a piece of land, especially for your livelihood, usually involves juggling several projects simultaneously which, like juggling balls, requires extra concentration. Few people are smallholders in isolation. They will have other responsibilities, roles and perhaps other employment. It may be necessary to integrate the demands of the land and its livestock alongside domestic duties, another job, or looking after dependents such as children or elderly relatives.

As the number of 'balls' which are in the air increase, so do the mental demands of the project and above a certain threshold, the stress of 'keeping them in the air' starts to become apparent. This threshold varies greatly between individuals. Some people like to focus on doing one or two things well, while others enjoy the diversity of managing multiple enterprises simultaneously. The latter seem to take a more relaxed approach to 'dropping balls', believing that the projects which are meant to succeed will survive whilst the others will fall by the wayside. For the former, it can be a cause of stress if too many projects are taken on and 'letting something go' involves a patch of garden getting covered in weeds or an animal's routine being neglected. They may sacrifice their own needs (to rest or spend time with the family) to the needs of their farm, only to realise too late that their health or relationships have suffered.

Mental energy should not be seen in isolation from physical energy. Stress in itself is not harmful, but prolonged stress results in the body producing copious amounts of stress hormones called cortisols. These clog up cells and result in a lack of well-being and that 'tired all the time' feeling, which even sleep will not resolve. Our judgement becomes clouded, we become less efficient and we are prone to make mistakes and faulty decisions. Such mistakes can result in more work and stress, drawing the overtired smallholder into a vicious cycle of crisis and reaction. Continuous flooding of the body with stress hormones may impair the immune system, and render the individual vulnerable to a host of diseases.[3]

Such mental and physical disintegration can be avoided when a positive mental attitude is cultivated and the smallholder knows when to take a break and re-evaluate the situation. By consciously observing energy levels, it is more likely that stress or exhaustion is noticed in its early stages, and action can be taken to alleviate it, by re-organising responsibilities or asking for help.

Emotional energy

The way we feel undoubtedly affects our energy levels and zest for life. When we feel happy, optimistic or fulfilled, we are likely to have more energy than when we feel disappointed, frustrated or overwhelmed. Other emotions, such as anger or anxiety, seem briefly to intensify high energy levels before leaving a person feeling tired and 'spent'. Hence, our feelings or emotions are an important influence on the overall amount of energy we are able to invest in the land. Cultivating the necessary conditions to encourage 'energy-creating emotions' can increase the likelihood of the project being successful and long-lived.

The optimal conditions for promoting emotional energy for most people include healthy and nurturing relationships with friends, family and work colleagues; a pleasant environment; meaningful work; and security of home or land tenure. Feeling appreciated and loved by those around you, the sense of achievement from doing a job well and the enjoyment of a bright spring day or a beautiful view, all contribute to positive emotional energy reserves.

Our emotional and mental states are also influenced by diet.[4] Hence, food can affect motivation and the way we relate to others. Food assumes great importance when doing physical work, due to its role as a fuel providing the energy for labour. People unused to fresh air and physical work often comment on how their appetite and enjoyment of food increases when they help out on a farm or smallholding. Seasonal food picked fresh from the garden or produced by a local friend, provides not only nutritional benefits but also deep pleasure and satisfaction, due to the connection we have with its source.

Spiritual energy

I would add a final category – spiritual energy – to my definition of human energy. In the same way that all physical energy in plants, animals and the soil comes ultimately from the sun, some people believe that there is a spiritual force that provides all things with energy. Such energy has different names in different cultures, and belief systems vary about whether it exists in just humans, all living things or inanimate objects too. It might be seen as emanating from an external god or creator of life, or be an all-pervasive force that exists simultaneously in all creation, described by some Native American tribes as 'The Spirit that Moves through All Things'.

It is important to acknowledge that many people are motivated by their spiritual beliefs, adding another dimension to the interacting combination of physical, mental and emotional energy. For some, ecological protection is a moral issue, and the reduction of environmental impact is a vocation powered by spiritual energy. Others feel the influence of spiritual energy, or inspiration, when they allow themselves to be creative, whether they are making a chair, cooking a meal or building a compost heap. Most gardeners and farmers have experienced the sense of wonder prompted by the germination of a seed or the birth of a lamb, calf or piglet. Direct daily contact with such miracles enhances quality of life, and living in close contact with nature feeds people's souls. Another manifestation of spiritual energy is evident when groups of people live and work together harmoniously, overcoming the challenges of personal difference to become a community.

The demands on human energy

Farming – conventional or organic – has never been a profession that can be contained within the conventional working hours of nine to five, five days per week. As any farmer will tell you, theirs is a lifestyle rather than a job, and involves a 365-days-a-year commitment, and a willingness to rise early and work late in certain seasons. Organic farming is by its very nature even more labour-intensive than non-organic farming. The replacement of artificial fertilisers and pesticides with a more complex system of fertility recycling, crop rotation, natural pest control and physical removal of weeds, creates greater time demands and skill requirements. Organic farms tend to be more diverse than their non-organic counterparts due to the need to combine animals or green manures with arable crops in rotations, and require a wider range of skills. The knowledge and problem-solving attitude required to farm organically provide a degree of interest and challenge appreciated by many who have converted from conventional farming. For businesses that are too small or new to employ other people, the demands of running the farm will fall on the shoulders of one or two people, and careful planning is required to maintain energy and enthusiasm throughout the year. The demands on those employing others to work on the land are also continual, since the workforce must be supervised, often trained and cared for so as to sustain motivation.

A few organic producers are endeavouring to cut their carbon emissions further by minimising fossil-fuel use, which increases the demands on their own energy. Substituting human and animal power for machinery brings home the reality of the knowledge, skill and physical strength developed by our forefathers, who managed for centuries to produce enough food to survive without access to oil. Few people today possess the skills to live without fossil fuels, yet if we are to cut carbon emissions on a scale significant enough to curb climate change, we must find less 'oil-dependent' ways to produce our food. The incentive to do this may come partly from oil price rises, as global supplies of oil start to decline, but we need to act now if we are to combat the imminent effects of global warming. My experience of living in a community that has not used fossil-fuel-powered combustion engines since 1994 was enlightening. The practical skills and strategies I developed over my four years there, in response to the absence of mechanised alternatives, give me hope that we have the capacity to survive and thrive beyond 'peak oil'. However, much refinement is needed, since at times the combined demands of long hours, physical work and community life become overwhelming.

Those who are producing food for local consumption are likely to become engaged in some form of marketing their goods directly to the consumer. This creates an additional set of tasks on top of food production and land management. The extra margins gained from direct marketing, as compared with selling wholesale, are hard-won, owing to the time spent preparing produce and interacting with customers. Direct marketing of organic produce often includes an educational element, since many consumers are so disconnected from how their food is produced that they are unaware of seasonality, the variety of fruits and vegetables it is possible to grow in a temperate climate, and the costs of producing food organically. Convincing them that the higher prices demanded for organic food are not only justified by increased quality, but also bring environmental benefits, requires tact, imagination and patience.

Even those who are not producing food commercially have an educational role. People pioneering low-impact subsistence lifestyles on the land increasingly attract interest from a public hungry to learn more about how they can reduce their ecological footprint. Many projects host visitors, who may want to participate in daily life and learn land management skills. Hosting of visitors can take place formally, through WWOOF or an apprenticeship scheme, or informally. It requires the willingness to offer a friendly welcome and perhaps meals and accommodation, to interpret what the visitor is seeing while looking around, to answer questions (often repeated by every visitor!) and to provide some form of teaching. On the whole, hosting visitors is a pleasure, since they usually bring a fresh face and interesting insights to the project. However, at busy times of year, finding the time to show people around can be difficult, and at the end of a hard day many individuals or families want to relax alone. The media is also fascinated by people who have had the courage and foresight to develop ground-breaking environmental projects. Discerning which requests for television, radio or newspaper coverage will result in genuinely informative material, rather than just entertainment, is a skill in itself.

Since livestock need daily care, vegetable crops need watering, frost protection, weeding and harvesting, and customers expect continual, reliable service, it is difficult for people living on the land to go away. It is hard to find people with enough detailed knowledge and experience to look after a farm and direct marketing enterprise when the smallholder takes a holiday. Most other people with the necessary skills are too busy running their own farms. Yet farmers are only human and need breaks sometimes, like everyone else. Continuing year in, year out without respite can eventually lead to chronic exhaustion and loss of enthusiasm.

The domestic demands of living a low-impact lifestyle also add pressure. Cooking on a wood-fuelled stove or open fire takes extra time, forethought and skill. Heating both space and water with wood is also time- and energy-demanding, especially if it is all cut by hand. In the absence of a washing-machine, clothes must either be taken to a launderette or washed by hand. Not that low-impact living necessitates the avoidance of washing-machines. One community I visited was powering their washing-machine with electricity from a wind generator, and I have heard of several examples of pedal-powered washing-machines. However, the maintenance of renewable electricity equipment requires more effort than being connected to the grid, and usually at the most inconvenient times!

Then there is a whole plethora of green-lifestyle issues that affect non-land dwellers, but may be exacerbated by living in a low-impact home. An example is car use. A good environmentalist will try to minimise car use by cycling and using public transport. Yet in rural areas bus services are often less frequent, railway stations can be a long way away, and the distances involved in regular, functional journeys make cycling impractical because it would take so long. Another example is nappies. Washing terry towel nappies is generally agreed to be more environmentally sound than using disposable ones, but without a washing-machine nappy management can be very time-consuming or results in carbon-emitting trips to the launderette. As a friend of mine said, "Trying to live simply is really quite complicated!"

The above factors all contribute to a potentially exhausting lifestyle, and it is not surprising that most people compromise on some aspects of trying to live sustainably. Energy levels will vary according to the time of year and the amount of work being done, as well as from person to person. In an ideal situation it is possible to regulate your energy levels by working when you feel energetic and resting when you feel tired. However, when trying to juggle the multiple demands of a land-based business, the needs of family and friends and a green lifestyle, something usually has to give. Most often the need to rest gets neglected in the rush to get everything done – feeding animals, keeping on top of the weeds, maintaining a supply of produce for customers, getting meals on the table for the family, fixing the fence so the animals don't escape, cultivating while the weather conditions are right – there's never a time when 'it's all done'. Yet forgetting to rest can lead to chronic exhaustion or poor judgement, resulting in costly mistakes.

The psychological demands of being responsible for land and animals, staying in business and integrating into the community are also a frequent source of pressure. Prolonged stress may cause conflict amongst couples or communities, emotional problems and ultimately burn-out. Any family of a farmer will be involved in the farm to a large degree, but when long hours or emergencies regularly take parents away from the home or chronic stress makes them irritable, resentment can build. When land-based activities and environmental values consistently reduce quality of life, it must be questioned whether they are truly sustainable

People are as valuable a resource as water, soil, plants and animals, when it comes to creating social change, which is what the environmental movement must do. In permaculture, a design concept used for creating sustainable human environments, 'People Care' is viewed alongside 'Earth Care' and 'Fair Shares' as one of the three core principles that underpin permanent systems. Patrick Whitefield, one of the leading permaculture teachers in the UK, points out that whilst it is possible to care for the Earth without caring for people, in a free society a design which is perfect ecologically but does not meet the real needs of people will not succeed.[5]

If more people are to be encouraged to produce local, organic food whilst living low-impact rural lifestyles, the quality of life to be enjoyed from doing so must be seen to be equal to, if not greater than, their current quality of life. In its Living Planet Report, the World Wildlife Fund sets out possible scenarios for reducing the Global Ecological Footprint to a sustainable level by 2030, but points out that the political feasibility of achieving any of these targets is not proven. It concludes that "One Planet Living is possible and compatible with meaningful and rewarding lives for all. High rates of material and energy consumption are not necessary to support a decent standard of living."[6] As Meadows *et al.* state in *Limits to Growth: The 30-Year Update*, "We don't think a sustainable society need be stagnant, boring, uniform or rigid. It need not be, and probably could not be, centrally controlled or authoritarian. It would be a world that has the time, the resources, and the will to correct its mistakes, to preserve the fertility of its planetary ecosystems. It could focus on mindfully increasing the quality of life rather than on mindlessly expanding material consumption."[7]

A deeper cause of exhaustion

As well as the practical reasons described above, I believe that there is a deeper explanation for the weariness experienced by some of those striving to live ecologically sound lives on the land. These people are in fact shouldering a disproportionate share of responsibility for the well-being of Planet Earth and its future inhabitants. Joanna Macy, an environmental activist writing from a Buddhist perspective, speaks of the need to be "in league with the beings of the future".[8] Many of her workshops bring participants into a wider consciousness of the interconnected web of life to which they belong. Not only do an individual's actions affect other people, creatures and environments on Earth today, but the way we choose to live our lives will leave a legacy for future beings.

Much of Joanna Macy's work focuses on the issue of nuclear waste and the inadequate provision for protecting generations far into the future from its radioactive effects. The toxicity of the waste generated through nuclear power and weapons production requires that it must be kept out of the biosphere for many times longer than recorded history. Yet officials at one of the two main waste repositories in the United States admitted that the site would be safe for one hundred years or so, but seemed unconcerned by the risks to people encountering it after that. Researching the genetic damage caused by ionising radiation, Macy learned that the damage would accelerate over time, with the hazardous life of plutonium spanning a quarter of a million years. This discovery prompted her and others to establish the Nuclear Guardianship Project, to ensure that containers are monitored and repaired and technical knowledge of the dangers of radiation is passed on from generation to generation. What a responsibility to pass on to our descendants, who may well find it hard to believe that the people of today could knowingly generate and leave behind materials that could cripple and kill far into the future.

Reading about the Nuclear Guardianship Project gave me a new perspective on other environmental threats created by humanity and renewed my motivation to act. Why should future people and other species suffer from a destabilised climate, water shortages, infertile soils and polluted rivers, just so we can live a life of convenience and choice? Many have responded to such a question by choosing to live the lives of voluntary simplicity that this book is about, but they are still very much in the minority. They are thus carrying more than their fair share of the burden of duty to future generations, and that is hard work. Moreover, they are doing so within a culture that appears so oblivious to the environmental repercussions of modern consumer lifestyles, that the institutional and economic barriers described above make their task all the more difficult. People trying to live in a low-impact way on the land and produce food for their communities are swimming against a sometimes overwhelmingly strong current, and it is not surprising that they sometimes get exhausted.

Occasionally the accumulated stress, weariness and despair at the enormity of the challenges faced by the world result in paralysing depression. Depression is becoming increasingly common in today's society, but that doesn't make it any more bearable or less isolating when you are the individual experiencing that 'dark night of the soul'. As an environmentalist, an additional problem can be that many health care professionals simply don't understand the profound motivations that drive people to choose low-impact lifestyles. When in a state of confusion and disarray, being urged by a counsellor to compromise on deeply-held principles to make your life easier can deepen the sense of being utterly alone that is part of the territory of depression. Yet despair is a natural and healthy response to the threats to our global environment. By learning how to embrace depression and use it as a force for positive transformation, it becomes an experience that can be valued rather than dreaded. Joanna Macy's writing on despair work [9] combines psychological theory with a spiritual approach to environmental issues to provide practical guidance for jaded activists.

It is not just the front-line anti-road protesters, nuclear guardians and GMO campaigners who are activists. Those who are working to create an alternative system of food production and distribution, rebuilding local communities and pioneering low-impact lifestyles are activists who are just as vulnerable to despair. We may not be exposed to the trauma of confrontation experienced by those practising nonviolent direct action, but the stamina required to continue building a sustainable society year in year out requires deep reserves of emotional resilience.

The human energy equation

I set out on my journey around land-based projects with the question, 'How do people who earn their living from the land in an environmentally sound way manage to maintain sufficient human energy?' In order to answer this question, I decided to look at the problem in terms of a formula in which several variables contribute to a particular outcome in terms of human energy use. The ideal, on one side of the equation, is sustainable human energy use, and this can be achieved by different combinations of variables. As my most recent experience had been living in a community and managing the land without the use of fossil-fuel-powered machinery, my starting point was to look at the different social structures and kinds of technology that other people were using. However, as I explored the subject of human energy further, I came to discover other variables. These include different livelihood strategies; the layout and design of the smallholding; attitudes to work; patterns of work, rest and celebration; and the influence of age and role in life upon the time and energy people have available for their land project. I am sure if I continued to study human energy, several more variables would come to light. The main body of this book outlines how each of the variables listed above influence the ability of the people involved to sustain their physical, mental and emotional energy.

Before embarking on a description of the variables in the human energy equation, it is worth considering what we can learn from our farming forebears. Chapter Two, 'Energy Use Through the Ages' charts the history of agricultural development, highlighting the interplay between different technologies and rural social structures. Chapter Three goes on to ask 'What is the role of smallholders in twenty-first-century Britain?', and discusses the environmental and social issues which motivate people to farm organically on a small scale and produce food for local people. Chapter Four provides an overview of the projects I studied during my journey around France and the UK, which form the basis of this book.

The next three chapters focus on the role 'Tools and Technologies' play in reducing carbon emissions whilst balancing the human energy equation. Chapter Five discusses the role of design and choice of production system in the efficient use of energy. Chapter Six compares hand tools, horse-drawn tools and tools powered by an internal combustion engine. Chapter Seven considers different options for domestic energy use, including house design, firewood management systems and off-grid electricity generation.

Chapter Eight considers economic variables, such as how people can generate a livelihood from the land, ranging from pure subsistence to commercial operations; and the issue of buying or renting land. I then turn my attention to the variable of social structures. Chapter Nine, 'Living and Working Together', looks at various aspects of communal living and different ways of working the land in a group. Chapter Ten compares the experiences of people living and working alone, as couples or in families, in communities and in clusters of independent but co-operating smallholdings. In Chapter Eleven I examine how people of different ages manage to combine their changing roles in life and energy levels with working on the land. Chapter Twelve considers the final variable – attitudes to work, rest and play. The last chapter, 'Surviving or Thriving?', draws together all the variables, as I compare the different case studies and analyse why some are struggling, some are thriving and some are merely surviving.

So, I invite you to join me in reliving my journey of discovery into the subject of human energy. I have benefited enormously from the encounters I have had with the many smallholders featured in this book. I hope they will inform and inspire you to find ways that you can thrive on your land for many years into the future.

Chapter Two

Energy Use Through the Ages

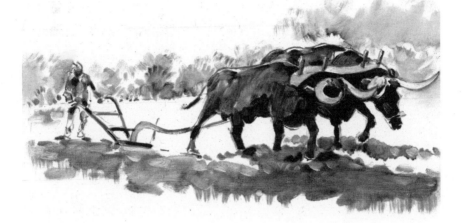

"Probably from very early times the history of agriculture in England has been largely that of change from semi-communal usages to a system of severalty, under which each individual owner or tenant could cultivate his individual plot of land in such fashion as best pleased him." – W. E. Tate[1]

Today's extravagant use of fossil fuels is the result of a long evolution of agricultural systems and tools. History can teach us many valuable lessons, and in trying to find solutions to our current predicament of fossil-fuel dependency, it is helpful to understand how people have used energy through the ages. Agricultural history reveals a number of striking trends that bear relevance to the subject of human energy. Firstly, there has been a movement over the last thousand years from semi-communal management of land to private ownership and management, which has allowed individuals increasing authority over the way in which they choose to farm.

Secondly, increased agricultural productivity has been brought about by a combination of improving yields on existing cultivated land and bringing previously uncultivated land (forest and scrub, wetlands and sandy heathland) into use. In the beginning, increases in yield were the result of observation of natural processes and ingenuity in adapting them to man's advantage – for example, folding sheep so their manure was concentrated where it was needed, and selectively breeding farm animals for advantageous characteristics. In the last two hundred years, many of the increases in productivity have been a result of fossil-fuel use. Early mechanisation of processes such as threshing were powered by coal-fuelled steam engines. Then in the twentieth century, oil-fuelled tractors and petroleum-derived agrochemicals further increased productivity per person involved in agriculture.

A third trend is the decrease in the proportion of the population engaged in farming, despite overall population growth. This was caused firstly by the severance of people from the land during the enclosure movements, and secondly the development of agricultural technologies, which replaced manual labour with machinery and, latterly, chemicals. In Britain in the twenty-first century, less than 2% of the population work in an agricultural industry that is highly dependent on fossil fuels.

Today we are faced with rising oil prices and the imperative to cut our carbon emissions. Yet, so far, very few farms have risen to the challenge of working the land without fossil-fuel-powered machinery whilst maintaining financial viability and sustaining human energy. History demonstrates that there is a close relationship between rural social structures and the kind of energy used in agriculture. Understanding this relationship could help achieve the goal of combining energy-efficient, sustainable agriculture with a quality of life which is acceptable to those working the land.

The measurement of energy

Work is measured in foot-pounds, and is done at different rates. It requires the expenditure or use of energy. The term 'power' refers to the rate at which work is done and/or energy is expended.

Since horses have been used for agricultural traction for much of history, the power of an average horse is the standard unit for measuring power. One horsepower-hour (hp-h) is the capacity to do 33,000 foot-pounds of work per minute for one hour, and is based on the ability of the average horse to lift 33,000 pounds one foot per minute for an hour. The maximum work capacity for a horse per day is about 10hp-h or a 10-hour workday.[2]

A comparison of the work capacity of a horse with that of a man and of a gallon of petrol gives a graphic insight into why technology has developed in its current direction, given the resources available. In a study of energy in 1979, it was stated that one man working a 10-hour day produces the equivalent of only 1hp-h, meaning that one man-power hour equals only about a tenth of a horsepower-hour.[3] Interestingly, 24 years later in 2003, Heinberg puts the average sustained human power output at only one twentieth of a horsepower-hour.[4] It is unlikely that this discrepancy reflects a genuine difference in the manual work capacity of human beings over a 24-year period. However, it is interesting to note how it corresponds with the decreasing importance of manual labour in industrial countries and perhaps reflects the corresponding enfeeblement of human beings. While humans appear weak alongside horses, the power of both is dwarfed by the capacity of oil to fuel work. A litre of petrol contains a tremendous concentration of energy – 8,200 kcal, to be precise. A mechanical engine is only 20% efficient in converting heat energy into mechanical energy, so only 1,640 kcal of work can be achieved with a gallon of petrol. Even at this low level of efficiency, this is still equivalent to 2.56 hp-h worth of work.[5] Table 2.1 provides an indication of how much energy is required by a human to perform various levels of work.

Sitting	19
Walking	130-240
Cycling	180-600
Swimming	200-700
Running	800-1000
Running very quickly	1240
Washing dishes	60
Washing clothes	125-215
Joinery work	195
Coal mining (average for shift)	320
Sawing wood	420

Table 2.1 – Energy requirements for various activities (kcal/hr).
(abbreviated from Pimentel and Pimentel 1979, p.31)

When considering energy efficiency in agriculture, a useful concept is the Energy Ratio (E_r), which measures the edible energy output divided by the energy input.[6] An E_r of greater than one indicates that more energy is harvested from a particular operation than is expended, whilst an E_r of less than one shows that the operation has not even managed to recoup the energy that was invested. Table 2.2 compares the energy ratios of farming systems across the world, and shows how industrial farming compares very poorly with subsistence and hunter-gatherer systems. This inefficient use of energy for producing food has been made possible by the availability of fossil-fuel energy that was cheaper than human labour throughout the twentieth century. Oil and other fossil fuels have made it possible for people to dramatically increase the amount of work they can perform in a given unit of time. Whilst during one hour a !Kung bushman of the Kalahari desert (hunter-gatherers) can gather 4.5 megajoules of food energy, a fully industrialised cereal farming system can produce 3,040 MJ. On average, the UK food system (1976) produced 30-35 MJ per hour.[7]

Er	Food Production System
0.13	Battery eggs, UK
0.34	All agriculture, UK (1968)
0.37	Milk, UK
0.85	Peas, UK
1.3	Allotment garden, UK; Rice, USA
2.5	Barley, UK
4.2	Sugar beet, UK
5-10	Tropical crops – some fertiliser and machinery
13-38	Tropical crops – subsistence, hand tools
42	Chinese peasants 1930s

Table 2.2 – Energy Ratios for Food Production
(abridged from diagram in Leach 1976, p.8)

It is also interesting to consider the relationship between land area, energy and different farming systems. For example, shifting cultivators have very low inputs and outputs of energy per hectare, and therefore need large acreages (10-140km²) to provide an adequate diet for each individual. In contrast, fully industrial farming systems growing staple crops such as cereals and potatoes, produce enough from a single hectare to feed 10-20 people on an all-vegetable diet. However, these systems are reliant on high inputs of fossil-fuel energy, and compared with shifting cultivation systems show a marked tendency towards diminishing returns.

A global comparison of farming systems on this basis reveals a couple of particularly interesting results. Chinese peasant farming systems display a very high output of energy per hectare, resulting from intensive manuring, inter-cropping and double cropping, showing that manual cultivation of very small plots (230m²) is a highly efficient and productive way of producing food. Although not quite as productive as Chinese peasant gardens, UK allotments showed energy outputs comparable with the best industrially cultivated farmland, for comparable energy inputs. The difference is that human labour rather than fossil-fuel-powered machinery constitutes 30% of the energy inputs into an allotment. Again, the high labour intensity and small-scale nature of allotments meant efficient use is made of space through inter-cropping, enabling a 250m² plot to provide all the protein needs and one-third of the energy needs of an average Briton.[8]

Early tool use

The use of tools is a feature that distinguishes human beings from other animals and enables them to utilise energy resources, and thus achieve greater productivity than they could using only their bodies. Whilst some animals are known to use tools, only humans have developed their use to the extent that modern society is dependent on a highly complex system of interrelated tools, including cars, medical equipment and computers. Archaeological evidence suggests that humans have been using tools for at least 100,000 years, and possibly longer.

Early tools were developed to assist in the harvesting of ever-greater amounts of energy from the environment. These started as adaptations of simple objects found in the environment, such as wood and flints, and evolved to meet the ever-more complex needs of the time. In his analysis of the interrelationship between energy, nature and society, Richard Heinberg provides a useful classification of tools relating to the energy that is used in their manufacture and the energy that they have the capacity to use:[9]

A *Tools that require only human energy for their manufacture and use.* Examples include stone spearheads and arrowheads, grinding tools, baskets and animal skin clothing. These sorts of tools are found in hunter-gatherer societies.

B *Tools that require an external power source for their manufacture, but human power for their use.* Examples: all basic metal tools, such as knives, metal armour and coins. These tools were the basis of the early agricultural civilisations centred in Mesopotamia, China, Egypt and Rome.

C *Tools that require only human energy for their manufacture, but harness an external energy source.* Examples: the wooden plough drawn by draught animals, the sailing boat, the fire drill, the windmill, the watermill. The fire drill was used by hunter-gatherers, and the wooden plough and sailing boat were developed in early agricultural societies; the windmill and watermill appeared at later stages of social evolution.

D *Tools that require an external energy source for their manufacture and also harness or use an external energy source.* Examples: the steel plough, the gun, the steam engine, the internal combustion engine, the jet engine, the nuclear reactor, the hydroelectric turbine and all electrical devices. These tools and tool systems are the foundation of modern industrial societies – in fact they define them.

Heinberg goes on to point out how this scheme of classification emphasises the cumulative nature of technological development. Whilst some Class A tools, such as flint blades, are still used in agricultural or even industrial societies, on the whole Class D tools did not exist in hunter-gatherer societies. Even though the categories do overlap to an extent (for example a Class D tool, the metal plough, pre-dates industrial society by three millennia), the scheme shows a trend over time of increasing capture of energy from sources external to the human body. In turn this captured energy was used to fashion even more sophisticated energy-capturing and energy-reliant tools and tool systems.

Some of the key developments in the capture of external energy in social history include: the use of fire; the domestication of animals for draught power; the invention of the wheel; wind and water power; the transfer of dependence on wood to coal (1300-1600) and the meteoric rise in the use of oil, beginning in the late 19th century.

Like animals, early humans had only their own energy available for the gathering of plants and hunting of other animals. Evidence suggests, however, that they used it so efficiently that they had time for leisure and were able to lead a rich cultural life.[10] Fire was one of the first tools with which primitive man started to colonise his environment. It was about half a million years ago that humans began to conquer their fear of fire and instead control it and use it to ward off large animal predators and clear vegetation.[11] Domestic fires also provided warmth in cold climates and the means to cook food, increasing the digestibility of certain grains and destroying micro-organisms responsible for food spoilage. With fire it also became possible to dry surplus meat and plant foods, thus stabilising the availability of food supplies for a long time after the harvest. Swidden agriculture, which uses fire to clear areas of forest for cultivation leaving a flush of fertility in the ash, is still practised in many parts of the world, whilst open fires or wood-burning stoves are used for cooking throughout the world.[12]

Harnessing animal, wind and water power

The earliest records of animals being used as beasts of burden come from Egypt, where donkeys were being used in 3000 BC. By 2500 BC oxen and water buffalo were being used to draw ploughs. This represented a major breakthrough in the efficient use of time, with one hour of ox-power substituting 3-5 hours of manpower in cultivating land ready for planting.[13] It was not until the 12th century AD that horses became used as draught animals in any great numbers, as a result of the invention of the collar.

The invention of the wheel around 3000 BC significantly increased the load of goods that could be transported, without any added energy input, either by man or other animals, thus increasing the efficiency of draught power tremendously.[14] As well as pulling carts and ploughs, animals (oxen, horses and mules) also provided power for machinery which included grain mills, pumps to drain mines, and textile mills.[15] During the medieval period human and animal power was gradually supplemented by power from watermills and windmills. Windmills were employed to drain water, thus reclaiming land in low-lying countries such as Holland. An early use of both types of mill was for grinding grain, but gradual innovations enabled them to be used to power saws and looms, to crush ores and to make paper.

The open field system

In the manorial open field system of medieval times, although land (arable strips and common pasture) belonged to the lord of the manor, it was farmed co-operatively by freemen and bondmen. The strips cultivated by each villager lay next to one another, with no fences in between. Sowing and reaping had to be carried out simultaneously, since before and after the crop, stock would be allowed on the land. Hence, whilst villagers lived in family households, they were obliged to co-operate in the management of their strips.

The manorial system was one of strict rules, which enabled a stable, sub-sistence society to maintain itself but did not lend itself to agricultural experiment and progress.[16, 17] The relationship between the lord of the manor and the villagers was one of mutual dependency, since muscle power was more essential to the prosperity of the lord than money rents. It was a system of self-sufficiency rather than commercial production, in which few manufactured articles were bought and the only market for farm produce was in neighbouring towns. At a time when the law was powerless to protect individual rights, the collective responsibility of the manor resembled a trade guild which encouraged mutual help and protection. "Communities grouped together in villages were less liable to attack than detached farmhouses and buildings; and common methods of farming facilitated continuous cultivation which otherwise might have been interrupted by the frequent absence of able-bodied men on military expeditions."[18]

Enclosure

The most significant factor in the transition from open fields to private land ownership was enclosure. Between the 15th and 19th centuries a series of enclosure movements extinguished the commoning economies, resulting in many of the landless poor moving to cities.[19] Those in favour of enclosure argued that it was necessary for national interest, since privatisation of farmland resulted in innovation and improvements in efficiency. Yet there is evidence that developments in agricultural methods, such as the sowing of fodder crops on the fallows, were made in common field farming in the run-up to the parliamentary enclosures of the eighteenth century.[20] Undoubtedly the century from 1700 to 1800 was one of great agricultural productivity, producing not only enough food for a population that doubled, and grain for three times the number of horses used in the previous century, but also cereals to export to Europe.

The technical advances which made these increases possible were due to the innovations of large landowners including Jethro Tull (1674-1740), Lord 'Turnip' Townshend (1674-1738) and Robert Bakewell (1725-95). Jethro Tull invented the seed drill, which made more economic use of seed as compared with broadcasting. He also advocated frequent tillage before and after sowing, to keep crops clean of weeds and increase the fertility of soil by admitting more air and water into the tilth.[21] Lord Townshend's contributions to agricultural history resulted from his attempts to increase the productivity of the light, sandy soils of his Norfolk estate. This he did by a combination of adding marl (soil consisting of clay and lime), inventing the Norfolk four-course rotation, which eliminated the need to leave land fallow every two or three years, and introducing the use of root fodder, to enable sheep to be folded and concentrate their manure on limited areas of land. Robert Bakewell concentrated his attention on stock breeding, selecting both for strength and activity in carthorses and weight of meat in sheep and cows.

The nineteenth-century family farmer

By the nineteenth century farming was a family affair, with a man's children being treated as his servants and remaining obedient to their parents throughout their lives. A typical farmhouse comprised not only the farmer's dwelling, but also a dairy, wood-house, brew-house, cheese rooms and servants' rooms. At this time comparatively little money passed between employer and employed, and payment for work was in kind, with beer and vegetables being a common currency. The labourers, of whom there were many, comprising both men and women, either lived in cottages in the village, which had previously been freeholders' dwellings, or built their own humble abodes as squatters on fragments of neglected land. The farmer, or united farmers of the village, ruled the labouring poor. "These labouring men, like his own children, must do as the farmer thought best. They must live here or there, marry so and so or forfeit favour – in short, obey the parental head. They did not use the power circumstances gave them harshly; but they paid very little regard to the liberty of the subject."[22]

With time the role of the agricultural labourer was diminished, as steam-powered machinery became more common, resulting in another exodus of rural dwellers to industrial occupations. One role that did remain right up until the second world war, was that of the horseman. The size of a farm was discussed in relation to the number of plough teams it supported, with a pair of Suffolk Punch horses being capable of cultivating about fifty acres of land during the year. Ploughmen were responsible for tending their horses, as well as working them, and took great pride in feeding and looking after their teams.[23]

The rise of fossil fuels

Whilst coal has been used for at least 4,000 years, compared with wood it is a smoky fuel, and it wasn't until the 16th century that its use became widespread in Europe. Growing populations in Europe were putting pressure on its renewable, but not inexhaustible, energy reserves – the forests. Between 400 and 1600 AD the amount of forest cover in Europe was reduced from 95% to 20%.[24] Initially coal was used primarily for heating, but innovations including the transformation of coal to extremely hot-burning fuel coke, meant that by the 18th century coal was able to replace man- and horse-power.[25] The invention of the steam engine enabled coal to power trains (previously pulled by horses), ships (previously powered by human rowers or the wind), and agricultural processes such as threshing grains (previously done by humans).[26] The use of coal represented a significant shift from renewable energy sources, such as animal power and wood, to a resource which could not be restored on a timescale meaningful to humans. It fuelled the 19th-century transformation to a more urban, mass consumer society and led to an unprecedented surge in population growth.

The first successful drilling of commercial oil occurred in Pennsylvania in 1859, and it quickly became widely available as a cheap and superior lubricant for the proliferating motorised machines of the 19th century.[27] People rapidly found other uses for oil derivatives, including lighting (kerosene), to power boilers and, most importantly, to fuel the internal combustion engine. In tandem with the increased use in oil was the development of electricity. During the late 19th and early 20th centuries, electricity use became widespread in lighting homes and streets, powering trams and underground trains and automating production tasks previously carried out by skilled labourers.[28] In the mid-1920s, farms were first electrified, substituting manpower and steam engines for jobs such as milking, cream-separating, chaff-cutting and water-pumping.[29] However, it was after the second world war in 1945 that the combination of oil and electricity brought about revolutionary changes in agriculture.

Fossil-fuel-based food production

The post-war era of agricultural modernisation in the UK was a response to wartime food shortages and an attempt to increase national food security. The 1947 Agricultural Act forced farmers to increase mechanisation and use artificial fertilisers and pesticides to increase the yield per hectare. Such changes were fuelled by the availability of cheap oil during the 1950s and 1960s. For example the Haber-Bosch process, which combines atmospheric nitrogen with hydrogen to make ammonia, was invented in 1909 and now provides more than 99% of all inorganic nitrogen inputs to farms.[30] It is a highly energy-intensive process, which relies on oil being cheap and readily available. Increased use of nitrate fertilisers led to lush plant growth, the abandonment of fertility-building rotations and the increased cultivation of monocultures. The result was that crops became more susceptible to pests and diseases, which were treated with petrochemical-based herbicides and pesticides. Whilst this era brought about huge increases in arable, livestock and dairy productivity, the costs to the environment have been great. These include problems such as nitrate leaching, pesticide accumulation in wildlife, soil erosion and biodiversity loss.[31, 32]

Mechanisation, electrification and increased chemical use to a large extent replaced human labour and the use of draught animals in agriculture. In the United States in 1776, 70% of power was supplied by animals and 20% by men. By 1850 animal power had declined to 53% and manpower to 13%. One hundred years later, in 1950, animal power and manpower had declined to only 1%, whilst fossil-fuel-driven engines provided 95% of the power.[33] In Britain, the number of farm workers declined from 880,000 in 1951 to less than 200,000 by 2003, a loss of 700,000 (79%) over 50 years.[34]

The recent history or agriculture is one of subsidy-led surpluses in the 1980s, giving way to low commodity prices and livestock diseases (BSE and foot-and-mouth disease) in the 1990s and the early 21st century. Farmers have been financially squeezed between the costs of inputs (seed, agrochemicals and animal feed) on the one hand, and prices dictated by globalised commodity markets or supermarkets on the other, resulting in the concentration of land into larger holdings and many more farmers leaving what is now considered to be an industry. This situation has resulted in a level of high dependency on fossil fuels for all involved in modern agriculture. Small family farms do still exist, but are often supported by a second livelihood, with many farmers' partners having to go out to work as well as playing a supporting role on the farm.

Dependence on a dwindling resource

With oil prices expected to rise as a result of peak oil, the fossil-fuel-dependent modern agriculture system is in a vulnerable position.[35] So, for that matter, is the global food system which depends upon cheap energy to transport, process and refrigerate food. In his book about peak oil and its consequences, Richard Heinberg predicts that "the lower energy economy of the future will be characterised by lowered productivity. There could be a good side to this, in that more human labour will be required in order to do the same amount of work, with human muscle power partially replacing the power of fossil fuels. Theoretically this could translate to near zero unemployment rates." [36]

The 2007 Annual Soil Association Conference, entitled 'One Planet Farming', focused on how the organic movement should respond to peak oil. Speaking at the conference, Richard Heinberg stated that instead of shedding labour to become more efficient, a reduction in the availability of cheap oil would require more people to work on the land.[37] He spoke of how Cuba, when cut off from imports of oil and agrochemicals by the collapse of the Soviet Union, found that organic practices required between 15% and 25% of its population to be involved in food production. It is unlikely that such a high proportion of the UK population would return to agricultural employment. However, research by Essex University found that by using labour rather than off-farm inputs, organic farms provide on average 2.5 times as many full-time equivalent jobs as non-organic farms.[38] Yet even organic farming is highly dependent on fossil fuels, since many farms are highly mechanised.

**Box 2.1: Climate Change and Peak Oil:
two sides of the same coin**

At last consensus is being reached between those in power that human-induced climate change is a serious threat to the world. The question now is how to negotiate significant-enough cuts in carbon dioxide emissions at a global level to stabilise the climate and minimise the potential devastation. To keep average global temperature change at below 2°C, it is necessary to stabilise concentrations of greenhouse gases (carbon dioxide, methane and nitrous oxide) in the atmosphere at, or below, the equivalent of 440 parts of carbon dioxide per million. Taking into account the increasing world population, the declining capacity of the biosphere to absorb carbon emissions and the need to allow people in developing countries to increase their emissions as they improve their living conditions, George Monbiot calculates that to achieve such stabilisation people in rich countries will have to cut their carbon emissions by an average of 90% by 2030.[39]

Whilst world leaders haggle over who should take what action, it is imperative that those with knowledge of how to cut carbon emissions set about making the necessary

Box 2.1 (continued)

changes straight away. First and foremost this means reducing fossil-fuel use, either by using it more efficiently or by substituting it with alternative sources of energy. Since most of the materials we take for granted in everyday life rely on fossil-fuel energy in their production and distribution, there are countless opportunities for cutting carbon emissions.

A related issue is the fact that the age of cheap and plentiful oil is drawing to a close. Globally, we have been using oil faster than the rate of discovery of new reserves since 1981, and in 2004 found one barrel of Regular Conventional Oil (that which is cheap and easy to extract) for every five consumed. The production of oil in any country normally begins to decline when half the total available has been extracted. In the 1950s, geologist M. King Hubbard was ridiculed for predicting that this peak production point for US oil would be reached in 1970. He was later proved correct. During the 1990s oil geologist Colin Campbell revived Hubbard's ideas, predicting that 'Peak Oil' for global oil reserves would be reached between 2006 and 2015, leading to significantly higher oil prices. Many claim that improved technologies will make it possible to extract the less accessible oil from rocks, sands and shales. However, the rate of innovation in the oil industry, which already uses very sophisticated methods, is unlikely to meet the demand for a diminishing resource. Not only are the demands of modern, industrialised societies exceeding the supply of oil, but rapidly industrialising countries such as China and India are requiring more oil to fuel their development each year. The advent of peak oil is likely to be a time of international tension as competing nations vie with each other for access to the remaining reserves.[40, 41]

Hence, one of the resources that has been a main cause of climate change is becoming harder to come by, just as the consequences of its use are beginning to show themselves. The solution to both of these colossal and impending challenges is simple – we must all dramatically cut our use of fossil fuels. Yet such a solution is painful to those addicted to the pleasures and convenience of a society fuelled by cheap oil. Whilst opportunities for cutting carbon emissions abound, at present too few people are willing to make the changes necessary for a peaceful and fair adaptation to the post-oil age. One opportunity lies in a radical restructuring of the modern food production and distribution system, whose extravagant use of world resources is a significant part of the problem.

Communal counter-movements

Enclosure was a highly controversial policy, and history books are full of accounts of the petitions sent by commoners and the enraged writings of their more literate supporters. Since then, others have taken a more practical stance against the trend towards privatisation and technological innovation, by setting up communes to reintroduce the principles of collective land ownership and simple technology. Their roots vary greatly, with some – such as the monastic tradition – being motivated by spiritual asceticism, whilst others – such as the Diggers of the 1650s – were overtly political. It should also be noted that in much of the world, including parts of Europe, a more common system of land cultivation still exists.

19th-century communities

The 19th and early 20th century are particularly rich in examples of rural communal experiments. These include the Owenite communities, which were based on utopian socialist ideas, and John Ruskin and William Morris's romantic socialist, craft-based movements. Robert Owen (1771-1858) wanted society reorganised into communes ranging from 500 to 3,000 people who would combine self-sufficiency with communal eating and child-care.[42] Ruskin and Morris's socialism aimed "to save people from the alienation of industrialism and to narrow the distance between humans and nature", by creating communities based on labour-intensive land cultivation and craft production.[43]

Concurrent with the above movements, but different in emphasis, was the Chartist Co-operative Land Society, founded in 1845. Chartism was a socialist movement which campaigned for the vote and other workers rights. A scheme was devised by the charismatic Irishman Feargus O'Connor to settle large numbers of working people on freehold properties, thus qualifying them to vote in county elections. The Land Plan involved people sending in weekly subscriptions until sufficient money had been raised to buy an estate. This would be divided into two to four-acre plots on which modest cottages would be built, and these holdings would be allocated to subscribers by means of a lottery. Rents from the smallholders would provide funds for the purchase of further land. Three settlements were established, giving working-class people access to land, which many continued to farm up until the second world war. Whilst more individualist than the Owen- or Ruskin-inspired communities, the Chartist Land Plan created settlements of smallholders who co-operated closely with each other and with local farmers, as they learned how to manage their land to provide for their needs.[44]

Later in the century Whiteway Community was founded in Gloucestershire (1898). Although at Whiteway collectivism was steadily forsaken in favour of private ownership, at the beginning members worked the land communally and shared all possessions.[45] One hundred years later Whiteway is more like a village, with people going about their lives separately, but there is one significant difference relating to land-holding. As soon as the original settlers received the title deeds to the land, they burned them. As a result, all 40 acres of the site are still communally owned and a person wishing to live there or buy an existing house must apply to the meeting for the land their house stands on. Over the years people have rebuilt and extended their houses, meaning that even here there is an issue of affordability, since people selling their houses wish to sell for a reasonable price to enable them to afford another elsewhere. Despite this, for those who are content to remain at Whiteway, however grand or humble their home might be, the common way in which the land is held is a great unifier – and some of the equality craved by the early socialist settlers lives on.[46]

Community movements abroad

Overseas, other political, social and religious movements have deliberately followed a pattern of communal living and land-ownership, against a background of concentration of land into larger private farms. Of these, the Kibbutz movement in Israel, which began in 1909, is probably one of the largest in scale, with over 250 villages inhabited by 150,000 people.[47] Equality, democracy and common ownership are central principles of Kibbutzim. In its traditional form, Kibbutz society is wholly collective, from land-ownership to meal-preparation and child-care, and many Kibbutzim operate large agricultural and light industrial enterprises. Decisions are made at weekly general meetings, and worker/residents are not paid a wage, being provided instead with accommodation, meals and other material necessities. Apart from a few Kibbutzim which have chosen to evolve into ecovillages, the movement has no explicit environmental agenda, and largely practises mainstream, industrial agriculture.

During the past two decades the movement has experienced a decline, with children leaving their Kibbutzim when they grow up, and few new recruits being attracted to the communal lifestyle. Recently, however, values have shifted to a more subtle balance between collective responsibility and individual freedom, resulting in a new surge of popularity. For example, residents can now buy and sell their apartments, people are paid for their work, and services such as child-care and the dining room are run as private businesses. Kibbutzim retain some of their socialist values, such as taxing high earners to help the financially weak. The new freedoms have attracted back old Kibbutz members, as well as new residents wishing to escape the 'rat race' of modern urban society.[48]

Gandhi saw self-sufficiency and self-governance at personal and village level as central to the Indian independence movement. In his view, Indians had no need to drive out the English, "They will go away of their own accord when we have driven out all the evils which oppress us and keep us enslaved." [49] The practice of Swadeshi, the principle of self-reliance, entails reducing personal needs to an absolute minimum and then endeavouring to meet those needs, ideally at family or village level, through agriculture and craft work. Gandhi believed that by reducing transport and trade of vital foodstuffs, cloth and other necessary items, people could be freed from exploitative, bureaucratic and over-complicated systems and thus be able to live simpler, more contented lives.[50]

In his later life Gandhi lived communally with those who had come to learn from him, practising Swadeshi and strengthening their resolve to live exemplary lives of simplicity, truth and nonviolence. Everyone ate together and participated in all aspects of communal work, including cooking, sweeping and emptying the latrines. Alongside the study of Gandhi's doctrine, members of the ashram became apprentices in one or more crafts, with all being required at least to card and spin enough cotton to make their own robe. When they were ready, students would be given charge of a poverty-stricken village, to win it over to the common causes of truth and nonviolence, and help it to achieve self-reliance. This involved reviving ancient village industries, co-ordinating various trades and rotating crops to enable the village to become self-sufficient. Any surplus produce was sent to the distribution centres of the Association of Village Industries, from where they were sent to shops in towns and sold at fixed prices.[51]

One of Gandhi's followers was Vinoba Bhave, who perhaps did more than any other person to spread and develop Gandhi's ideas of nonviolence and self-reliance. He established another ashram near Wardha in Madhya Pradesh. Barren wasteland was rapidly converted into green and productive agricultural land, providing a self-sufficient base from which workers could set out to work in service to their fellow human beings. This ashram, and the many that followed after Vinoba set out in 1951, on his pilgrimage to promote land redistribution, were characterised by the strict discipline and love of the Gandhian order. Whilst equality and service to one's fellows were key principles in these ashrams, there is no doubt that the influence of Gandhi and the leadership of Vinoba were central in drawing together a diverse group of people to work so harmoniously and productively for a common cause.

Inspired by the time he had spent in India with Gandhi (1937) and Vinoba (1954), the Italian Lanza del Vasto returned to Europe and established L'Arche, a movement to promote nonviolence. A number of communities were established to enable members of L'Arche to deepen their commitment to the Gandhian values of simplicity, service, sharing and self-reliance. La Borie Noble, the first of the L'Arche communities, was started in south-west France in 1948, and was followed by seven others in France, two in Spain, one in Italy and one in Canada. Life in the communities is characterised by a combination of manual work and spiritual search, aiming to allow individuals from all religions, and those without religious affiliation, to find their role in the task of building a nonviolent society. Living in community enables the aims of self-reliance in basic needs, food, clothing and accommodation, to be realised more easily, whilst creating opportunities for daily practice of sharing, reconciliation and other elements of personal development.

Lanza del Vasto died in 1981 but L'Arche lives on, as both a peace movement and a simple, self-sufficient way of life. The remaining communities publish a newsletter, campaign against arms, and host peace camps alongside their daily routine of prayer, meditation, farming and craft activities. While researching for this book I spent a week at the original community, La Borie Noble, and gained valuable insights into how the spiritual dimension of the community contributes to their ability to communally farm 120 acres of land without the use of fossil-fuel-powered machinery.

Back to the land in 1970s Britain

In the UK, the 1970s saw a peak in the development of communal land projects, which began in the 1960s with Findhorn and continues to this day. Whilst the reasons for the establishment of communities such as Laurieston (1972), Old Hall (1974), Lower Shaw Farm, Redfield (1978) and Canon Frome Court (1978) were often broader than pure self-sufficiency and environmentalism, these are themes that have remained to a greater or lesser extent, reflected by the practical activities of the communities.[52] Much of the motivation to live a greener, less consumer-based lifestyle came from the 1970s concerns about oil shortages, nuclear power and weapons, and conventional chemical farming. Usually a strong dose of socialism was blended with these environmental motives, with shared homes and incomes, collective child-care and non-hierarchical, consensus decision-making, forming a model for most of the communes. Old Hall appears to have been more focused on group living and socialist values than organic farming in the beginning, even though the community has successfully farmed its 60 acres organically since it began. Although most people at Old Hall have part-time jobs outside the community, they collectively farm a small herd of dairy cows, sheep, pigs, bees and vegetables, and attain a high degree of food self-sufficiency.[53]

Of the 1970s communities still in operation today, many have evolved away from the radical, communal model towards a more liberal, individualistic mode of life. For example, residents at Canon Frome Court now eat together formally only once a week, and in 1987 Laurieston Hall changed from being an income- and meal-sharing commune to a housing co-op and work collective. Few of the community members are entirely employed in land-based activities, with collective commercial activities tending to be education-based, and farming and forestry being purely for subsistence.

Not everyone in the 1970s' 'back to the land' movement chose to live and work communally. Inspired by John Seymour's books about self-sufficiency, many individuals and families also bought smallholdings during that era. They tended to settle in more remote areas of the UK, such as Wales and the south-west, where it was still possible to buy an affordable house with some land. Others started in a more communal vein, with two or more families sharing a house and land, but evolved over the years into privately owned holdings.

The modern-day ecovillage movement

The Global Ecovillage Network was founded in 1995, following the annual conference of the Findhorn Community in north-east Scotland. Its aim was to link the hundreds of small projects that were working towards a common goal but hitherto had not known about each other.[54] Their motivations combined social, ecological and spiritual aspects, with one usually being dominant over the others at first, but all three becoming equally important as the ecovillages evolved. Both in wealthy industrialised countries and developing countries, the idea of ecovillage development has been welcomed as a practical way of addressing environmental, social and economic problems. Yet, especially in Europe where planning laws and building regulations are strict, concrete examples of functional ecovillages have been slow to appear and the ecovillage movement is still in its infancy.

Ecovillages differ from communes, or intentional communities, in that they offer residents a greater degree of autonomy, a feature which makes them more attractive to people used to living independently. Some previously existing communities encompass many of the features of the ecovillage movement, including independent co-operating households, eco-design of buildings, growing and trading of food, a barter currency and care of the elderly or disabled. For example, Camphill Communities are a long-standing tradition of ecovillages which practise the philosophy of Rudolf Steiner. They grow and process biodynamic food for themselves and to sell, operate a range of craft workshops, offer live-in work opportunities for mentally handicapped people, and build or retrofit their homes to use natural resources efficiently.

Diane and Robert Gilman, who produced an early report on ecovillages, defined them as follows:[55]

1. Human scale – between 50 and 500 members.

2. A full-featured settlement, in which the main functions of life – food provision, manufacture, leisure, social life and commerce – are present in balanced proportions. This does not mean, however, that ecovillages should be totally self-sufficient or isolated from their surroundings.

3. Human activities harmlessly integrated into the natural world by adopting a cyclic approach to resource-use and aiming at a more equal relationship between humans and other forms of life.

4. Supportive of healthy human development by balancing and fulfilling human physical, emotional, mental and spiritual needs not just for individuals, but for the whole community.

5. Successfully able to develop into the indefinite future.

These principles relate closely to the theme of this book, which is the integration of people's social needs with ecologically and economically sustainable land-based lifestyles. Although the ecovillage movement covers a much broader range of domestic, commercial and educational activities, many parallels and areas of overlap will become apparent in the following chapters. Indeed, some of the communities I visited fit very closely with the ecovillage definition above.

Informing the future by learning from the past

Over the centuries the pattern of land-holding in Britain has moved away from communally held and managed land towards privatisation and the concentration of farms into fewer and larger holdings. Whilst this change was brought about by a series of parliamentary Enclosure Acts pushed through by the powerful to the detriment of the weak, it is interesting to ask the question, "Was such privatisation inevitable?". If you look at the history of intentional communities in the nineteenth and twentieth centuries, whose utopian aspirations were to hold land and other property in common, very few have survived in their original form, if at all. Either they have finished after an average life of about ten years or, like Whiteway (founded 1898) and Laurieston Hall (founded 1972), they have become less communal. Such trends reflect the profound challenges of living in close proximity with other people. It is no coincidence that today's ecovillage movement emphasises separate households and the concept of neighbourliness, rather than common ownership.

Yet there are significant benefits to sharing responsibilities and the daily details of domestic and work life. In today's individualistic society, many people long for a more practical and meaningful experience of community. It is not only the people living in communities who point out the advantages of sharing, but people who are working alone, who can see that in some respects communities offer improvements in quality of life.

Furthermore, when it comes to addressing the challenges of climate change and 'peak oil', it is interesting to observe that it is mainly communities, rather than single people and family farms, which are attempting to avoid fossil-fuel use altogether. This reflects the need for there to be more hands to undertake work when machinery is not being used, and in the absence of many willing hands, farmers and smallholders – especially those who are running commercial operations – have little choice but to employ machines.

Among the communities in this book, three – La Borie Noble, Steward Wood and Tinker's Bubble – are attempting to live and work with minimal or no fossil-fuel-powered machinery (See Chapter Seven, pp.145-8). Their reasons vary for abandoning a source of energy upon which so much of modern society depends. At La Borie Noble it is the avoidance of machinery, rather than fossil fuels, that is the aim, due to a Gandhian ethic of simplicity to counteract the negative social and economic effects of mechanisation (see Chapter Five, Wise Choice of Tools, pp.116-9). At Tinker's Bubble the policy of not using fossil-fuel-powered combustion engines is due to both the environmental costs of fossil-fuel dependence and a counter-reaction to the trend of fewer people managing larger amounts of land with machines. Steward Wood is more environmentally motivated in its non-fossil-fuel use and employs numerous modern technologies to harness renewable energy (solar, hydro and biodiesel). The only other people operating without fossil fuels are the smallholders in the Pyrenean Vallée de Mérens, where subsistence rather than commercial activities is a predominant concern.

Where one source of energy, such as oil, is eliminated, other sources must be found. If, as rural history seems to show, increased privatisation of land use is only possible with abundant fossil fuels, does that mean we all need to live and work in communities? Yet, as the history of communities demonstrates, there is a trend towards privatisation due to the challenges of living and working collectively. In my experience, living and working with other people both gives energy and takes it away. All too often people are tempted to subsidise their enterprise or community with their own energy and time, and this is sustainable only up to a point. A central question in this book is therefore, "What kind of rural social structures will enable people to manage the land sustainably and productively, reduce their dependence on fossil fuels, and sustain their own energy and enthusiasm into the future?"

Chapter Three

The Role of
the Modern Smallholder

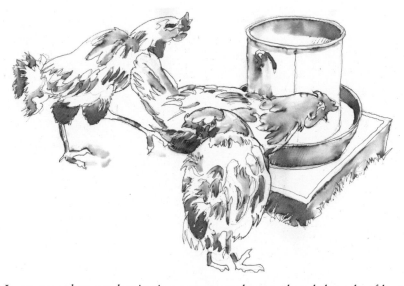

In an age when mechanisation appears to have reduced the role of human labour to an all-time low, the question of how to sustain human energy in agriculture may seem like a distraction from some of the more pressing problems faced by environmentalists. After all, hasn't technological innovation saved land-based labourers from hours of drudgery, digging, weeding and sawing?

The central decades of the twentieth century saw an unprecedented rate of technological change in all parts of industrial society. These changes were based on the availability of fossil-fuel energy in the form of coal, oil and natural gas. The increased mechanisation of agricultural processes and the growth in the agro-chemical industry were made possible by cheap and abundant fossil-fuel energy. It became possible and economically viable to transport food for long distances between the producer and the consumer, and to process basic commodities into countless products to catch the attention and add to the convenience of shoppers. Now climate change means we must find ways to cut carbon emissions, and the imminent decline in one of the most versatile fossil fuels, oil, is forcing us to seek other sources of energy. We would be wise not to forget that until the twentieth century, farming was largely dependent on the power of humans and animals (horses and oxen).

In this chapter I argue that smallholders have a role to play in helping adjust to a low-carbon society. Rather than being an anachronism from the past, hand tools, horse-drawn equipment and organic farming methods could contribute to providing basic food products for local people. These traditional technologies, enhanced by modern innovation, are most appropriately used at a smaller scale than their fossil-fuel-dependent equivalents. Were sufficient numbers of people to become skilled in managing land, cultivating crops and distributing food locally, the need for the huge industrial farms and centralised food systems would be diminished. Yet, compared with the fossil-fuel-dependent food production and distribution systems currently dominant in most industrialised countries, organic methods and direct marketing (when the farmer sells direct to the consumer) require a greater input of time, skills and effort on the part of the producer.

Gobbling up oil and belching greenhouse gases

The food production and distribution system upon which most people depend is one of the biggest producers of carbon dioxide in the UK. Agriculture alone contributes 8% of the UK's emissions of the greenhouse gases carbon dioxide, methane and nitrous oxide, not including the production and transport of agrochemicals or the management of food beyond the farm gate.[1] Modern agriculture is highly dependent on off-farm inputs, which generate carbon dioxide both in their manufacture and transport to the farm. The manufacture of farm machinery, compound animal feeds, pesticides and nitrate fertilisers all require large energy inputs, resulting in carbon dioxide emissions. Frequent ploughing and harrowing of soils stimulates the break-down of soil organic matter, releasing further carbon dioxide. A recently completed 25-year soil survey by the National Soil Resources Institute found that UK soils are losing 13 million tonnes of carbon each year, far more than previously realised. This means that the UK's soil is a major contributor to climate change, producing carbon emissions equivalent to 7.3% of the UK's official greenhouse gas emissions in 2005.[2]

After leaving the farm, most food travels long distances and undergoes extensive processing and packaging before it reaches the consumers. The relative carbon emissions resulting from sea freight and air freight are 2.74g carbon per tonne kilometre and 156g carbon per tonne kilometre respectively.[3] Whilst non-perishable foodstuffs such as grains, frozen meat and wine can be transported by ship, most fresh fruits and vegetables require rapid transport and are frequently air-freighted. In 2006, 29% of vegetables and 89% of all fruit consumed in the UK were imported.[4] Meanwhile, domestic transport of food by road is accounting for a growing proportion of energy use and carbon emissions in the UK. The Department for the Environment, Transport and the Regions stated in 2001, "Road transport is one of the fastest-growing sources of CO_2 and accounts for around a fifth of total emissions. Unless action is taken over the next two decades, car traffic could grow by more than a third, and van and lorry traffic is forecast to grow even faster."[5] There is no reason why a much greater proportion of fruit, vegetables and other basic foodstuffs cannot be produced in the UK, within a few miles of where it will be consumed. Smallholders, as we shall see later in this chapter, could play a significant role in substituting local produce for unnecessary imports.

Organic dividends

Organic farming methods have much to recommend them in terms of energy efficiency. One study comparing organic and conventional livestock, dairy, vegetable and arable systems in the UK found that the average energy saving for eight crops when produced organically, compared with non-organic crops, was 0.68MJ/kg or 42%. Fertiliser and pesticide inputs combined account for half the energy input in conventional potato and winter wheat production and up to 80% of the energy consumed in some vegetable crops.[6]

Instead of importing fertilisers onto the farm, organic farmers concentrate on recycling carbon-rich organic matter, by composting manure and crop residues, and rotating fertility-building crops with those that are net takers of fertility. Hence, compared with non-organic systems, organic practices result in higher levels of carbon-rich organic matter being stored in the soil.[7] The combined annual costs of carbon dioxide, methane, nitrous oxide and ammonia emissions from all agriculture in 2000 were £523.8 million. Whilst organic farming also produces greenhouse gases, were all of the UK to be farmed organically, Pretty *et al.* estimated that costs would be reduced to £204.7 million.[8]

Organic farming also brings social and economic dividends to rural areas. Studies have shown that it is creating more jobs than conventional farming, encouraging younger people into farming and bringing optimism and job satisfaction to this beleaguered sector. A survey of 25% of the organic holdings in the UK found that, on average, organic farms provided 3.08 jobs per farm, compared with 1.28 per farm on non-organic farms.[9] Small organic farms, with an average size of 36ha, supported the greatest number of jobs, providing an average of 5.23 jobs per farm. By substituting off-farm inputs with management practices such as rotation and mixed farming, organic practices call for a more diverse range of skills bringing more job satisfaction.[10] Furthermore, a study of the impacts of organic farming on the local economy found that organic farms generate higher sales values per hectare than non-organic farms.[11]

The past twenty years have seen a rise in the popularity of organic agriculture, with total sales of organic products growing from £1 million to £1 billion between 1984 and 2004. During this time the number of organic farms in the UK has grown from fewer than 300 to over 4,300.[12] This growth has accelerated, with sales of organic food and drink growing by 30% in 2005 to £1.6 billion, in contrast to a growth rate of 3% for non-organic food and drink in the same year.[13] The rapid growth in demand for organic food has outstripped UK supply for certain food categories (fruit, vegetables and arable crops) and supermarkets, which now sell 75% of organic food, have turned to imports to make up the deficit. The energy requirements of such imports threaten to dwarf the energy savings made by organic production methods.

Local food for local people

A growing local food movement is responding to the need to reduce the distances food is transported. Initiatives, ranging from farmers' markets, farm shops and box schemes to lobbying for the use of local food in school meals, have grown in prominence. Besides reducing food transport, and thus carbon emissions, bringing producer and consumer closer together through local and direct marketing enables food to be consumed when it is fresh and has its greatest nutritional value. This is particularly true for vegetables and fruit. Compared with mangetout peas that may have been flown from Kenya or plums picked in Spain, which will take at least a week to reach the consumer after harvest, vegetables purchased at a farmers' market or via a box scheme will probably have been picked only the day before.

The regeneration of local food systems keeps money circulating within the local economy. Retailers and service providers can multiply the value of each pound by a factor of over two, by spending it on local suppliers. Conversely, if investment 'leaks' out of a local economy, by being spent on external businesses, its value is diminished.[14] Bringing consumers into face-to-face contact with producers builds understanding about agricultural methods, seasonality and trust in food safety. For producers, regular interaction with customers not only provides valuable feedback about the product, but also social interaction, which may be a welcome change in an otherwise relatively solitary profession. Direct marketing tends to lead to greater collaboration amongst farmers, in order to meet consumer demand, building trust and friendships within farming communities.

Ultimately, local food production is necessary to ensure access for all to sustainably produced, affordable basic food products, such as fruit and vegetables, grains, dairy produce and meat. Gandhi taught that staple foods should not cross borders, since to do so leads to exploitation, corruption and dependence.[15] At present, however, it would be hard for the entire UK population to subsist purely on a locally or even nationally produced diet because key staples, especially seasonal fruit, vegetables and pulses, are under-supplied.

Tough times for farmers

The replacement of labourers and horses with machines and agrochemicals after the second world war led to an 80% reduction in the agricultural workforce.[16] Before the second world war around 15% of the UK's population was employed in agriculture, but today less than 2% of people work directly in the production of the UK's food.[17] The land left by those farmers and labourers was concentrated into fewer, larger holdings. Between 1956 and 2003 the number of farm holdings in the UK fell by 40%.[18] As a result, farming has become more specialised, with small mixed farms being replaced by large, solely arable or livestock businesses.

The legacy of specialisation has been devastating disease, economic instability and the narrowing of farm skills to chemistry, mechanics and the management of paperwork. Financial worries and isolation now top the list for causes of farm-related stress.[19] Over the period 1973-2004 there was a 39% decline in average income per person employed in agriculture.[20] Globalisation and farm subsidy reform have contributed to the financial uncertainty, whilst supermarkets have used their power to demand unreasonable levels of cosmetic perfection. One farmer now commonly manages the land of several farms on his own. Hence, these pressures often have to be born alone, because the farmer may see no-one but his family for days on end. Even traditional social meeting places like cattle markets are disappearing as produce is sold by telephone, eliminating opportunities to share joys and grievances with others in the same position.

Tragically these pressures have led some farmers to take their own lives. The combination of financial worries, family issues and work problems has led to high levels of stress and depression among farmers.[21] Between 1991 and 1996, 190 farmers, farm managers and horticultural workers committed suicide, averaging one death every eleven days during that period. In 2003, 55 farm workers took their lives, raising the average to one suicide every seven days of that year.[22] Furthermore, the poor pay and stressful, tedious nature of modern farm work mean few young people want to follow their parents into agriculture. Between 1993 and 2003 the proportion of farmers aged 55 and over rose from 48% to 56%, while the proportion of those under 35 fell from 6.8% to 3.7%.[23]

In contrast, organic farmers tend to be enjoying their work, with more of them stating that they would be happy to stay in farming as compared with their non-organic colleagues. Such job satisfaction appears to be feeding into the next generation, with 64% of organic farmers expecting a family member to take on their farm after them, compared with 51% of non-organic farmers.[24] The average age of organic farmers is 49, with the proportion of organic farmers aged under 55 years old being 69% compared with 48% of non-organic farmers. Organic farming is also attracting new entrants into the agricultural sector. In a study of one fifth of the registered organic farms in Britain, 31% of the farmers they surveyed were 'new entrants', meaning that they came from non-farming families.[25] Many of these people are leaving their professional jobs in cities to apply their business and marketing skills to farming enterprises.

Such statistics are in striking contrast to the picture of general agricultural employment in the UK. As non-organic farmers retire, they tend not to be replaced, which consolidates the decline in farmer numbers resulting from farms going out of business and farm workers seeking alternative employment. Yet the land still needs to be managed and people in Britain still need to eat. Some scientists and economists envisage an efficient future, involving a small number of highly specialised farmers. They would use industrial techniques to produce a narrow range of crops on large acreages of good land, while poor land is turned over to conservation.[26] Meanwhile, the rest of the food needed to feed the nation would be imported from abroad.

Diminishing national food security

We seem to be approaching a situation alarmingly akin to that faced by the nation at the time of the second world war – a situation of dependence on distant lands for the production of staple food crops. Comparing import and export data for twelve key food types, Jules Pretty discovered that only two (cereals and oil seed rape) were net exported, whilst the remainder were net imported.[27] For some, such as sheep products, imports and exports are almost balanced, whilst for others, fruit for example, the ratio of imports to exports was as much as 9.62:1. Between 1997 and 2006 the UK's self-sufficiency for all foods has gone from just under 70% to just over 60%.[28] Recent policies encouraging more farmland to be managed for conservation, while food production is concentrated in a few more fertile regions seem set to exacerbate this situation. Increasing our dependence on imported foodstuffs has two major implications – increased long-distance transport of food and reduced national food security.

To return large tracts of the UK to a more natural state, at the expense of increasing carbon emissions through increased food transport seems perverse. Organic farming enables environmental protection to be integrated with food production and has the potential to meet the nutritional needs of the entire UK population. At a large scale it does, however, produce lower yields per hectare when compared with certain conventionally produced crops, and therefore requires more land. In a calculation of the land requirements for feeding the present British population of 60.6 million using various systems (chemical, organic and permaculture farming with and without livestock) Fairlie concludes that mixed and vegan non-chemical farming could produce sufficient food, fuel and fibre, whilst leaving a tenth of the UK's land area for wildlife.[29] There is evidence to suggest that on smaller farms yields are often greater per unit area as a result of increased labour intensity and a greater diversity of crops being grown.[30, 31]

In 2003 the UK Government stated that, "National food security is neither necessary nor is it desirable", but many, including the Government's Sustainable Development Commission (SDC) disagree. The SDC emphasises that "encouraging the diversity of our food production system would increase our resilience to withstand the shocks and challenges posed by global insecurity." Such resilience, they state, will be necessary to address "the potential risks from climate change, global resource (e.g. oil) disruption and transport breakdowns."[32]

Finally, why should nations that are struggling to produce enough food for their own populations be using their land to grow staple and luxury products, as well as biodiesel crops, for wealthy countries such as the UK? Not only does production of crops for export take up land, but often the irrigation requirements of these cash crops lead to serious local water shortages. The pressure on farmland in tropical and sub-tropical countries is predicted to grow as a result of climate-change-induced droughts, floods and sea level rise. Is it right to expect these countries to continue growing export crops, while their own populations starve, or become displaced by environmental degradation, and farmland in the UK is turned over to nature reserves and golf courses?

The current scale of local, organic production

For organic agriculture and the local food movement to make a significant impact in cutting carbon emissions, reducing fossil-fuel dependence and bringing about fairer use of global resources there needs to be a dramatic increase in production. The £1.6 billion organic market represents only

1.3% of the £120 billion UK grocery market.[33, 34] Likewise, the area of land which is certified organic represents 3.6% of all UK farmland.[35] Only 4,285 (1.3%) of the 323,767 agricultural holdings in the UK are organically certified.[36] For organic farming to fulfil its potential to reduce carbon emissions, increase rural employment and draw money into local economies there is considerable room for expansion.

Another solution could be the more widespread, but partial adoption of organic techniques. Whilst the term 'organic' has a legal definition which requires that food which is marketed as such has been produced to a prescribed set of standards, many of the techniques of organic farming are transferable to mainstream agriculture. Systems like integrated crop management (ICM), which combines traditional and organic practices such as crop rotation with the reduced use of fertilisers and pesticides, could have a more significant environmental contribution than pure organic practices, if adopted by the majority of UK farmers.

The market share of local and regionally sourced products is only marginally larger than that of the organic market, at 3.3% of the UK grocery market, with total sales in 2005/06 being £3.97 billion.[37] In 2005 total sales from the 550 farmers' markets, at which 10-15% of stall-holders were selling organic produce, amounted to £220 million.[38] This represents only 0.12% of the UK grocery market, and shows how direct-marketed organic food is small fry compared with the types of food consumed by the majority of UK residents. All these figures point to the fact that if organic and local food is to bring the benefits outlined earlier, there needs to be a dramatic growth in the numbers of organic producers, the area of land managed organically, and the marketing channels through which locally produced food can be obtained.

Small is productive

How can smallholders help bring about such a massive expansion in the local production of organic food? It is commonly thought that large farms create economies of scale through increased production efficiency. In conventional agriculture, the cultivation of large, monocultural fields with powerful machines and agrochemicals has been found to produce higher yields of commodity crops than is possible at a smaller scale using organic methods. However, the measurement of productivity in terms of the yield per unit area of a single crop hides the fact that small farms, when viewed as a whole, are sometimes more productive than large ones. By their very nature, small, mixed organic farms tend to produce a more diverse range of crops than conventional ones. The total output per unit area of a small farm, which is often composed of more than a dozen crops and animal products, can be far higher than that of a large monocultural one.[39]

In developing countries the benefits of small farms, including higher total productivity, crop diversity and greater food security, are increasingly being recognised. In Latin America, small farms are three to fourteen times more productive per acre than large farms, while in Taiwan net income per acre of farms of less than 1.25 acres is nearly double that of farms over five acres.[40] An amalgamation of results from 293 different comparisons of organic and conventional methods of farming showed that small farms tend to produce more per hectare of land. This result led them to claim that an increase in the number of small farms would enhance food production.[41] Such high productivity amongst small-scale, subsistence and commercial farmers in tropical countries is partly due to the prevalence of poly-cropping. This is the practice of cultivating several different crops on the same piece of land, either simultaneously or in rotation, which increases sunlight capture, makes more efficient use of soil nutrients and reduces pest and disease problems. Yield advantages for poly-cropping systems can range from 20% to 60%, whilst the crop diversity means smallholders are buffered against variations in crop price and weather conditions.[42] Such poly-cropping systems operate best on small farms, because more labour per area is required and farmers are able to put greater effort in the precise management of small areas of land.

In a densely populated country like Britain, the pressure on land for farming, wildlife conservation, house building and leisure pursuits (e.g. golf and horse-riding), is very great. For a truly sustainable future, it is necessary to combine high agricultural productivity with ecologically sound land management, to reduce food transport, increase national food security and accommodate multiple land-use requirements. It would be unwise to directly extrapolate the findings of higher agricultural productivity on small-scale farms in developing countries to the UK, due to different climatic and socio-economic conditions. However, it is worth challenging the assumption that in temperate, industrialised countries, large-scale non-organic agricultural production is always more efficient.

An analysis of data from the United States Department of Agriculture (USDA), showing the relationship between farm size and output per acre in the United States, indicated that the smallest farms, those of 27 acres or less, have more than ten times greater dollar output per acre than larger farms.[43] This is largely due to the higher value crops, such as vegetables and flowers, in which small farms tend to specialise. However, it also reflects the increased crop diversity and greater labour intensity and application of inputs per unit area. The appropriate scale of production varies greatly between crops, and will be influenced by the location and quality of land. Rough upland is better suited to low intensity grazing, over a large acreage, than intensive horticulture, and it is hard to be commercially competitive growing cereals on small acreages. Certain kinds of enterprise, for example organic vegetable, fruit, poultry and pigs, can be competitively produced at a small scale, and, when managed in an integrated system, make efficient use of the land.

Small farms bring wider benefits to the environment and rural communities. It is easier to manage a diverse range of habitats at a small scale, and to provide the attention to detail necessary to care for natural resources such as soil and water. When areas, dominated by large corporate farms were compared with those characterised by smaller family farms, researchers found that in the former, nearby towns were in decline. Fewer local people were employed and agricultural revenue was drained off into larger cities. In contrast, where family farms predominated, income circulated among local businesses, generating jobs and community prosperity. In the Amish areas of the eastern United States, where small farmers eschew bank credit and much modern technology, agricultural communities thrive. One such area, Lancaster County in Pennsylvania, is the most productive farm county east of the Mississippi River, receiving annual gross sales of agricultural products of $700 million. Although they are renowned for being self-reliant and trading actively within their communities, the Amish are also market-orientated and do substantial trade with the outside. "Their economies are highly diverse, and integrated rather than fragmented, co-operative rather than competitive, based on value added rather than commodity products and dedicated to reciprocity more than dominance." [44] If we are interested in developing truly sustainable rural economies and becoming less dependent on fossil fuels, we would be wise to learn from the example of the Amish.

People are often better motivated when working for themselves, when they can experience directly the fruits of their labour, rather than for a big land owner. If every village in the UK had four or five small farms producing vegetables, fruit, eggs and meat for local consumption long-distance food transport would be reduced dramatically. Farmers would have a direct relationship with their customers, and consumers would gain a greater understanding of the way in which their food is produced. Other food products, such as cereals, dairy produce and meat could be produced on larger farms, and processed locally or even on-site. An integrated local food network might include a diverse range of artisan cheese makers, bakeries with in-store mills to grind grain from local farms, weekly markets which attract a dozen different fruit and vegetable stalls, and facilities for processing surplus produce into jams, pickles and pies. In some parts of the UK, the development of such networks is already underway. However, local and organic food are still viewed as niche products for the environmentally aware and well heeled. For a network of diverse and integrated small-scale producers to develop to the necessary scale requires a massive increase in the number of skilled and motivated farmers, growers and smallholders.

The question "Can organic farming feed the world?" has been debated repeatedly over the years. I firmly believe that it can, but only if we change the way we view agricultural productivity. The provision of fresh, tasty, nutritious food for local people must be seen as a primary aim, and integrated with the management of a diverse and beautiful landscape, wildlife conservation and stewardship of natural resources, such as water and soil. Smallholders are well positioned to provide all of these benefits and could play an important role in the transition to a low-carbon economy.

Low-impact living

The extravagant use of resources by the modern food system is only one aspect of our climate-altering dependence on fossil fuels. The lifestyles enjoyed by the majority of people in wealthy countries such as the UK also rely heavily on oil for heating, electricity, transport and the manufacture of most consumer items. Living in rural areas results in particularly high car-dependency, due to poor public transport provision and the dispersed nature of schools, shops and social networks. In order to maintain the ecological benefits of returning to the land to increase the production of local, organic food, it is necessary to minimise domestic resource use and need to travel.

For a farmer or smallholder, the options available for reducing environmental impact include:

- Living in a small, well-designed and insulated house, built from local/recycled materials.
- Providing electricity with renewable sources such as wind, hydro or solar power.
- Cooking and heating space and water with wood, or wood products such as pellets or wood chip, burned in a fuel-efficient stove.
- Walking, cycling or using public transport to cut down/eliminate car use.
- Stopping flying altogether!
- Choosing locally produced, minimally packaged food when supplementing produce grown on the farm.
- On-site composting of organic waste.
- Water conservation through rainwater harvesting, recycling of grey water and use of dry composting toilets.

Several recent studies have shown that living in communities or ecovillages can result in people significantly reducing their ecological footprints, while retaining a high quality of life. As well as adopting the measures for sustainable lifestyles listed above, living communally enables resources such as cars, renewable-energy infrastructure and washing-machines to be shared. Furthermore, where residents eat together regularly or live in the same building, energy use is reduced when compared with that used by many individual households. Having a social support network within walking distance cuts down on the need to drive to see friends or gain access to child-care, while many community members are able to work from home and thus avoid commuting.

The ecovillage at Ithaca in upstate New York was found in two separate academic studies to have a footprint 40% lower than the national average for the USA. Closer to home, a study of Findhorn community in north-west Scotland found that its residents have a footprint of 2.71, which is just over half the UK national average, of 5.4.[45] Co-operating with each other has enabled residents at one of the communities featured in this book, Keveral Farm in Cornwall, to reduce their ecological footprints to 2.29ha/person, 38% of the UK national average. However, even this lower level of environmental impact exceeds global ecological capacity to supply all materials and absorb all wastes, which has been calculated to be 1.8ha per person.

The website www.myfootprint.org enables people to calculate their ecological footprint, by answering a series of 15 questions about their lifestyle. For a person who is combining the measures for reducing environmental impact listed above, the Ecological Footprint can be reduced to between 1.3 and 1.7 global hectares. This is below the 1.8 ha which is available for every person on Earth, and would therefore be reasonably sustainable if the majority of those living rurally reduced their environmental impact to this extent.

Rising to the challenge

The truth is that human society needs to change radically if we are to avoid the ravages of climate change and related environmental degradation. We have a choice.

Either we can delay the pain by adopting technological fixes, which enable life to continue as usual for a limited amount of time. Such a future could include building more nuclear power plants to meet current demand for electricity. Many scientists also advocate cropping the best agricultural land ever more intensively, employing the latest agrochemicals in combination with genetically modified plant and animal species. This approach, they argue, would provide sufficient food for the growing global population, whilst freeing up marginal land for conservation of wild species. Enabling land to revert to wilderness would have the benefit of strengthening the Earth's ability to regulate its climate thereby moderating the effects of global heating caused by human activities.[46]

Alternatively, we could re-organise our lifestyles to be radically more energy-efficient, tailoring our consumer needs to what it is possible to produce locally. One element of such a re-organisation would be that more people would become directly involved in managing the land to provide for their basic needs. Many new entrants into organic farming are attracted not by potential financial success, but because they believe that they will enjoy a better quality of life than previously. All the people I interviewed whilst researching for this book were either new entrants themselves or the children of new entrants. Among their reasons for choosing to live and work on the land, quality of life issues featured highly. The reality is not always so rosy and some aspiring food producers fall by the wayside as a result of unremitting hard work, stress and ill health. Even if parents survive the rigours of farming, if their children perceive sustainable production as offering a quality of life inferior to that of the parents of their peers, they are unlikely to want to continue running the farm after their parents.

Not surprisingly, politicians favour the 'technological fix, to enable business as usual' approach, since they doubt the willingness of the electorate to change their way of life enough to cut carbon emissions on the scale necessary. The challenge is to prove that living on or earning a livelihood from the land in an environmentally sound way can result in increased happiness and health benefits as well as being economically viable.

With the public beginning to wake up to the severity of climate change, the lunacy of long-distance food transport and the health risks of industrially produced food, the market for local, organic produce is expanding rapidly. A large-scale expansion of this sector is necessary both to meet the demand and make a significant cut in carbon emissions. It is essential that existing local, organic producers are able to sustain their activities over the long term and share their skills with new entrants. The rural idyll which attracts so many to the countryside must reflect genuine improvements in quality of life, and not be tarnished by unreasonable long working hours, exhaustion, ill health and continuously high stress levels. It is possible to produce fresh, healthy food for local people whilst minimising your ecological footprint and sustaining your energy and enthusiasm. In this book I will introduce you to some of the people who are succeeding at doing it.

Chapter Four

Land-based Livelihoods
and Low-impact Lifestyles

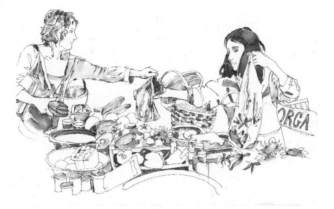

The case studies on which this book is based are a very small sample of the land-based ecological projects operating in the UK and France at present. They include forestry initiatives as well as food producers. Whilst many are commercial at various scales, some are managing land purely for their own subsistence and enjoyment. They are connected by the fact that all are trying to gain at least a proportion of their basic needs by managing land in a way they perceive as being relatively environmentally sound. Apart from that the sample is fairly diverse in terms of scale, enterprise mixture, social structure and the degree to which they integrate their environmental values into their personal lives.

Having embarked on this project as a personal mission, the criteria for selecting the case studies were far from scientific. In France, I chose to visit projects that were using horse-drawn tools to grow vegetables, where people were living communally or in a low-impact way, places where I could improve my French and ones that were en route on my cycling trip. Back in the UK, I chose certain projects I had been meaning to visit for years and others I was told about by people I met along the way. At each place I conducted interviews with one or more of the people who have a significant role in the operation. Through a mixture of questioning and observation I hoped to understand the aspects of the project which were making it work in terms of human energy. Hence, I combined questions about the project itself (enterprise mixture, scale, technology employed etc.) with questions about how each individual experiences life in relation to the project (see Appendix 1 for interview questions).

As I settled back into life in south-west England and started sifting through my findings and trying to arrange them into a meaningful order, other projects suggested themselves to me as illustrating specific points I wished to make. Hence, my visits continued and I spoke with people running successful projects and ones which had failed, people working alone to realise their vision and others working in community. Altogether I studied 28 different projects, and the material on which this book is based is the result of many people generously sharing their time and experiences. In addition, over the last ten years I have worked at or visited a number of other, similar holdings and I draw on casual observations from these places as well.

Whilst not statistically representative, I believe these examples are illustrative of a range of land-based initiatives being developed by new entrants into small-scale agriculture and forestry. Most are being run by either new entrants or first generation farmers, and all are adhering to organic or permaculture principles in their management of the land. Another common feature of the case studies is that they are either consuming their produce themselves or selling at least a proportion of it locally either through direct marketing channels (box schemes, farmers' markets, farm shops) or wholesale to shops, restaurants or marketing co-operatives.

In this chapter I will introduce the case study projects, which will become familiar as the book progresses. Table 4.1 summarises some of their defining features and is followed by an overview of the enterprises they illustrate, the different scales of operation and social structures encountered, and the variety of lifestyles and attitudes adopted by the people running the projects.

This is a book about people, upon whom the success of any farming or forestry project depends, and how they can sustain their energy to meet the ongoing demands of a land-based lifestyle. The key to maintaining motivation lies in finding work that is meaningful and provides regular pleasures to temper the frustrations and times of low energy that usually arise. The final portion of this chapter therefore addresses some of the reasons why interviewees chose to live and work on the land and examines the pleasures that they experience in daily life.

Social and economic features

The 28 case studies include 11 family farms, four projects being run by single people, nine communities and two community-supported agriculture schemes. The remaining two are what I call 'clusters'. They are groups of

	Project name and location	Date est.	No. adults	No. acres	Land-based activities
Single people (4)	Dun Beag (Argyll)	1995	1	30	Forestry, veg, fruit
	Ourganics (Dorset)	1999	1	5	Vegetables, fruit, eggs
	Briggs Farm (Dorset)	2003	1	12	Vegetables, pigs, sheep
	Jade Gate (Gower, Wales)	1995	1	5	Vegetables
Family Farm (11)	La Fermette (Loire, France)	2002	2	60	Vegetables, eggs
	Les Jardins de Mondoux (Limousin, France)	2001	2	19	Eggs, cereals, veg & fruit
	Little Farm (Devon)	1997	2	8	Vegetables
	Pentiddy Woods (Cornwall)	2001	2	27	Craft, courses, veg
	Tamarisk Farm (Dorset)	1960	4	600	Cereals, meat, veg
	Sea Spring Farm (Dorset)	1986	2	15	Indoor vegetables
	Longmeadow Organics (Dorset)	1986	2	9	Vegetables
	Galingale (Somerset)	1997	2	23	Veg, sheep
	Trading Post (Somerset)	1999	4	5	Veg, fruit, eggs
	Meadows Farm (Dorset)	'86-94	2	18	Veg, pigs
	Wood White Farm (Dorset)	2003	1	5	Veg, eggs, charcoal
CSA (2)	Earthshares (Nairnshire, Scotland)	1994	2	23	Vegetables & fruit
	Stroud Comm. Agric. (Gloucestershire.)	2001	2	23	Vegetables, fruit & meat
Cluster (2)	Vallée du Merens (Ariège, France)	1978	30	200	Veg, fruit, dairy, meat
	Fivepenny Farm (Dorset)	2003	4	43	Veg, eggs, meat, craft
Comm-unities (9)	La Sorga (Dordogne, France)	2002	4	43	Vegetables
	Brockhurst (Kent)	1997	6	35	Veg, fruit, goats, willow
	Brithdir Mawr (Pembrokeshire)	1994	10	85	Veg, goats, seed-saving
	Tinker's Bubble (Somerset)	1994	10	40	Veg, fruit, forestry, cows
	Laurieston Hall (Dumfries & Galloway)	1972	20	123	Camps, veg, meat, dairy
	Steward Woodland (Devon)	2000	10	32	Courses, forestry, veg
	Mulberry Tree Farm (Herefordshire)	2001	4	16	Veg, sheep, forest craft
	La Borie Noble (Cevennes. France)	1948	30	120	Cereal, veg, dairy, craft
	Keveral Farm (Cornwall)	1973	15	30	Veg, campsite, compost
28	**Total case studies**				

Table 4.1 – Overview of the case studies.

two or more smallholdings which are run independently, yet are close enough to each other (within a mile radius) to be able to co-operate and help each other out when the need arises.

The interviewees' economic dependence on their land-based activities varied considerably. Whilst for some self-sufficiency in food, fuel and other basic needs is their primary objective, for others commercial production is a defining feature. Only three projects (Longmeadow, Briggs Farm and the Trading Post) are mainly economically dependent on their land. These are market gardens which sell their vegetables via box schemes and in two instances farm shops. Even here the incomes of all three are supplemented by some vegetables and other produce being bought in and retailed. At eight of the farms run by families or single people, the farm income is being supplemented by off-site employment or state subsidies. In some cases this employment relates to the land work, for example tree surgery, hedge laying or running a photographic library of horticultural pictures. For others, off-site work is unrelated (child-minding, care work and teaching) or indirectly related (running a local Healthy Living Centre and working for ADAS).

The pattern at most of the communities is self-sufficiency supplemented by off-site employment. The exceptions are La Borie Noble in southern France, Tinker's Bubble in Somerset, and Laurieston Hall in south-west Scotland. At La Borie Noble, self-sufficiency is so complete that the income gained from selling surplus produce provides individuals with all their needs. All income is shared and individuals must make a request to the treasurer for money to buy personal items if they are needed. One of the primary aims of Tinker's Bubble is that residents earn their livelihood from the land. Although most residents are not yet 100% dependent on the land, a mixture of individual and collective land-based enterprises contributes significantly to their incomes. Many of those who live at Laurieston Hall are employed to a greater or lesser degree in running the 'People Centre', which hosts courses and camps, whilst others work part-time off-site.

Enterprises and scale of operations

As tables 4.1 and 4.2 show, the size of each holding ranges from as few as five acres in three instances, to as many as 600 acres in the case of Tamarisk Farm. The latter started as a 60-acre smallholding and has grown over the years as more land has been bought or rented. I have chosen to include it since it is the farm I have been working on whilst writing this book. Hence I have been able to study how the people running it have managed to sustain their energy and evolve their enterprises over a period of 47 years. Most of the holdings in the study are less than 50 acres.

Acreage of project	No of projects
10 acres and less	6
11-20 acres	5
21-50 acres	11
51-100 acres	2
101-200 acres	3
More than 200 acres	1 (600 acres)
Total no. projects	28

Table 4.2 – The distribution of holding sizes.

Acreage of holding is a poor indicator of the scale at which most projects were working, as it does not reflect the area of land actually being cultivated or even managed. For example, one couple who owned 15 acres of land are only using one acre for their horticultural operation, while much of the rest is grazed by horses. Two of the places with between 100 and 200 acres comprise considerable areas of woodland or scrub which are used extensively, for firewood collection and wild food foraging, if at all. The acreages of the other two larger holdings represent land used for arable, grazing animals and hay-making. The 600-acre family farm is managed with the help of fossil-fuel-powered machinery, whilst the 120 acres of La Borie Noble is farmed by a community who use hand tools and horse-drawn machinery.

Food is the most immediate resource people think of when earning a living from the land. This is reflected by the fact that all the projects discussed here contain an element of food production. However, many are producing more than food from their land. Water and firewood spring immediately to mind as subsistence resources upon which the people in my study depend. Nine projects also use their own timber, either for building or craftwork. Other ventures include the growth and processing of medicinal herbs, a commercial seed-saving enterprise and the hosting of camps and courses. In nine cases the land is also being used as a venue for courses and camps, which rely on the food and renewable energy resources being produced on site.

Vegetable production features centrally in this book. 20 of the 28 case studies are commercial horticultural operations, whilst the remaining eight grow vegetables for subsistence. Since I am a market gardener myself, I have to admit to a certain bias towards visiting horticultural projects! However, fruit and vegetables are nutritionally important, and two of the most accessible to cultivate of all land-based products. They are also the food type which is currently most under-supplied in the UK organic market and therefore are frequently being transported over long distances or even imported. Since quality deteriorates from the moment a plant is harvested, there are nutritional as well as environmental reasons for prioritising horticulture as a way of producing local food.

The scale at which vegetables were being grown ranges from half an acre to eleven acres, and the kind of technology employed generally became more mechanised as the size of operation grew. Those who are producing for subsistence – mainly communities – tend to cultivate vegetable patches by hand. At one end of the commercial spectrum are Tinker's Bubble, Mulberry Tree Farm, Sea Spring Farm, Ourganics, Jade Gate and Wood White Farm, whose horticultural operations use less than two acres each. The focused attention on small areas results in high productivity per square metre, and the techniques these small-scale producers use vary greatly. The majority of Sea Spring Farm's horticultural operation takes place in polytunnels mulched with black plastic and fitted with drip irrigation pipes, while Ourganics and Wood White Farm combine outdoor raised-bed systems with the use of one or two polytunnels. The grower at Jade Gate cultivates his two-acre market garden using a small horse, using tools bought from farm sales, and produces enough vegetables to supply up to eighty families with weekly vegetable boxes.

On the other end of the scale, Longmeadow Organics, Galingale, Briggs Farm and Meadows Farm cultivate between two and eleven acres of vegetables using tractor-drawn tools such as ploughs, harrows, steerage hoes and planting platforms. At its peak, Longmeadow Organics were producing 140 vegetable boxes per week, as well as selling to a few retail and catering outlets from 6.5 acres, whilst Briggs Farm is currently delivering 80-100 boxes per week, produced from 3.5 acres of cultivated land.

An enterprise that works well in tandem with horticulture is free-range egg production. This is because chickens are good scavengers and convert food waste and problematic insects into highly fertile manure. Seven of the holdings run commercial egg enterprises, with chicken flocks ranging in size from 20 to 300 birds. A further seven keep hens for domestic consumption of eggs and occasionally meat.

Other initiatives involving animals include sheep (5 case studies), pigs (5), beef cattle (2), dairy cows (5 case studies), milking goats (4) and llamas (1). Flocks of sheep range in size from 10 to 170 ewes, and pigs are limited to one or two breeding sows. The only places in my study keeping cattle for beef are Tamarisk Farm, which keeps a herd of 25-30 Red Devon breeding cows and followers, and Fivepenny Farm, where one family breeds from a couple of suckler cows. The llamas were kept at a small-holding at the head of Vallée de Mérens. The main justification for keeping them was their ability to produce prolific amounts of manure in concentrated heaps, thus making it easier to collect! This manure, in addition to that produced by the couple's 30 goats, was a valuable resource at the sandy-soiled holding, high in the French Pyrenees, where bringing in extra manure was impractical.

As for dairy production, this was mostly small-scale subsistence production, with between five and 30 goats being kept and hand-milked, and between one and six cows. All of the dairy cows and goats were kept predominantly for home milk consumption, with processed produce, such as cheese, being sold occasionally when in surplus. One producer is intending to start making yoghurt commercially when the processing rooms which are being built on her farm are complete. She is also intending to produce cured meat products from their pigs, and butcher the meat in their on-site meat-cutting rooms.

Only three farms – Tamarisk Farm, La Borie Noble and Les Jardins de Mondoux – are producing cereals. This reflects the fact that, compared with vegetables, under current economic conditions cereals are harder to grow in a financially viable way on a small scale. Modern cereal cultivation is highly dependent on machinery, including tractor-drawn ploughs, harrows and seed drills, combine harvesters and balers for the straw. To justify investment in such equipment, or even to make it worth hiring in a contractor in the UK, it is necessary to have a large acreage.

Tamarisk Farm grows wheat, rye and oats on about 25 acres as part of a four-year rotation on 70 acres of land, which by modern standards is small-scale. A few years ago the decision to buy a small, second-hand combine harvester was prompted by the difficulties they experienced in finding a contractor willing to operate on such a small acreage. Apart from some of the ploughing, which is also done by contractors, the rest of the field work is performed using the farm's 100 horsepower tractor. The oats are used as animal feed and about a quarter of the wheat and rye are milled at the farm, using a 2.5kw electric mill capable of processing 50kg per hour. The resulting flour is sold at the farm's own shop, as well as at several other local outlets. The remainder of the grain is sold to two local water mills associated with commercial bakeries – Town Mill Bakery in Lyme Regis and Ottery Mill in Devon.

The other two cereal farms are in France, and neither could be considered to be commercially competitive as commodity producers. However, through keeping production costs down by using simple technology, milling the grain themselves and baking bread which they can sell locally at a premium (due to its organic, 'artisan' status), they are able to gain a reasonable return on their efforts. The smallest, Les Jardins de Mondoux, hires a contractor for ploughing and combine-harvesting their two-acre field, to supplement the farm's own 30 horsepower Massey Ferguson tractor. The farmer, Gitta Wulf, mills her own wheat in 3kg batches using an electric table-top mill. She bakes about 20 loaves per week, which are sold at local markets and at the farm gate, bringing in 15% of the farm's income (€3,500 per year).

In contrast, no diesel-powered machinery is used in the bread production at La Borie Noble. All cereal cultivation is done using horse-drawn tools, but mains electricity (probably nuclear-powered!) is used for milling. Large sourdough loaves are kneaded by hand, in an operation akin to judo, and baked in a large, wood-fired oven. The bread is mainly for the community's own consumption. A neighbouring Buddhist community buys 50kg bread per week from La Borie Noble, but this is only possible because extra flour is bought in to supplement that which is home-grown.

Providing a venue for, or actually running, courses and camps is a form of diversification which is arguably land-based when the resources for catering come from the land or the course content is directly related to the land. At some places, such as Laurieston Hall, visiting courses and camps are offered a professional service of accommodation and catering. Elsewhere, course participants visit for the day or camp in tents, whilst instruction in subjects such as permaculture design, rustic furniture making and the cultivation of chilli peppers is offered by those who run the project.

At the seven woodland enterprises I encountered softwood forestry, coppice work and the conservation management of mixed deciduous woodlands. Initiatives include the restoration of native woods by removing alien species such as Sitka spruce and sycamore, the cultivation of future high-quality timber trees, and coppicing both for firewood and green-woodworking materials. Two places have very different facilities for planking saw logs. At Dun Beag in western Scotland, a lightweight petrol-powered mobile Lucas sawmill is used to convert low-quality sitka spruce into building materials, which are being used to create affordable housing. In contrast, a seven horsepower 1937 single cylinder, mobile steam engine, fuelled with wood powers the 1921 Stenning rack saw-bench at Tinker's Bubble. It is used to cut Douglas Fir and Larch logs felled on site, to meet the community's needs for building materials and fence posts, along with the occasional order from outside the community.

A more refined style of adding value to wood was in evidence elsewhere, such as using traditional green-wood working techniques to make a range of furniture and bowls. Two interviewees were charcoal burners, alongside other occupations. One uses the wood which is a by-product of his tree surgery business, and supplies charcoal as well as free-range eggs and vegetables to a range of local shops and garages. The other is restoring coppice on his land and uses the smaller quantities of charcoal he produces in blacksmithing workshops at community festivals and schools.

The variety of scales of commercial production amongst the farms and smallholdings I studied is graphically illustrated when the annual sales of each holding are compared. The turnovers range from £4,000 to £95,000 and bear little relationship to the acreage of the holding.

Lifestyles

While all the projects I visited exhibited care for the environment in their management of the land, the degree to which their ecological values influence their lifestyles varied. On the one hand families and communities were trying to minimise their environmental impact by living in small, self-built eco-homes serviced by renewable energy and compost toilets, sharing cars with their neighbours and reducing their consumer needs. Other people limited their ecological efforts to the, nevertheless valuable, activities of recycling and thoroughly insulating their otherwise fairly conventional homes.

Trying to live, as well as work, in as sustainable a way as possible adds extra demands on personal energy use, especially in today's society which often seems biased against greener lifestyles. For example, trying to live without a car in rural areas is difficult due to the poor public transport and dispersed nature of modern life (friends, family and services usually requiring a journey of at least three or four miles). Yet the beliefs of many of those I interviewed motivated them to incorporate, at some inconvenience, more sustainable practices into their daily lives in order to cut carbon emissions, reduce pollution and conserve biodiversity. The ways people are attempting to live more sustainable lifestyles are an important variable in this analysis of the human energy demands of different smallholdings.

In comparing the environmental credentials of the lifestyles of the case studies I focus on the following features:

- Design and size of house
- Domestic energy supply (fuel and electricity)
- Car use
- Shared resources

Design and size of house

I encountered a wonderful variety of living accommodation, ranging from simple benders, caravans and a shepherd's wagon to wooden and straw bale eco-cabins and round houses. Many had designed and built their own houses to meet their combined needs for affordable housing and the desire to minimise resource use. Common features therefore included the use of locally available and recycled materials (wood, straw bales, stone, re-used windows, pallets), high insulation (straw bales in walls and roof, sheep's wool and rock wool), thermal mass (cob and stone) and natural light. In trying to minimise visual impact, some had chosen turf roofs, whilst others had opted for imitation or reconstruction of traditional buildings.

In contrast to these self-built dwellings, some of my interviewees were living in more conventional houses. These too varied greatly and included old farmhouses, a Victorian terraced house and a modern brick bungalow. Five out of the nine communities I visited were using buildings from old estates and farms, including a large elegant hall dating back to 1893 and a modern pebbledashed farmhouse. Such houses have the benefit of being surrounded by farm buildings and sometimes workers' cottages, offering opportunities for conversion into additional accommodation. At Brithdir Mawr and Keveral, farm-buildings had been converted into comfortable flats enabling residents to combine the privacy of their own accommodation with the benefits of living and working in close co-operation with others.

Domestic energy supply

Again, the sources of energy utilised for cooking, heating space and water ranged from mains electricity, gas and oil, to a variety of renewable energy options. Wood was frequently used for heating space, even in houses that also had fossil-fuel-powered heating, whilst at a number of places it was used exclusively for cooking, space and water heating. These projects also tended to provide all or most of their electricity from renewable energy systems, including wind generators, solar panels and micro-hydro generators. Apart from two exceptions, the communities and single people were using renewable energy sources more than couples and families, who tended to be living in houses attached to the grid.

Car use

Living rurally, all the projects were using cars for transport to some extent. The main efforts to reduce the environmental impact of driving were car-share schemes and the use of biodiesel made from recycled chip oil. The car-share schemes were all operating in communities and varied from formal arrangements in which a limited number of cars were owned by the whole community, to informal lending of private cars to fellow community members. At Tinker's Bubble, two cars are shared by the community of ten adults and all the costs of tax, insurance, running and maintenance are combined into a mileage cost of 25 pence, payable by each person whenever the car is used, on top of a £1 start-up fee. Such an arrangement makes the cost of driving more visible, deters people from making very short or long journeys (which could be undertaken by walking, cycling or public transport) and encourages people to share journeys to cut costs.

Shared resources

Generally speaking, those who were living communally tended to share resources more than people living independently. Such communal resources included renewable-energy systems (wind generators, solar panels, and batteries), washing-machines, farm animals and equipment. A couple of smallholders were sharing farm machinery (a tractor, a topper and a steerage hoe), but those who had tried to share hay-making equipment had struggled when they both wanted to make hay at the same time. Shared resources bring the benefit of reduced consumption of purchased goods, but must be balanced against the possible inconvenience of items being poorly maintained or misplaced when they are needed.

Reasons for choosing to live and work on the land

The first question I asked everyone during their interviews was why they had chosen to live and work in their particular way on the land. Interviewees gave varied responses, which are ranked in order of the frequency with which each theme was mentioned, in Table 4.3.

By far the most common reason for choosing to live and work on the land was a desire to live in a more environmentally sustainable way. This was expressed both as a political statement and a profoundly practical response to the destructive impact of many aspects of modern, Western lifestyles, as these responses demonstrate:

"To help a small part of the planet."

"I spent a lot of time in Thailand and saw how people lived, saw ancient culture (2,500 years old) and how western culture was affecting it. I was very impressed by the people. When I returned to the UK I got the biggest culture shock and realised it was quite illusory and unsustainable. For several years I pottered about and travelled in the UK. Western culture was crazy. I needed to be where my roots were and exist on the land in a more sustainable way. I wasn't willing to engage with mainstream society, had very few possessions, couldn't engage working as an engineer and needed to find another way to live."

"I had an increasing awareness of resource use, climate change, corruption in the world and didn't feel I could continue living like that. I needed to start taking responsibility for my life, how I live, where I live."

"As I became older I became more aware of environmental issues. It became

Rank	Frequency with which theme mentioned (n=67)	Theme
1	23	Political – to take positive environmental action
2	16	Reasons relating to children
3	15	Directed by circumstances/opportunity arose
4=	14	To live with like-minded people (C.D.*) Previous experience of living on land
5	11	Wanted to work on land/be a farmer or grower
6=	10	Wanted to be close to nature Land-based lifestyle was long-held dream
7=	9	Didn't choose to live like this – it just happened I needed a change from previous lifestyle – stress Wanted to be self-sufficient/have control over resources
8=	8	Housing issues (affordable, desire to self-build) To have greater independence/control over life
9=	7	To live in a pleasant environment/the countryside Influenced by upbringing
10	6	Wanted to work outside
11=	5	Attracted by healthy and fulfilling lifestyle To share resource (*C.D.) Belief in common ownership (*C.D.) Did a permaculture course
12=	3	Seeking stability/security I needed to live like this
13	2	To do something real/tangible
14=	1	I was needed by community/elderly parents Attracted to non-hierarchical (*C.D.) Financial reasons To be with my partner more

Table 4.3 – Ranked responses to the question,
"Why did you decide to live and work on the land?"
*C.D. = Community Dweller

clear that engendering a wider awareness of natural cycles of nature and our interdependence with the natural world was maybe one of the most important changes we needed to make as a civilisation. The reason why I grow organic vegetables and dabble in renewable energy systems is because I wish to promote and demonstrate these ideas as well as live in a way which is less harmful and feels right."

"I wanted to take responsibility for that which I used. I saw so many ways the world and its wildlife were being damaged by Western culture and global trade."

"Living my politics as much as possible. I wanted to provide for myself."

Connected to these more political environmental reasons, were a large number of responses where people were attracted to the pleasant environment of their current home or wanted to live in the countryside generally, be closer to nature and spend more of their time outside. Whilst some people had grown up in rural or even agricultural settings, others came from a more urban or suburban environment. Another strong motivation for a number of people was the desire for their children to enjoy a rural upbringing and to understand where their food came from, as well as wanting an occupation that enabled them to spend more time with their families:

"To be with the children whilst working in the garden."

"Here I could live and work and be with the family."

"I grew up on a smallholding. I wanted to bring my children up like that, so they could grow up outside, lots of space, natural surroundings."

"I wanted to have kids. I had had an upbringing here (at community) that had benefited me and I thought it could benefit my children."

"When we had children we wanted them to have the space, contact with animals and grow our own food."

Some people had returned to a land-based livelihood via a circuitous route:

"I was brought up on a conventional arable and pig farm. I didn't feel much of a connection with it. I studied and picked up some environmental ideas, sustainability, organic farming and became vegetarian. I went on a permaculture design course, which opened up my ideas. I saw the way forward was to produce food for people and get the message across that way. I wanted to find a way of living on the land, making a living out of it, contributing to community, live a relatively simple way of life. Interesting that I've come full circle from my agricultural background – now I eat meat and raise pigs again.

> "I grew up with it (agriculture) as a child and I didn't want to do it and it wasn't in my game plan. It's a damn hard life. Then I met my husband."

A third important motivation for choosing a land-based livelihood and home was the independence it provided, compared with conventional modern life. Nine people cited the desire to have direct control of the resources with which to meet basic needs such as food, shelter and electricity, rather than having to earn money with which to buy them. Another eight stated that they wanted the independence of being self-employed, which gave them the power to choose how to use their time.

> "Primarily self-empowerment. To directly get the things you need, rather than going out to do other work to get money to buy things. Life is increasingly ruled by accountants etc, who have the power, yet put them on a desert island and they'd starve."

> "We're moving towards self-sufficiency to be out of the rat race and in control of how much we work."

> "I like self-employment. I can work when I choose to work."

> "Having worked for other people, which I found frustrating at times, I wanted to work for myself."

> "I wanted more independence with schedules."

A very specific attraction of certain set-ups was the affordable housing they offered or the opportunity to self-build. Such reasons were cited mainly by community dwellers, although a single person and a family farmer also mentioned being able to build their own house as key reasons for their choices:

> "We definitely wanted to build a house."

> "I've always wanted to build my own home."

> "Affordable housing and land were major reasons for joining the co-op."

> "I'd always felt uncomfortable in a flat – much more space, comfort, convenience than I wanted. I resented that there was no choice of another way to live, and it had to be paid for. At (the community) I was able to build a house appropriate to my needs."

It was interesting to observe how, for many people, their current living and working arrangement was not a conscious choice, but rather the result of circumstance. For instance, one family who had started selling their surplus garden produce tapped a market which led to continuous expansion of their market garden until they were growing several acres of vegetables. Others had followed partners into a communal or land-based lifestyle and found that they liked it. In contrast, for many their lifestyle was the end result of a long-held dream or simply a natural progression from the outdoor profession they had been practising previously.

> "I had never decided to live any other way."

> "It wasn't really a decision. It's something I've always wanted to do."

> "It was the idealistic sixties, back-to-the-earth thing. I grew vegetables, used to preserve food. I wanted to try the market-garden thing."

> "I'd had inspiration since very young (5 or 6 years old). I grew up in Swaziland and had trouble with the school system. Seemed to be lies – very dodgy. I was looking for alternatives to what was around me and dreamt of self-sufficiency."

A number of reasons for lifestyle choice related specifically to communal living, the most frequently cited being the desire to live with like-minded people and enjoy the benefits of mutual support.

> "I love being close to the earth and close to nature, but I couldn't do this on my own. I want to live with other people who share my beliefs and have them help me bring up my children."

> "My main reason for choosing a community was to get social support with the children, when my partner was away. I wasn't an activist or anything."

> "I wanted to have other adults and kids around."

> "I found 'normal' life, in a house, on my own with a full-time job unsatisfying. I yearned to live in community and have a deeper connection with people."

> "I've always like the idea of living co-operatively. It's preferable to isolation. Before living here I had lived on traveller sites and liked group living."

For others, the motivation for living in a community ranged from the ideological (a belief in common ownership and co-operative working), to the practical (greater security and stability in a community compared with tenancies, squats and nuclear families).

Happiness, and the vitality and human energy that flow from it, is closely related to achieving personal aspirations. Whilst interviewees had various reasons for choosing to live and work in their particular way, whether their expectations were born out seemed to be an important factor in determining the success of the project. The fact that so many of the themes mentioned as motivations for choosing a land-based way of life recur in the following section as pleasures experienced whilst living out that lifestyle, is an indication that on the whole people's expectations were fairly realistic.

Main pleasures

The second question in the interviews was, "What are the main pleasures you gain from living like this?". Many of the answers I received echoed and amplified the reasons given for choosing their particular way of life. For example, frequently mentioned pleasures were the social environment, the beautiful surroundings and the sense of freedom people felt about how they used their time. The responses to the pleasure question are ranked in table 4.4, according to how frequently each theme arose.

It was very interesting to see how many people valued the social context of their land-based lifestyle, which was often the first pleasure they mentioned. All but three of the 29 who cited social environment as being a pleasure, were community dwellers. As we will see later on, living in close proximity with others was also seen as the source of many problems including enervating conflict and time-consuming meetings. However, the enjoyment of sharing meals, responsibilities and resources such as land, housing, cars and agricultural equipment, as well as the stimulation and friendly support of living close to others clearly outweighed the drawbacks of communal life for a number of people. On a deeper level, the sense of belonging, resulting from being part of a community, was specifically mentioned as an enriching and psychologically important aspect of life:

> "There's the pleasure of sharing. I don't think anyone should sit alone with their meal. It's fun meeting people, exchanging things (culture, experiences), stimulating mentally, constantly discussing, questioning. There's always someone to cook a meal."

> "The moments of hysterical laughter around the kitchen table, or group hug. Feeling of being loved and being part of something. Moments of human contact. Almost everything is pleasurable."

> "Pleasures to do with social – feeling of belonging."

> "I enjoy living with a bunch of people with whom I'm in equal relationships."

> "Knowing there are people around, though not actually interacting directly with them."

> "Having both people around and my own space."

The last two quotes illustrate the point that whilst having people nearby is valued, most people also need to have their own private space. The scale at which privacy is needed varies. Some are content to simply have their own room, others need a house even if it is very small and simple, whilst many need to own their land, and take pleasure from the wider community as these non-community dwellers demonstrate:

Rank	Frequency with which theme mentioned (n=67)	Theme
I	29	Social environment
2	22	Quiet or pleasant environment
3=	21	Control over time and being self-employed Sense of realness, connection, meaning to life
4	13	Access to opportunities
5=	12	Sense of achievement/challenge Hosting visitors Eating home-grown produce
6=	11	Sense of belonging Being outside
7=	7	Building our own home Sharing resources and responsibilities
8=	6	Sense of living in the 'right' way Other people's appreciation of what we produce
9=	5	Lifestyle for children Quality of life
10	3	Flexibility Not having to commute
11=	2	Variation and diversity of experiences/work Developing land-based knowledge and skills Being creative When co-operating works/achievement as a group Sharing cooking and eating Escape from conventional life

Table 4.4 – Ranked responses to the question,
"What are the main pleasures you gain from living like this?"

"Living in a quiet place with a good social environment of neighbours and friends."

"People around are ever so friendly, but it's nice to have your own patch."

This theme of having control over land, use of time and decision-making was one that re-emerged strongly as a pleasure, mentioned by single people, family farmers and community dwellers:

"Being in control of our lives more – control of physical environment."

"It's very rare that I have to do anything I don't want to do" (C.D.)

"Being in charge of my own schedule and having flexibility and diversity in what I do."

"I love the freedom of being able to not work if you want to, and go and pick blackberries."

"To be busy when my energy is high in the summer and not busy when it is low in the winter."

Having control over your time-management and the power to make independent decisions about land-management is a form of freedom. The appreciation of this freedom reflected the disempowerment some people had experienced in mainstream life, prior to living as they are now, when they had had to work to other people's schedules, perform meaningless tasks and exist in a way that was disconnected from natural cycles. An equal pleasure was the sense of 'reality' and meaning that people's lifestyles gave them, along with the feeling of 'this is the right way to live'.

"Being able to go to sleep every night and think that whatever we did was worth something."

"The 'being out there' with the mud, wind, trees, animals etc. A real, earthy sort of existence."

"Key part – being in the elements in a strong way – fire, wind, mud, rich depth of beauty to it. Being in a warm bender on a cold night with a big stack of wood."

"Everyday things take more time to do, so you get more pleasure from things like a cup of tea or having a bath because you can't get it at the flick of a switch."

"I've really enjoyed knowing that whatever I put in I get something back – sowing seeds results in food, cutting firewood enables me to have a fire, collecting water leads to a cup of tea."

"Feeling like we're living more responsibly, realistically, sustainably."

Thirteen respondents mentioned the specific opportunities that their lifestyle provided. These included an enjoyment of sharing their pleasant environment with visitors, cooking food for friends over a fire and living without mains electricity. Some community dwellers considered that they were able to enjoy a better quality of life and more opportunities on a low income in a community than they would if they lived alone.

The constant challenges and sense of achievement derived from a land-based livelihood were mentioned as a pleasure by 12 people, and the satisfaction of eating fresh, home-produced food on a regular basis was valued highly. People also enjoyed watching other people appreciating both the produce of their land and the experiences gained by a visit:

"It's a challenge. Making it work is quite pleasurable. When customers come in and say 'Wow, this is fresh.' We're providing an alternative for people."

"When everything in the boxes was mine and had been harvested that day. The produce was fine, fresh, no one could find fault. This year it's even better. I find that amazing."

"The satisfaction of the People Centre – seeing people come for the week as individuals and then join as a group together. We're good at that. Feeding them wholesome meals."

"The food – growing, harvesting and eating your own food is a real privilege. Harvesting salad and eating it 15 minutes later."

"Seeing people be inspired and provoked by what we have done here."

Many, many more pleasures were mentioned and the sense of the richness and diversity of people's lives in the places I visited shone through in most responses to this question, even when other aspects of life were tough. As one couple I interviewed observed, "Even when we're extremely tired we still can take pleasure in things like a beautiful sunset," to which his wife responded, "It's a life skill, being able to get up and go out to enjoy a sunset when you're that tired!"

Such a comment reflects a crucial ingredient in the successful sustenance of human energy – attitude. The ability to recognise and remember the pleasures and privileges of one's chosen lifestyle is as important, if not more important, than political motivation when times get tough. However, developing a healthy attitude to work and leisure is a refinement that will be addressed towards the end of this book. Before that it is necessary to explore some of the more practical components of sustainable systems, such as choice of tools, social structures and livelihood strategies.

Chapter Five

Energy-efficient Design

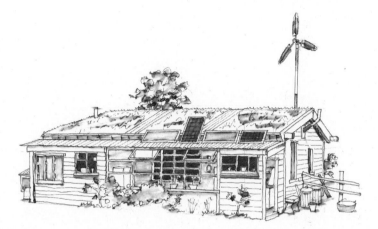

A well planned or designed system can make a significant contribution to the energy efficiency of a farm, smallholding or forestry project, and general energy efficiency facilitates the wise use of human energy. In this part of the book I will look at methods for designing sustainable ways of living on the land from a human energy perspective. Physical layout and choice of production system are two aspects of design that can influence the energy input which is required, and will be examined using the case study holdings to illustrate the discussion.

Several of the projects I visited were designed using permaculture principles, which offer a useful basis for creating sustainable living systems. Other projects had naturally arrived at permaculture style solutions without labelling them as such. Many more of the places I visited were employing organic principles on their gardens and farms and the second half of this chapter will compare organic production systems with permaculture design to show how each can contribute to balancing the human energy equation.

The role of permaculture

Permaculture is "the conscious design and maintenance of agriculturally productive ecosystems which have the diversity, stability and resilience of natural ecosystems."[1] Its name comes from the fusion of the two words, "permanent" and "agriculture", implying that systems designed with permaculture techniques are likely to work for a very long time. There is much debate about the value of permaculture between permaculturists and other land managers. Some see it as repackaging of old ideas and common sense. Even permaculturists don't claim many of the concepts used within permaculture to be new, but state that it is the deliberate application of patterns and ideas observed within nature to create low-input man-made systems, that distinguishes it from other land-management practices.

As part of the research for this book, I went on a permaculture design course to make up my own mind on the value of permaculture as a design technique, and to find out how it could help conserve human energy. Although many of the ideas on the course seemed very familiar to me after eight years of working on farms and market gardens and studying agriculture, I came away with a useful set of tools for designing sustainable systems. I wouldn't say that permaculture training is imperative for anyone wanting to live sustainably on the land – there are many valuable pathways to this knowledge, not least of which is experience. However, as a framework for working out solutions to ecological problems and bringing together complex ideas, permaculture design is a valuable skill. I would recommend it be used to complement other more specific skills, such as market gardening, forestry or green building.

In his book *The Earthcare Manual*, the permaculture teacher Patrick Whitefield makes the point that good designs come from 'listening' to the land and the people who will be affected by the design.[2] Listening to the land involves mapping, surveying and observing it, ideally for a full year. This enables a greater understanding of how the land responds to different weather conditions (e.g. wind, frost, rain, drought), variations in light and shade, and seasonal changes in flora and fauna. Listening to the people who will be part of the system is an active process, which entails asking questions (verbally or via a questionnaire) and being prepared to hear all their responses before making design suggestions. When all the necessary information (base map; site survey; questionnaires) has been gathered, it is evaluated and analysed before the actual designing begins. At this stage it can be helpful to identify strengths, weaknesses, opportunities and constraints (SWOC) or use the key planning tools outlined in the 'Layout' section below. In making design proposals it is a good policy to revisit the aims of the project, before outlining general suggestions and fleshing them out with details.

Layout

The layout of a farm or smallholding can help life run smoothly and efficiently, or sap people's energy and cause endless frustration. The latter was evident in the response to a question about the main problems experienced in day-to-day life, by one community member:

"There's the weariness of being up the hill, so everything has to be hauled up. The fact that poor design leads to extra energy wastage every minute of the day. You could have two lifetimes with all the energy wasted."

A member of another community also made reference to the inconvenience of living up a hill and the difficulty of getting her three-year-old son up and down it. Clearly the choice of location for your home and its related facilities is of primary importance when designing the layout of a holding. It is not surprising therefore that the concept of zoning, one of the permaculture planning tools which will be discussed below, centres on the home.

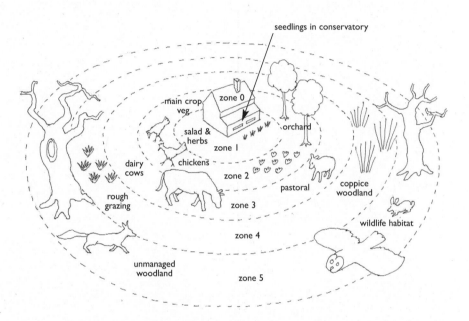

Figure 5.1 – Permaculture zoning.

Together with networking, sector and elevation, zoning is used by permaculturists to find the best placement for elements in a design.[3] Patrick Whitefield defines the four words as having the following meanings in a permaculture context:

- The zone in which a piece of land falls reflects how much human attention it receives, or how close it is to the back door. For example, whilst a herb garden would need to be easily accessible, and hence near to the house, a plantation which only requires occasional visits can afford to be much further away.

- Network analysis looks at the relationships on a site where there is more than one centre of human attention.

- A sector is an area affected by an influence coming onto the site from outside, such as wind, sunshine, flows of water, pollution, neighbours and views. The principle of sector is to place things so they have the best possible relationships with these influences.

- The elevation characteristics of the site include the degree of slope, the direction in which the slope faces (its aspect), its height above sea level and its height relative to the surrounding land.

One of the two holdings at Fivepenny Farm in Dorset is a good example of zoning being used to manage the needs of a working farm alongside parenting responsibilities. The farmhouse (Zone 0) was (until it had to be moved to a less visible place) located within the market garden (Zone I), right next to a polytunnel. On the front of the farmhouse, a conservatory provided a warm, easily accessible place for raising seedlings. Having the polytunnel so close to the house, meant that on a wet or cold day Jyoti, the farmer, could still be within hearing distance of her young children if they wanted to stay in the house while she worked. The orchards, chicken run and main crop vegetables (Zone 2) are all slightly further from the house, but still within hearing distance of a fox attack. The sheep, cows and pigs are rotated around the outer fields of the farm (Zone 3) but are still less than five minutes walk away from the house, so daily feeding and milking is convenient. A mixed woodland (Zone 4) has been planted down the hill at the far southern edge of the land and a network of mature hedgerows on ancient banks around the farm provide a valuable habitat (Zone 5) for wild mammals, birds, insects and plants.

Pentiddy Woodland Project in Cornwall has two centres of operation, the barn and the homestead, illustrating the principle of network. The family were fortunate that, when they bought it, the land already had a barn up near the road. This has provided a valuable covered area where deliveries of logs, straw and other materials can be stored. Half of the barn has been converted into a workshop, home to Anthony Water's furniture-making business, Heartwood Designs. However, being exposed and highly visible the barn area is not an ideal site for a house, so they have tucked their mobile home into a more sheltered spot further down the field. The two sites are joined by a track winding up through the newly planted hazel coppice, and each has overlapping zones of activity around them. The vegetable garden is conveniently close to the mobile home and the sheep are kept in a field just beyond. Up near the barn, a children's playhouse has been constructed, providing a focus for the children's play if Anthony is watching them whilst working in the workshop.

The concept of sector is demonstrated by the irrigation system at Ourganics, a permaculture project in Dorset. The low-lying location of this mixed smallholding (salad and fruit garden, orchard and free-range hens) might be seen as a disadvantage due to the flood risk from the adjoining river. However, Pat Foxwell who owns the garden has adapted the traditional system of irrigating meadows to improve grass-growth, to create a low-energy irrigation system for her market garden. Water flows around the nearby village and surrounding fields in a system of gravity fed leats. By creating a pond at the top of her garden, near to where the leat enters her land, Pat is able to divert and store water for use in the garden when she needs it. During dry months, the pond sluice is opened daily at 4pm to flood the garden. Thus the water table is raised to near the surface at the top of the garden and at the bottom, where there is a system of raised beds, the paths between the beds become miniature canals. The water backs up against a bung, which when removed enables it to drain into a lower pond and from there flow back into the leat. This irrigation system simply requires the daily opening and closing of the sluices, and a little annual maintenance of the pond banks, and makes good use of a natural resource which flows through the land anyway. Compare this with the time spent watering plants by hand or the high technical input and investment involved in buying automatic irrigation, and the system scores highly in human energy, ecological and financial terms.

The forestry permaculture project at Dun Beag makes use of its position on the side of a Scottish mountain to demonstrate the elevation principle. The house and workshop are located where light reflected from the sea can penetrate horizontally through the trees. Working on a hill it is wise to work with gravity wherever possible, and the slope is used for the easy movement of wood from the plantation area down to the road. At the time of my visit, a mobile sawmill was being operated in the plantation above the house and milled planks were being moved downhill in a plastic chute. The community composting scheme at Dun Beag also uses gravity to help turn the compost down the slope.

The four concepts can be used to analyse the existing set-up of a smallholding, farm, community or project; to develop a new design or as a way of evaluating a new design proposal. It is critical that the four are used together, because it is the interactions between them which give the full benefits. However, it may be found that there are conflicts between the ideal locations suggested by different tools. Part of the creative process is to reconcile the results from applying all the tools to find the 'best fit' for that particular situation.

Unfortunately sometimes the power of one influence over the others can skew the outcome of the design exercise and result in a layout that is far from ideal. I am thinking particularly here of planning authorities, which could arguably be described as a sector influence, since they come from the outside. Like neighbours, planning authorities will be concerned with the visual impact of any new development and will want to minimise it if they allow it at all.

For example, the residential settlement at Tinker's Bubble is on top of a hill, 5-10 minutes walk from the road, where it is hidden by a conifer plantation. The shade of the trees surrounding the houses makes cultivating vegetable gardens outside the back door impractical. Renewable-energy equipment (solar panels and wind generator) has to operate outside the plantation, at some distance from the settlement. This leads to efficiency losses as electricity travels along long wires to reach where it is needed. However, whilst the hill and the dispersed nature of different elements of the community cause frustration to all its members at some time or other, the layout has also brought benefits. Being high up, on free-draining soils covered by a layer of pine needles, winter mud is less of a problem than it would be in a low-lying open space or deciduous woodland. The trees also provide welcome cool shade during the summer and seem to reduce the prevalence of flies and midges compared with the open areas down the hill.

One consequence of the residential part of Tinker's Bubble being located at a distance from the farm land is that various alternative centres of operation have developed, illustrating the principle of network. At the bottom of the hill, near the road and the car park is a communal barn, which was originally built to house the sawmill. It was built there to enable timber to be extracted downhill, and near its point of departure when it is planked up and stacked to be seasoned. The barn is also used as a fruit and vegetable store and packing shed, being conveniently near both some of the gardens and the car park for transporting produce to market. Another centre of operations is the stable/tool shed, which is located in a field cut off from the rest of the open space by a small wood. It serves as a winter animal shelter, milking parlour and source of manure for the communal garden, which is next door. The different collections of buildings are joined by a well-trodden network of paths along which milk, vegetables and firewood are transported regularly. Although the overall layout is far from ideal, an attempt has been made to cluster complementary functions.

Production systems

In case 'production systems' sounds too industrial, here is what I mean in this context. I am using production in a broad sense to mean all 'products' which are gained from the land including wildlife conservation and the pleasure of having a green place to share with other people as well as subsistence and commercial goods. All farms, smallholdings and forestry projects are systems in that they are an assembly of components connected together in an organised way.[4] A farming system is "a group of interacting components, operating together for a common purpose, capable of reacting as a whole to external stimuli and centred on the farming family." [5]

It is important to include human beings in the design of any farming or forestry system, for it is they who are responsible for making the decisions and carrying out the work. When I was studying for my MSc in Sustainable Agriculture, we spent time discussing what exactly was meant by 'sustainable agriculture'. A definition which I liked was that "agriculture is sustainable when it is ecologically sound, economically viable, socially just, humane and adaptable, and is a dynamic concept which allows for the changing needs of an increasing global population."[6] Such a definition goes to the heart of what this book is about – namely, the importance of placing the well-being of the workers on an equal footing to that of the environment and the finances of the farm.

The main production system I encountered at the projects I visited was organic farming, a system centred around the maintenance of a healthy, living soil from which strong, disease-resistant plants and animals can grow. Successful organic farming relies on the knowledge and observational skills of the farmer, and as such requires a high input of mental energy, whilst being a low-input system in terms of external materials. The application of permaculture principles to farming and forestry, which I witnessed on at least ten holdings, has the potential to reduce the human input required to produce food and other goods by replicating self-perpetuating natural ecosystems. The remainder of this chapter will focus on organic farming systems and systems based on permaculture principles, comparing the contributions each can make to the sustenance of human energy.

Organic farming

Organic farming is a production system which uses crop rotation, the recycling of organic matter, nitrogen fixation by leguminous green manures and aspects of biological pest control instead of depending on synthetically compounded agrochemicals to maintain soil fertility and control crop pests and weeds.[7] It is a term legally defined by European legislation and to sell produce as organic, producers must be certified by a body whose standards comply with those of Europe. This seemingly tiresome bureaucracy is necessary to protect consumers, who are typically separated from the producer by a long supply chain. To obtain certification a farmer must abide by the detailed production standards of a certifying body, such as the Soil Association or Organic Farmers and Growers in the UK, be inspected annually, be subject to spot checks and pay a registration fee.

All the case studies in my survey were using organic production practices, but only ten out of the twenty-eight were officially certified organic.

This is mainly because; unless you are commercial, the cost of certification (with the Soil Association, between £420 and £620 per year depending on acreage) is not worthwhile. Furthermore, any processing of raw materials requires additional fees. Some projects, especially those using permaculture principles, also find organic standards restrictive of certain practices which make sense ecologically. For example the use of well-composted human manure and wood ash, both of which complete the nutrient cycle, are prohibited as soil additives.

Organic farming is different from non-organic agriculture in that it replaces off-farm inputs like nitrogen fertilisers, pesticides and herbicides with processes involving on-farm resources, such as the people, the soil and natural predators. As such, it is a cyclical system, as opposed to the linear nature of conventional farms which receive inputs (agrochemicals, feed, medicines) on a large scale, apply them to plants and animals to produce food which is sent on to, often distant, consumers. Looking more closely at the cyclical nature of organic farming it is possible to identify several processes at work:

- *Recycling of organic matter* – Organic matter, the basic building-block of soil fertility is a farm's most valuable resource. Care is therefore taken to recycle it at almost every opportunity (except human waste!!) by composting plant residues and animal manure and sowing green manures as a catch crop to prevent nutrient leaching.

- *Leguminous green manures and off-farm organic matter* – Nitrogen-fixing plants, or legumes, are sown as green manures to replace some of the nutrients lost to the farm when produce leaves the holding. It may also be necessary to import some compost or manure to make up for lost nutrients.

- *Rotation* – Both plant crops and livestock are rotated between different parts of the farm to prevent the build-up of pests and diseases.

If the soil is healthy, then the plants and animals that depend on it will be healthy. This is the underlying philosophy in organic farming. In theory it sounds straightforward, but the practice involves considerable knowledge, skill and attention to detail. Hence, the farmer is one of the farm's greatest resources. Whilst some processes on organic farms require more manual labour than conventional farms (for example weeding), management and observation also require a significant input of human energy. This was commented on by two of my interviewees, who said:

"People (as opposed to machines) pay attention to detail – if there are any problems with a crop you can sort them out. One of my workers always tells you if there's a problem (not everyone's like that). I try to walk round every day. With organic, if you spot a problem straight away you can deal with it more easily."

"We believe passionately that if you're going to grow vegetables you've got to live where it is – don't even begin to think about it if you can't. With the exception of being very large scale, mechanised, but at our scale you've got to live there. Badgers on the sweetcorn, blight on the potatoes – you've got to be observing it all the time."

The message is clear – thorough knowledge, detailed awareness and timely intervention can prevent small problems turning into big ones and often save a lot of work.

It would be wrong to assume that the use of fossil-fuel-powered machinery is reduced for organic farming systems because no sprays need to be distributed. Mechanical operations such as ploughing, harrowing, brush weeding and ridging up are frequently used on commercial organic farms to control weeds. Some even argue that organic systems require greater use of machinery than non-organic ones. 17 out of my 28 case studies use a tractor or rotavator for market gardening, arable cultivation, pasture management or hay making.

Therefore, organic systems employ natural processes and organisms (e.g. nitrogen fixation, earthworms, predators) to do much of the work of growing and protecting crops, but they also require skilled and careful management. Of course, the humans involved also have ongoing work, caring for animals; planting, weeding and harvesting crops; making hay; mending fences . . . the list is endless. However, a good farm manager or gardener will time operations to minimise work. For example, by hoeing before the weeds get too big or mending the fence before the animals escape.

Permaculture systems

Whilst organic systems use natural processes to help them, permaculture systems go a step further, trying to mimic ecosystems to create 'edible landscapes'. In theory, a well-designed, mature forest garden could be self-regulating and require no input of human energy, whilst providing a harvest of fruit, nuts, roots and leaves. As Patrick Whitefield says, "Permaculture is a low-energy approach, making minimum changes for maximum effect, working in co-operation with both natural forces and human communities."[8]

Bill Mollison and his colleagues, who pioneered permaculture in Australia in the 1970s, observed and analysed natural ecosystems to try to understand why they are so productive. They identified a number of features that contrast with industrial agricultural systems, as shown on table 5.1.[9]

Natural ecosystems	Industrial agricultural systems
• Diversity of species	• Monoculture
• Perennial and annual plants live together side by side	• Highly dependent on annual crops
• Multidimensional climax ecosystems (herb layer, shrub layer, canopy layer)	• Unidimensional
• Cyclical flows of energy and matter	• Linear flows of energy and matter
• Soil naturally fertile and covered by organic matter	• Nutrients supplied by fertilisers and soil often left bare
• All elements form an integrated whole and beneficial relationships arise between organisms	• Elements of system operate in relative isolation
• No tillage	• Tillage

Table 5.1 – Comparison of some defining features of natural ecosystems and industrial agricultural systems.

It is upon these features of natural ecosystems that permaculture design is based. For example, permaculture combines the principles of diversity, mixing perennial and annual plants and uses the concept of multidimensional design, by mixing tree crops, fruit bushes and edible herbaceous plants in forest gardens. Companion-planting makes use of the beneficial relationships between certain plants, such as marigolds which attract hoverfly which eat aphids on tomatoes. The idea of linking the outputs and inputs of different elements of a system and trying to make sure that each element produces more than one output, mimics the processes of ecosystems.

When combined, these principles have the potential to create a system in which human input is minimised, an objective which tallies well with that of trying to sustain human energy. During my travels I observed permaculture principles being applied individually and in combination, whether or not the project or farm identified itself as being a follower of permacultural ideas. This illustrates how permaculture is simply a modern name for the conscious practical application of common sense, based on observation of natural systems. Whether old or modern, permaculture principles applied to food production and land management have the potential to maximise energy efficiency and I witnessed them being used advantageously at several projects. To demonstrate this I will use some of the case studies to illustrate the application of the following permaculture principles:

- Diversity
- Input-Output (Linking and Multiple Outputs)
- No-Dig or Minimum Tillage
- Energy Flows

Diversity

As species diversity enhances the stability of ecosystems by increasing their capacity to adapt to change, so economic diversity enhances the stability of farms, smallholdings, or forestry initiatives. In practical terms this means spreading your effort between different enterprises, rather than relying on the production of one product or the whims of a single market. Hence, the losses caused by crop failure or the price of milk dropping are less likely to cause financial ruin because there are other income streams. Operating more than one enterprise can also enhance quality of life by varying work and encouraging the development of a range of skills. Involving the local community in a project can enrich it introducing social and cultural diversity, bringing a wider range of skills and outlooks.

You can have too much of a good thing, though, including diversity. The more enterprises a farm contains, the more it is necessary to spread your attention between them, which can be mentally tiring. The number of different projects a person can juggle varies greatly between individuals, and it is worth looking realistically at your own capacity to concentrate on different enterprises simultaneously before diversifying your attention too widely. One man I spoke to, who combined land work with off-site community development work, described his method of finding a balance between too much and too little diversity as follows:

> "I never take on more than three off-site contracts at the same time. I can juggle with three balls, but struggle with four or five balls, both literally and metaphorically."

All the permaculture holdings I visited consisted of several interlinking enterprises catering for a number of different markets. Mulberry Tree Farm, a two-family community in Herefordshire, consists of a one-acre market garden supplying vegetable bags to local families; a coppicing, charcoal making, green-woodworking and blacksmithing business; a mixed orchard; small flocks of sheep and free-range hens and a willow plantation to supply one resident who works as a sculptor and landscape gardener for community initiatives. From the start their projects have been firmly rooted in the local and regional community and the volunteers who help with the garden and craft workshops, run by the group at community festivals, ensure that fresh ideas and inspiration are constantly flowing into the community.

At Mulberry Tree Farm, the involvement of four co-operating adults spreads the responsibility for managing a great diversity of enterprises. Two other permaculture projects I visited were run by single people, yet still succeeded in keeping several micro-enterprises in operation. Pat Foxwell at Ourganics specialises in supplying salad and eggs to restaurants, shops and box schemes, but also grows a range of other vegetables which she sells at a monthly market in the village and to a handful of box scheme customers. She also runs permaculture courses, using her field as both a teaching aid and to supply food for the catering. David Blair, the forester at Dun Beag in Scotland, also uses his woodland as an illustration during permaculture courses, whilst running a woodland restoration and timber business, operating as a depot for a community composting project and growing his own food (fruit, vegetables and eggs).

Input-Output (Linking and Multiple Outputs)

Simply increasing the number of enterprises which make up a whole project could be very stressful unless the different components are linked. "The essence of what makes an ecosystem work is the network of beneficial relationships between its components. In order to allow these relationships to happen it is necessary to place things so that the output of one can become the input of another. This is linking." [10] Usually the different elements of a land-based system aren't chosen at random, but because they integrate with each other. For example, Fivepenny Farm comprises two market gardens, free-range egg and pig enterprises, a small herd of Jersey cows and another of mixed beef and dairy cows. The livestock (chickens, pigs, sheep and cows) contribute manure for the gardens. In turn, waste vegetables from the gardens and the market stall contribute food for the chickens and pigs. At certain times the chickens help to control pests and utilise crop residues in the garden and provide another product for the market stall – eggs. In the future, when the dairy enterprise starts up, whey and buttermilk will also help to fatten the pigs.

Another permaculture principle is that every plant, animal and structure in a design should serve as many functions as possible – this is the principle of multiple outputs. The community at Mulberry Tree Farm first started keeping sheep to manage their species-rich pasture, but the annual sale of lamb to friends and students in a nearby city now provides a valuable contribution to the project's income. In addition, the sheepskins of the lambs can be cured to make beautiful rugs.

'No-Dig' or Minimal Tillage

'No-dig' gardening has the potential to reduce energy use compared with a system based on inverting the topsoil. It is an example of how imitating natural ecosystems can improve efficiency, and is a central feature of permaculture. Its large-scale counterpart, minimal or no-till farming, is gaining popularity amongst conventional cereal farmers as a means of soil and energy conservation. However, it is harder to control weeds without herbicides at field scale than in a domestic vegetable garden, and most organic cereal farmers continue to plough. At an intermediate scale are the commercial organic market gardens described in this book, which range in size from a quarter of an acre to 11 acres. Some of those cultivating a smaller area (up to two acres) used no-dig systems, whilst the larger growers used tractors and rotavators to plough and cultivate.

Conventional wisdom is that weeds are best controlled by inverting the soil surface by digging or ploughing. The resulting exposed topsoil can then be kept clear of weeds by regular hoeing or harrowing, whilst the crop benefits from the rapid release of nitrates resulting from organic matter being oxidised. In a natural ecosystem, however, such regular, widespread disturbance of the soil rarely occurs, yet the soil remains fertile and aerated due to the organisms – earthworms, microbes and mycorrhizas (symbiotic fungi which help plants to access nutrients) – which are active within it. Inverting the soil by digging or ploughing, results in many of the soil microbes, 80% of which live in the top 5cm of the soil, being buried and thus destroyed.[11] Exposure of the soil to the air causes the rapid break-down of organic matter, upsetting the delicate balance between aerobic and anaerobic conditions which are a necessary part of the regulation of plant pathogens. Bare, cultivated soils are more vulnerable to erosion from water and the wind, and the mechanical action of ploughing or rotavating can compact lower layers of the soil, making them impenetrable to plant roots. The aim of minimal tillage or no-dig gardening is to allow the soil organisms to operate without disturbance, thereby maintaining the open structure and long-term fertility of the soil whilst eliminating the energy-intensive processes of ploughing or digging.

In a no-dig garden the natural tendency of the soil to be covered with either vegetation or leaf litter is imitated to control weed growth. Growing plants in dense stands so they out-compete weed growth or using natural or artificial mulching materials to block out light are common permaculture practices. Mulching not only saves time digging out weeds or hoeing, it also conserves water by reducing evaporation, and thus reduces the need for irrigation. At Sea Spring Farm, a couple run a successful business growing chilli peppers in ten polytunnels whilst also pursuing careers in editing, photography and horticultural journalism. They save time on weeding and watering by using black plastic sheeting to mulch all their tunnels and placing drip irrigation pipes underneath the mulch. Thus they are able to maintain the business on a part-time basis.

Laying mulch over grass or weedy ground for a few weeks or months is an effective way to start a garden. The initial enthusiasm of new gardeners is often dampened if their first job is several hours of back-breaking digging, as recommended by many gardening books. Instead, start in the autumn by creating a layer of well-rotted manure over the area of your bed. Cover it with cardboard or old newspapers (thickly layered) and weigh them down with a thick layer of damp straw, hay or old carpet. During the first season, vegetables raised in pots or potatoes can be planted through the cardboard, which after a winter of rain will be starting to disintegrate. By the time the first crop comes out the mulch will have mostly rotted away, and can either be removed or supplemented with more mulch for subsequent crops. I am constantly surprised by the light, friable quality of the bare soil that is revealed when the mulch is lifted.

On a small scale, preparing beds by mulching is a relatively easy way to create a clear patch of soil, but I add a note of caution to those wishing to scale up the process. The hardest work is usually accumulating the mulching materials, and when mulching is expanded to larger areas the quantity of materials needed can be quite staggering. I decided to start my quarter-acre plot at Tinker's Bubble using straw and cardboard as mulch. After a morning telephoning businesses in the local town to find out where I would be able to collect waste cardboard, and then a whole day travelling around collecting it in a large van, I was dismayed to find that it only covered a fraction of the area I wished to mulch. Amassing enough straw seemed almost as difficult, since I tried to use spoiled (damp and mouldy) straw and thatching rubbish (the old thatch which is removed before a roof is re-thatched), both of which were free. I ended up having to plough over half the garden with our horse to prepare it in time for the growing season, and concluded that unless you have space to stockpile the materials when they become available, there is a limit to the area it is sensible to try and mulch at one time. If you are committed to no-dig, I would recommend opening up smaller areas one season at a time, whilst for those who are in a hurry to start a large garden I would recommend cultivation with a machine or horse-drawn tools.

Fixed or raised beds are the other main feature of no-dig gardening. To conserve the natural aeration caused by soil organisms and avoid compaction, it is best not to walk on the soil and to create a system of access paths that enable you to reach all parts of the bed. Such paths can be straight lines between four-foot-wide beds, or wind between more irregular shaped beds. A classic permaculture idea is the keyhole-shaped bed, which enables the gardener to stand on a peninsular of compacted ground, surrounded by productive beds.[12] At Ourganics, this idea had been extended into three dimensions, with domes covered by netting, up which climbing plants can grow, shading the beds. By standing in one place the gardener can harvest climbing beans and shade tolerant salad leaves and strawberries, without compacting the soil in which they are growing.

Again, scale needs to be considered. Whilst raised beds with vertical sides constructed of planks, slab wood or woven branches have the benefit of preventing weed encroachment from the paths, they take time to construct. For a small family garden or a school growing project, such beds are ideal because once built they are easy to keep clear of weeds without too much bending. If larger-scale food production is your aim, the substantial input of labour and materials for a very limited productive area does not seem worthwhile. This was made very clear to me when I visited the community of La Sorga in France, where two weeks previously 14 volunteers had spent a week constructing beautiful raised beds with sides woven from branches, creating a growing area of about 50 square metres. The amount of labour input to create such a small growing area was in marked contrast to the farm I had just left, where one couple were cultivating 4 acres of vegetables with the help of a horse.

This is not to say that commercial growing in beds is impossible. For two years I worked at The Trading Post, a very productive five-acre market garden which is managed on a system of fixed beds, roughly level with the ground. Blocks of four-foot-wide beds, with mulched paths and wooden planks inserted at the ends to stop grass encroaching, contain beautiful soil and occasionally get cultivated with a rotavator if weeding has been neglected for some reason.

Another inspiring example of fixed beds, managed the no-dig way, is Charles Dowding's very successful commercial salad garden. When I visited briefly in September 2007, I was impressed by the abundant and immaculate rows of healthy plants, with not a weed to be seen between them. Attentive weed control is central to Charles' system. Before establishing raised beds he meticulously removes perennial weeds, such as docks, stinging nettles and couch grass, and remains vigilant for shoots that indicate remaining root fragments. Rather than incorporating compost, he lays it on the surface of the new beds, leaving earthworms and other soil fauna to mix it into the soil below. After planting, he recommends pulling out stray clumps of grass or chickweed throughout the winter to prevent them seeding in the spring, thereby multiplying themselves a hundredfold. By refusing to dig, he is neither burying weed seeds that are lying on the surface nor exposing buried seeds to daylight which would trigger their germination. He is also managing to make a good living from a small acreage of land without using fossil-fuel-powered machinery or tiring himself out with a harsh regime of manual work.

Energy flows

Ecosystems are very efficient in their use of energy, which in all instances can be traced back to the sun. Plants capture the sun's energy through photosynthesis and store it as carbon-based sugars. Through complex food webs, this energy is passed along from one creature to another, with a small amount being lost as heat during each transfer, until it has all been broken down into its constituent parts of carbon dioxide and water.

Energy cannot be recycled; it can only pass through a system, so it is important that in man-made systems, as in nature, it is used as efficiently as possible. In permaculture this is done by maximising the number of ways that the energy of each element in the system is used. For example, rather than viewing chickens solely as a source of eggs, the additional ways in which they use their energy (as body heat and by foraging for insects) can be turned into an advantage. A classic permaculture idea is that of combining the chicken house with the greenhouse, so that the warmth given off by the chickens at night helps raise the temperature in the greenhouse. Chicken tractors are a concept which uses the chicken's foraging instinct to clear ground of weeds and insect pests prior to cultivation, by confining them in a small area and then moving them on to the next area. Such a system is used on a commercial scale at Fivepenny Farm, where chickens are also brought into the polytunnels for intensive periods to clear old crops and the pests that have accumulated during their cultivation.

I witnessed another example of using foraging animals to harvest energy in the French Pyrenees. The mountain farm where I was staying had very sandy soils, which required a high input of compost to keep them fertile. Bringing compost in from other farms was out of the question, since the only access to the holding was via a steep mountain path. The manure generated by the farm's 35 milking goats was therefore as valuable a resource as their milk. In addition, 16 llamas were also kept for their manure. All the animals ranged throughout a 30-acre fenced parkland each day, and were folded at night, hence concentrating the plant energy from the mountainside in the barn. The resulting manure, when composted, produced sufficient organic matter to replenish the fertility of the sandy soil in the garden each year.

Two compatible systems?

Organic farming and permaculture design are two environmentally benign ways of managing land to produce food, fuel and fibre. Whilst the two sets of ideas and principles can be combined to create systems that are productive and energy-efficient, it is common to find people focusing more on one method or the other. One of the reasons for this is that it is harder to apply certain permaculture principles, for example 'no-dig', on a large scale.

Many organic producers, including several of those included in this book, operate at a relatively large scale and use machinery fuelled by fossil fuels or biodiesel to plough and cultivate their land in fairly conventional ways. They produce bulk volumes of a limited range of crops, for which, whilst they gain a premium for being organic, cannot be sold for a particularly high price. Others go to the opposite extreme, operating at a small scale (one sixth of an acre to one acre) and focusing on smaller quantities of diverse, high-value crops cultivated with hand tools and no-dig techniques. As noted earlier, it is difficult to find enough mulch to operate a hand-tool-based no-dig system at much more than the family garden scale. Although minimal tillage is becoming an increasingly popular way of preventing soil erosion and compaction on conventional farms, particularly in the United States, it is hard to control weeds without the use of herbicides or a plough.

However, the two systems need not necessarily be seen as mutually exclusive. As we shall see in the next chapter, I came across two farms that were managing to apply the principles of minimal tillage to organic vegetable production using shallow cultivations with horse-drawn tools. Furthermore, experiments are being carried out both in the UK and in the US to find ways of producing organic cereal crops with minimal tillage techniques. One method is bi-cropping an under-storey of low-growing white clover with cereals. The idea is that the clover will not only fix nitrogen to supply nutrients to the cereal, but its ground-hugging growth habit will subdue the growth of weeds.[13] At Wakelyns Farm in Suffolk, successful organic bi-cropping trials have been carried out with winter oats, wheat and triticale, but the technique is still at experimental stage.[14]

More radical ideas for reducing tillage include those suggested by Fukuoka and Wes Jackson. Fukuoka, a Japanese farmer and scientist, evolved an organic system that involved sowing pelleted grains of rice or barley into a permanent sward of white clover before the previous crop had been harvested. By flooding the field once a year he weakened the clover enough to prevent it out-competing the cereals. Over 25 years of development, Fukuoka's Natural Farming system became able to achieve yields comparable with those of conventional farmers in his locality.[15]

Wes Jackson is an agricultural scientist from Kansas, USA, who became alarmed by the soil loss resulting from modern cereal production. He observed how the natural vegetation of North American plains, the prairie, is a perennially productive ecosystem that preserves the soil. He established the Land Institute at Salina, Kansas, to undertake research into how prairie ecosystems could be imitated to form 'domestic prairies' consisting of mixtures of perennial plants which could produce edible grains and seeds. After studying the remnants of native prairie, his research team embarked on programmes of plant breeding and experimentation with different combinations of grasses (including domestic cereals), legumes (to provide nutrients by nitrogen fixation) and composites (members of the daisy family, such as sunflowers). The research is still in its early days, it could take fifty to a hundred years to determine whether the idea will work. However, early results have shown high total productivity compared with monocultures and success in out-competing annual weeds, due to the advanced state of growth of the perennial plants in early spring. Furthermore, lack of soil disturbance by cultivation enables the development of very effective networks of mycorrhiza (roots and fungal bodies) to transfer nutrients from legumes to other plants.[16, 17]

Whilst good design, incorporating natural principles, can go a long way towards reducing the work of producing food, fuel and shelter, human effort is required to implement the design and maintain it over the long term. A variety of tools are available to help create and manage gardens, farms and forestry systems and the next chapter examines the different options which are available.

Chapter Six

Wise Choice of Tools

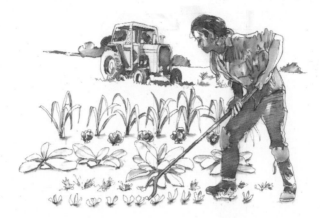

The modern agricultural systems which have brought people in wealthy countries a continuous supply of cheap and varied food are heavily dependent on fossil-fuel-powered machinery. It is commonly assumed that, in today's world, mechanisation is the only way in which it is possible to run an economically viable farming business. Indeed, with the high cost of living in modern society it is difficult to be commercially competitive if fossil-fuel power is replaced entirely by human labour. Yet, most people are now aware of the urgent need to reduce carbon emissions. One way to do this is to explore ways in which human labour and animal traction could be combined with mechanisation to produce food, fuel and timber in an efficient and economically competitive way.

The farms, forestry projects and smallholdings I visited used many different combinations of tools. Whilst some avoided the use of fossil-fuel-powered machines altogether, others used tractors or chainsaws and mains electricity on a daily basis. Most used a combination of fossil-fuel-powered machinery and human labour or animal power. It is in studying these systems of compromise that clues can be found as to how to realistically reduce fossil-fuel use, whilst remaining economically competitive and sustaining human energy. In this chapter I will first examine three of the options for horticulture, agriculture and forestry: hand tools, horse-drawn tools/machines, and machinery powered by fossil fuels or biofuels. I will then describe some of the systems which combined the use of two or three of these technologies. I will also look at the human energy implications of eliminating fossil-fuel-powered machinery altogether.

I have chosen to use the word 'tool' to represent any equipment that helps a person to do the job in hand. Hence in this context, not only spades, ploughs and chainsaws are considered to be tools, but also animals, such as sheep dogs, or the harness that enables a horse to be put to work. As Richard Heinberg points out in his classification of tools, outlined in Chapter Two (p.31), some tools require an external (or non-human) energy source, such as fire or oil, only in their manufacture, whilst others require an external source for their operation as well. Machines are more complex tools, which are made from a system of interacting parts. They can still be powered by human energy, as in the sewing-machine or the bicycle, or may employ an external source of power such as petrol, biodiesel or electricity. The latter are sometimes referred to as power tools, and here I refer to them as fuel-powered machinery. Alternatively, machines can be powered by draught animals, falling water or the wind. Although the point at which a simple tool becomes a machine is difficult to define, for the purposes of this chapter, all machines can be considered to be tools.

Hand tools

Using hand tools is as much a matter of engaging the mind as using muscles. A well designed and maintained hand tool, employed intelligently, can be a pleasure to use. Unfortunately, all too often poorly designed, badly maintained tools, used without skill, lead people to the conclusion that manual work is too difficult. The result is that many jobs that could easily be done by hand are performed by machines, resulting in inefficient use of fossil fuels. Gardening is the area where hand tools are most commonly used today, so I will start here, before moving my attention to activities where hand tools are less commonly seen in action.

Horticulture

The scale of a horticultural operation will determine the choice of tools, with manual operations gradually being replaced by mechanical ones the larger the acreage under cultivation. Various combinations of technology were being employed on the farms I visited, but hand tools were always present to a greater or lesser extent. On the whole, it was those places where gardening was solely a means of subsistence where hand tools were used exclusively, whilst most of the commercial operations were using them in combination with a rotavator, tractor or horse-drawn implements.

There is an excellent account of using hand tools for horticultural work in Eliot Coleman's classic book, *The New Organic Grower*. Whilst he does not use hand tools exclusively, his system of small-scale commercial growing combines the best modern designs of hand tools with moderate use of a walking tractor or rotavator. The premise of his book is that it is possible to make a good living from horticulture on five acres of land. Whilst for tilling (preparing soil, incorporating manures and crop residues and creating seed beds) he recommends a two-wheel walking tractor, for weed control he advocates cultivation with hand tools. His weed-control philosophy is one of prevention rather than cure by agitating the surface soil to cut off small weeds and prevent the appearance of new ones. "Weeding", he says, "deals with the problem after it has occurred. Weeds should be dealt with just after they germinate. Small weeds are easy to control, and the work yields greatest return for the least amount of effort. Large weeds are competition for the crops and the grower." [1]

Coleman's choice of tool for preventing weed growth is the wheel hoe, which he considers to be the most efficient implement yet designed for extensive garden cultivation. His favourable comparison of the small-wheel model with large-wheel alternatives gives an insight into the level of detail that is worth considering in the pursuit of human energy conservation. The diagram below (Figure 6.1) shows how, in a well-designed tool, the force exerted by the operator is transferred directly to the working part. In the case of a wheel hoe, this is the hoe part of the tool, not the wheel. A small-wheel design results in a much higher percentage of the effort being applied to the cultivating blade, because the force from the operator is transferred directly rather than via the wheel.

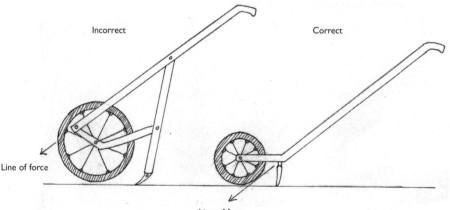

Figure 6.1 – Wheel hoe.

A similar application of basic physics can be used when filling wheelbarrows. By placing the load directly over the wheel, effort is saved compared with placing the load further back which results in the operator having to lift more weight himself. Such correct use of a simple tool like the wheelbarrow will not only save the gardener's back from being strained, but will also reduce the energy he needs to push the load. Hence, transferring multiple loads of manure, sand or wood-chippings becomes less strenuous and maybe even enjoyable.

When I was a student at Newcastle University, I used to be a conservation volunteer. I remember a task we undertook in the Scottish borders, laying footpaths in a stunningly beautiful country park. This involved wheel-barrowing gravel down from the road along a series of zigzagging paths. Once I had got the hang of it, I vividly remember the exhilaration of running down the hill with barrows of gravel, controlling it around corners and safely delivering my load to the path at the bottom. A couple of years later we did a similar job, laying paths alongside the River Tyne. This time we were moving gravel along the level, but by filling the barrows over the wheel and working steadily through the day (fuelled by cups of tea and biscuits) we moved seven tonnes between about twelve of us. A friend commented that the task could have been completed more efficiently with a machine. However, since it was a beautiful spring day, with the May blossom out and the river flowing gracefully alongside us, the quiet work of pushing a well-loaded wheelbarrow was a pleasure and was probably performed using less calories of energy in total than would have been used by a machine.

Another detail of wheelbarrow design is the height of its handles. With a good wheelbarrow it should be possible to keep your arms straight whilst holding the handles and pushing it along. With some barrows the handles are so high that it is necessary to bend your arms to hold the barrow off the ground, making the process of pushing it more strenuous. The solution lies in adapting the tool to suit the user, a principle which can equally be applied to other tools. For example, a barrow with high handles can be adjusted by carefully bending the handles to suit the height of the main user.

Choosing the suitable weather conditions for each task also saves energy, as well as protecting the soil from compaction. Where soils contain a high proportion of clay, wet weather quickly leads to soil clinging to tools and boots, making them heavier to lift. Such mud clogs up the wheels of barrows making them harder to push, and significantly increasing the total amount of energy required to complete a job as compared to drier conditions.

To achieve maximum efficiency with hand tools, they should be an appropriate weight and well maintained. Coleman points out that when a field worker with a cultivating hoe is making an average of 2,000 strokes per hour, the weight of the tool is an important consideration. "If a tool weighs even a few ounces more than necessary, the effect of moving that weight over a day's work results in the unnecessary expenditure of a great deal of energy. A well-designed cultivating hoe (otherwise known as a draw hoe in Britain) should weigh no more than one and a half pounds. A modern wheel hoe should weigh no more than 15 pounds (6.8kg)." [2] Likewise, Coleman estimates that even a moderately dull edge on any hoe can lessen efficiency by 50% and recommends that a small file is carried in the back pocket and used regularly to hone the hoe blade. The same goes for other cutting tools, including spades, which are noticeably easier to use when sharpened.

Whilst Eliot Coleman sings the praises of well-designed modern tools, I would emphasise the value of traditional, hand-forged tools. Early in my time at Tinker's Bubble I invested in a new spade and proudly arrived home with my purchase. Two friends soon disabused me of my enthusiasm by pointing out the shortcomings of my modern, mass-produced tool – namely the uniform width of the blade from top to bottom and the weak join between spade and handle. I have since become an equal connoisseur of old tools, whose craftsmanship makes them a pleasure to work with, as well as being better designed for the job. Features of hand-forged tools include finer, tapered tines on forks, which allow them to move more easily through the soil, and similarly tapered profiles to spades (see Figure 6.2). The presence of foot-treads on the top of spade blades also increases comfort when digging for long periods. The more you work with hand tools the more you come to notice and appreciate the subtleties of design that came so naturally to our forefathers.

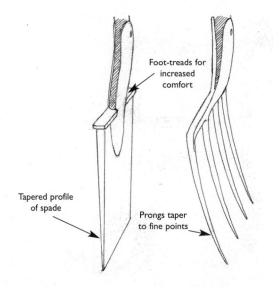

Foot-treads for increased comfort

Tapered profile of spade

Prongs taper to fine points

Figure 6.2. – Profile of spade/fork to illustrate dimension of taper.

Along with correct use of well-designed tools, a thoughtful approach to the task in hand pays human energy dividends. For standing jobs, try to maintain an upright position, rather than bending your back to get closer to the ground. This is easier said than done, and I have constantly to remind myself not to edge down the tool handle into a position where my back is bent. Coleman observes that with a draw hoe, body position is determined by hand position. He recommends holding the handle with both thumbs pointing up to ensure the kind of upright position that enables you to continue hoeing for long periods without getting a sore back. Different types of hoe and other hand tools require varying approaches, but it is worth experimenting with hand positions to discover ways of moving that are more comfortable and can be sustained for the duration of the task. Repetitive strain injury can be avoided by changing your grip on the tool intermittently and learning to work on both sides of your body, rather than relying solely on your dominant hand.

Sometimes it can be easier to fragment tasks into two actions rather than combining them into a more strenuous motion. Where I currently work, the head gardener is very fond of ridging up vegetables to control weeds and strengthen them against being blown over. I was finding ridging up broad beans with a mattock very hard work until I started loosening the soil that was to be drawn up the ridge in a separate action to the actual ridging up. Going down the far side of the row with a crone (a bent-over fork used in a raking action) to loosen the soil involved less bending than trying to combine it with the upwards pulling motion and gave me more power to break it up. I was interested to observe the paradox that in this instance fragmentation of tasks was beneficial to the individual worker as well as to the efficiency of getting the job done. In industrial terms, fragmentation of tasks is often seen negatively as it makes individual jobs meaningless to the people doing them. However, when the fraction of a task can be seen as part of the overall whole, particularly if the same worker is carrying on with the next stage, it can be wholly beneficial.

I love gardening with hand tools, but it has its limits. At Tinker's Bubble I met those limits whilst trying to cultivate a quarter-acre, commercial garden, part-time. Whilst I believe I could have taken it further had I been able to work at it full time, the battle against docks and couch grass was ongoing. I became increasingly interested in the possibilities of horse-drawn tools as an appropriate technology for small- to medium-scale horticulture. As a rule of thumb, an acre is considered to be the maximum area it is possible for a full-time grower to cultivate by hand. However, it is hard to produce competitively priced vegetables solely with hand tools. There are however, many intermediate possibilities between hand tool and tractor-based systems, and these will be examined later in the chapter.

Mowing

Anyone interested in keeping grazing animals will need to store forage for the winter. These days in the UK, haymaking – mowing, turning and baling – is most commonly done by tractor. Few smallholders can justify the capital costs of buying their own haymaking equipment and since everyone wants to make their hay when the sun is shining, there is great competition for the services of contractors during summer dry spells. Mowing by hand, using a scythe, is one alternative, if only a small number of animals need to be kept in hay for the winter. The community of Tinker's Bubble have been making hay by hand since 1994, to feed a Shire horse and one or two Jersey cows. Starting with a motley selection of heavy old English scythes and pitchforks, handled by inexperienced haymakers, both tools and technique have been honed over the years to significantly increase efficiency and enjoyment. The two main developments which have made haymaking more pleasurable and less time-consuming are the introduction of high-quality, modern Austrian scythes, and reconditioned horse-drawn tools for tedding (turning and aerating the hay) and raking it into windrows.

Like other hand tools, the ease of use and efficiency of scythes relies on their careful design and proper maintenance. The replacement of heavy 'traditional' scythe blades with lightweight ones imported from continental Europe is bringing about a resurgence of interest in the scythe as an alternative, non-fossil-fuel-powered mowing tool in the UK. Austrian blades differ from English ones due to the tension incorporated into the steel during manufacture, which enables them to be lightweight whilst retaining their shape in use.[3] Yet the blade is only half the scythe. Without a snath, or handle, the blade will be useless. The fitting of the snath to both the blade and the mower can make the difference between a tool which is a pleasure to use and one that frustratingly skids over the grass rather than cutting it. In his addendum to *The Scythe Book*, 'The Scythe Must Dance', Peter Vido discusses blade fitting in great detail and identifies the 'hafting angle' and the 'lay' of the blade as the two features that distinguish a well matched blade and snath (handle) from a poor one.[4] The hafting angle is the distance relationship between the centre of the upper grip of the snath, the blade's beard and the blade tip (see Figure 6.3). The lay of the blade refers to the way the blade meets the ground when held in front of you as if you were mowing.

Maintaining a sharp edge on a tensioned continental blade involves peening and honing. As a blade is sharpened, the thin concave cutting edge is worn down until it acquires a convex bevel (see Figure 6.4). Peening is the process of hammering the blade upon a small anvil to draw out the steel a tiny bit with each blow, to thin out and thus sharpen the cutting

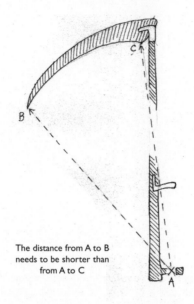

The distance from A to B
needs to be shorter than
from A to C

Figure 6.3 – Hafting angle on a correctly fitted scythe blade.

edge. It takes 10 to 20 minutes, and should be repeated every 12 hours of blade use. Peening can also be carried out to straighten accidental dents in the blade.[5] Honing, or whetting, the blade with a stone is carried out more regularly, in the field, to maintain the even, 'keen' edge which enables the blade to slice easily through grass. It should be repeated every five minutes or so, and this 30-second pause will result in a tidier cut, requiring less effort.

As with gardening, mowing with a scythe is a practice that benefits from the thoughtful development of technique. In *The Scythe Book* by David Tresemer, useful guidelines are given for those who seek to use a scythe for haymaking, clearing weeds and the small-scale harvesting of grains. In the chapter on mowing technique, it becomes clear that using a scythe is an art which depends on the combination of relaxed and mindful use of the body, with a mental attitude of steady, unhurried intention.

Tresemer suggests a twisting exercise to begin each mowing session, to remind the mower of the shape of the movement. From a relaxed, but erect standing position and becoming aware of and releasing any unnecessary tension in the body, "I begin to twist my torso from one side to the other, to face my right, then my left, letting my arms swing free. There is twisting movement in my ankles, knees, hips and all along my spine. The energy that issues in the mowing stroke is stored in our tendons and muscles as we mow. When I am at one extreme of a twist in the body, my tendons are

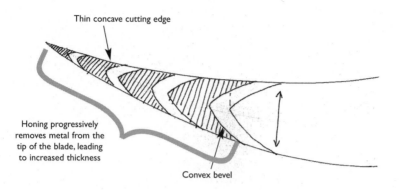

Figure 6.4 – Convex edge of blade resulting from sharpening (see pp.105-6).

storing energy, as a wound rubber band does. This energy is released to aid the contraction of muscles when I twist to the other side. The best stroke uses all the tendons in all the joints." [6] Keeping this motion in mind when starting to mow, the movement of the scythe across the swath can be likened to a pendulum, rhythmically slicing through the grass from right to left. Hence, mowing becomes a self-perpetuating action, the body moving the scythe like a spring, and can be maintained for hours.

Later in 'The Scythe Must Dance', Vido adds four guidelines to help develop efficient, easy on the body and enjoyable use of the scythe:[7]

- Do not carry the weight of the blade. Let it slide forward and back in continuous contact with the surface. "On an obstacle-free terrain the only reason to lift the blade is to hone it."

- Attempt to cut equally to the left and right of your body's centre

- Direct the blade so as to leave all the cut grass on the clean stubble of the previous strokes.

- Shift your weight from one foot to the other to create a sideways rocking motion whose natural velocity helps move the scythe through the grass.

Such technique requires practice, however, and a novice often finds himself investing more energy than necessary in a stroke by lifting the blade with his arms and hacking at grass or becoming bent over into a tiring stoop.

I have merely skimmed the surface here on the subject of scything styles and recommend further study of *The Scythe Book* or attending a scything course for anyone seriously interested in developing this skill. My purpose in covering the use of the scythe is to illustrate how the mindful use of the body can make the difference between a short-lived, physically draining manual activity and one that is a pleasure and can be sustained until the task is complete. Tresemer speaks of the altered sense of time when mowing is going well and the worker forgets herself in the rhythmic motion of the scythe. He quotes a farmer who says, "I come to feel indolence in action, letting the scythe do it, and a force that is not me takes possession of us both and we swing, swing." [8] He notes the Zen paradox that if you give up the hurried intention of 'getting the hay in', you will in fact cut better. This is because a hurried mower will have forgotten the best use of his or her body in his or her rush to achieve the final goal. Instead, focus on inhibiting habitual tensions to let the body move in its natural rhythm and the scythe will follow. This motion, once mastered, turns the scythe into an efficient and highly flexible tool that can accommodate changes in terrain, different types of grass lying in varying directions and unexpected obstacles, better than most machines. Scythes have the added advantage of enabling smallholders to mow in awkward corners, which are inaccessible to machines yet may still yield significant amounts of hay.

Forestry

At Tinker's Bubble, the policy of not using internal combustion engines prohibits the use of chainsaws. The two-person saws, axes, crowbars and ropes that are used instead to fell Douglas Fir, Larch, Ash and Sycamore trees require skill, experience and a knowledge of physics to be employed effectively. Although I have only occasionally been part of the forestry team, the predominant impression I have gained is of the importance of maintaining an alert, thoughtful attitude to the task in hand. I should add that an alert attitude is also vital to use a chainsaw safely and efficiently, and many of the same techniques apply. My aim here, however, is to illustrate how the application of mindfulness can save both time and energy when felling with hand tools

The tree to be felled should have a clear, uphill path along which to fall. It is a good precaution to tie a rope around the tree about 20ft up, with which to pull the tree down if it gets caught in the branches of neighbouring trees. A 'gob' cut, or wedge-shaped notch, is then made to create a hinge which will control the direction in which the tree falls. This is made by sawing a horizontal cut about a foot from the ground with a two-person saw and then cutting a diagonal line down towards to the first cut. The initial cut should be made at a perpendicular angle to the direction in which you intend the tree to fall. A useful trick is to check that the handles of the saw are pointing exactly in the direction you wish the tree to fall. Use of the two-person saw will also be made easier if the blade is kept level and straight in the cut, rather than becoming bent, and the operators should aim for an alternate rhythm of pulling and being pulled back. This cut should reach one third the way across the tree on the side of the trunk it will fall towards. The upper line of the 'gob' can be cut either using an axe or the two-man saw. Swinging the axe to cut the gob requires practice to increase power and accuracy. It is important to cut away all the wood above the saw cut, so that the 'hinge' is narrow enough to allow the tree to fall when the fibres on the opposite side are cut.

The two-person saw is used to fell the tree, by making a cut on the opposite side to the gob, again keeping the saw perpendicular to the felling direction. This third and final part of felling can be either exhilarating, if the tree falls in the direction you want it to, or highly frustrating, if it gets hung in a neighbouring tree. The outcome depends on the accuracy of your cutting angles. If the tree gets hung up, and you are lucky, hauling on the rope which was tied onto the tree before felling will dislodge it. An iron bar or a sturdy branch can be used to lever the trunk off the tree stump once they have been fully severed. Sometimes, however, a winch or a horse is necessary to drag the base of the tree away from the stump and allow its upper branches to slide to the ground.

Once on the ground, the side branches are cut off with an axe or bow-saw to leave a log which must be crosscut into suitable lengths for extraction to the saw mill. This in itself can be a challenge if the ground is uneven, and the application of basic physics is vital in propping up the log to ensure that the saw is not pinched. Using a crowbar, or long, strong piece of timber as a lever can magnify human strength, enabling one person to lift a log while the other slides something (usually another log) underneath to hold up the log which is to be sawn.

The importance of mindfulness

As illustrated above, far from being a mindless activity, manual work using hand tools employs the brain just as much as the body. Time and again I have been reminded of this fact in all areas of physical work. Sometimes, when I have become tired and gone on working too long, it has resulted in time-consuming mistakes or minor injury. Attitude, it seems, is everything when it comes to using any hand tool effectively and is a skill that is being rapidly lost in this age of 'labour-saving' machinery. Yet the sense of achievement and exhilaration that results from mindful operation of hand tools is a pleasure that must be experienced to be believed.

Skilful use of any particular hand tool requires far more detailed instruction than I have included here, combined with considerable practice. I have aimed to provide an overview of the potential efficiency and pleasure that can be gained from the thoughtful use of hand tools. I thus hope to have sparked the interest of people who may not previously have considered many of the finer aspects of manual work, considering it too energetic, primitive or inefficient to count as a viable option for managing the land.

Box 6.1 Guidelines for enjoyable use of hand tools

- Keep tools sharp
- Choose strong but lightweight tools
- Well-designed tools directly transfer effort into work
- Apply knowledge of basic physics to work and tools (conscious forces, levers, pivots etc.)
- Early cultivation of weeds saves time and effort
- Work with the weather
- Learn how to use your body without straining it
- A steady, mindful approach will maintain energy and quality of work better than a hurried, end-gaining one.

Horsepower

I first became seriously interested in the potential of horse-drawn tools when I was living at Tinker's Bubble, where a Shire horse was used to perform traction work. The horse, Samson, was regularly employed to extract logs, draw a plough or chain harrow and to cart anything from manure to apple-juice bottles around the farm.

Having been fortunate enough to have spent a childhood riding and becoming accustomed to the ways of horses, it wasn't long before I started to work Samson too, mainly for carting. It took me longer to become convinced of the benefits of using him for horticultural work, as I was a firm advocate of minimal tillage gardening as a way of caring for the soil and its organisms. However, when I first took on my garden, I was faced with a quarter of an acre of weedy land, and the challenge of mulching at this scale forced me to rethink my plans. I decided to experiment by ploughing some of it and mulching the rest, as described previously in the section on 'no-dig' gardening. Whilst our early efforts at ploughing were somewhat hit and miss, as we learned to regulate Samson's speed, direct the plough in straight rows and ensure that the weeds were buried, it still proved to be a more time-efficient way of reclaiming the land than the mulching.

Furthermore, our single-furrow horse-drawn plough is a very different tool from a multiple-furrow plough pulled by a powerful tractor, as it cuts to a depth of only 10-15cm and hence inverts less of the fertile topsoil. Although it is possible to shallow plough with a tractor, the tendency is to use the power of tractors to bury weeds at a greater depth than might be possible with a horse plough.

I continued in subsequent years to plough parts of the garden, whilst continuing to experiment with mulch in other parts, but gradually realised that if I wanted to scale up my market garden I needed to look beyond hand tools and mulch. At this stage most people would start thinking about employing a tractor, or at least a rotavator, but the prohibition on using fossil-fuel-powered combustion engines at Tinker's Bubble ruled out this option. The other factor which pushed me to find out more about horse-drawn equipment was my lack of skill and interest in working with machinery. I had observed the hours spent tinkering with old machinery to keep it working and realised that when you start using such technology you either need to enjoy mending machinery or have enough money to buy reliable new equipment or to pay someone else to mend it.

There are at present only a handful of people in the United Kingdom using horse-drawn tools to produce vegetables commercially. According to the editor of the magazine *Heavy Horse World*, there are eight farms in the UK that use heavy horses predominantly to undertake arable fieldwork and daily tasks, such as carting manure and forage for other livestock. More people use draught-horses alongside tractors for odd jobs around the farm, such as harrowing grassland, but the majority of heavy horses these days are kept for breeding and showing. Since the government removed draught-horses from the annual farm survey, no data exist for the numbers using horses for practical land management.

One farm which continues to depend on horses is the 200-acre Northumbrian Farm of Sillywrea, where teams of Clydesdales are used for cultivating 18 acres of arable and for transporting manure and winter fodder for 200 ewes and 30 cows and calves. Whilst agricultural contractors are now used to combine the barley and bale the hay, horse-drawn implements are still used for ploughing, harrowing, drilling seed and cutting 40 acres of hay.[9] All these operations are carried out using old horse-drawn tools, acquired over many years at farm sales. Other people have adapted modern, tractor-drawn machinery to be pulled by horses by employing a hitch-cart. These versatile carts enable tractor-trailed implements to be attached behind and powered by a small generator, to perform tasks such as hay-cutting, muckspreading and other jobs that would otherwise require a tractor PTO (the power take off, a linkage with the tractor engine that drives machinery with moving parts).[10]

The everyday use of draught-horses is more common in continental Europe and the United States, perhaps because, being less crowded than the UK, there is less pressure to maximise the financial return on acreage. In many Eastern European countries, such as Romania and Poland, horse traction is still a central part of a more traditional, peasant agriculture. In the United States, the Amish tradition, which now spreads across several states, may have influenced other farmers who follow a low-impact, low-technology agricultural philosophy. The *Small Farmers' Journal*, published in the US, has several regular contributors who use working horses and in some states it is possible to undertake apprenticeships on organic farms which employ horses.

Horse-drawn horticulture

On my cycling trip around France and the United Kingdom, one of my aims was to explore the possibility of using horse-drawn tools for commercial organic horticulture, and I visited several places where this is happening. Whilst in France I discovered PROMMATA, a small intermediate technology company which specialises in designing simple animal-traction tools for use in developing countries. Their designs have become popular amongst small producers in France, to whom they have sold about 150 of the tool systems. A year later I enrolled on one of PROMMATA's three-day courses to learn how to use their simplest tool, the Kassine, for market gardening with donkeys. The Kassine is a lightweight, adaptable frame, with wheels and a handlebar, onto which a variety of tools can be fitted to undertake different cultivations.

The cultivation system for which the Kassine has been designed avoids ploughing, replacing it instead with shallow cultivation to create a surface tilth. The tilth, which contains considerable grass, weeds and roots at this stage, is then ridged up, composted *in situ* over winter and then harrowed and prepared for planting as ridges or furrows. The hands-on PROMMATA course gave ample opportunity to experiment with the different tool attachments, which included fixed and spring tine harrows, duck's-foot hoes, a shallow sub-soiler, a ridging plough and an innovative tool which uses two discs to create ridges. The attraction of these tools over the traditional tools found at farm sales in the UK is that they are lightweight and therefore less tiring to operate and the attachments are specifically designed for horticulture. (See Appendix 2, p.305, for PROMMATA.)

The farm where I first discovered PROMMATA tools was La Fermette, in north-west France. The farmers, Laurent and Gudule Cuenot, spent six years travelling around Europe in a horse-drawn caravan before settling at their 50-acre farm. They decided to transfer their horse skills to horticulture, and invested in a modern system of tools designed by PROMMATA specifically for minimal-tillage market gardening. They do have a tractor and rotavator, which they use for opening up pasture to start vegetable plots, but on the whole they manage their five-acre garden with the PROMMATA tools and a traditional fixed tine harrow. These tools were used to cultivate moderately weedy ground, to hoe between rows of crops and to earth up potatoes. When I visited in 2005 they had been growing for two and a half years and were supplying 14 vegetable boxes per week to residents in a nearby city. They were also selling vegetables off the back of a horse-drawn cart in the local village, as described in Chapter Eight (Livelihood Strategies, p.157).

Another holding I visited briefly was Jade Gate Organic Produce in south Wales. Ed Ravell, the grower there had already established a thriving five-acre market garden using a Massey Ferguson '64 tractor before he bought Thorn, a 14.2hh cob, to reduce his dependence on fossil fuels. First Thorn took on the weekly 12-mile circuit to deliver vegetable boxes, and he and his lightweight cart became a well-known feature of neighbouring Swansea. To shorten the original door-to-door van delivery round, a system of 12 drop-off points within easy walking distance of customers was devised and deliveries were undertaken on Sundays, when the roads were at their quietest. Hence, the length of time spent delivering (9 hours), remained the same whilst the task of delivering became more interesting, enjoyable and sustainable.

The cultivation system prior to Thorn's arrival had involved annual ploughing to control weeds, causing nutrient-leaching in the wet Welsh climate. After a few years of experimenting, Ed arrived at his current system of minimal-tillage cultivation. A tractor is still used for muckspreading, ploughing and setting up ridges after a fallow period. Thereafter, from year to year the ridges stay put and weeds are controlled with just two horse-drawn tools, both found at farm sales. The first is a scuffle hoe, or 'scuffler', and is like a small, width-adjustable, fixed-tine harrow with blades on either side. It is used to cut the roots of weeds and knock down the sides of the ridges, leaving the crop growing on top of the ridge undisturbed. Immediately after the 'scuffler', a ridging plough is taken between the rows to rebuild the ridges. These operations are repeated every month or so, when the weeds are no more than 12cm high. The ridges remain fixed, meaning that compaction from horse and driver is limited to the paths between them and crops benefit from an aerated, weed-free soil. The period of exposure to leaching is significantly reduced by only ploughing once every few years and keeping the ground covered with crops. Furthermore, compared with a tractor-drawn steerage hoe, with a horse it is possible to continue controlling weeds when the crop is bigger.

A small and hardy horse like Thorn can be kept outside on grass, and needs little extra feed beyond winter hay and grade-out carrots. The only other costs are shoeing and the occasional vet's bill. The business is financially viable without any subsidies, and provides good value, organic vegetables to 80 households for ten months of the year, as well as meaningful employment for Ed.

Horse logging

A more common use for working horses in the UK is log extraction, or 'snigging'. Whilst there are only 15 full-time horse loggers working in the UK, there are many hundreds of people working horses for log extraction part-time or as a hobby. They operate in public and private woodlands, extracting coppice poles, soft- and hardwood thinnings and large saw logs.[11]

Horse logging has distinct benefits over other timber-extraction systems. Horses are able to navigate difficult terrains, such as steep slopes and rocky ground that would be inaccessible to machinery. They also do less damage to the surrounding woodland, its ground flora and the soil, where heavy machinery causes soil compaction and churns up large, muddy ruts. Logging equipment ranges from simple chains and a swingletree (a metal bar with chains connected to both ends which run either side of the horse and attach to the collar) to Scandinavian logging arches. The former drags one or more logs along the ground with chains attached to the swingletree, whereas the latter lifts the front of the log off the ground onto an arch on wheels making it easier for the horse to drag and enabling the movement of heavier logs.

Horse logging varies greatly in the different countries where it is practised, with the size and breed of horse, and equipment used, being chosen to fit the forest management system and terrain.[12] It is skilled work, since it requires good horsemanship and an obedient and responsive horse, as well as an awareness of where the log is likely to roll as you weave between the trees. However, horse logging is economically competitive when compared with mechanisation, since it requires less infrastructure (such as stoned roads) and reparation of the damage caused by machines.

The pros and cons of horsepower

Using working horses appeals to the romantic, as well as the environmentalist, in many people, since it combines quiet and aesthetically pleasing technologies with a close relationship between humans and animals and a reduction in fossil-fuel use. However, in evaluating their place in a land-use system that aims to sustain human energy as well as the environment there is a trade-off to be considered. For whilst horses have many advantages over tractors, such as eating grass, hay and oats rather than using oil; providing valuable manure rather than diesel fumes; and having the potential to replicate themselves; they do have to be looked after and they require land to support them.

Although, on an immediate farm level, horses require more land than a fossil-fuel-powered tractor to provide grazing and forage, from a broader perspective the point is debatable. From an ecological footprint point of view, fossil-fuel use requires forested land or ocean to sequester its carbon emissions, so, whilst little land is required in its production, diesel nevertheless requires 'shadow acres' to make its use sustainable. As for biodiesel, which is being heralded by some as the saviour that will enable internal combustion engines to be used without producing net carbon emissions, the land requirements for this are considerable, and are discussed in the following section – machinery.

From a human energy perspective, a downside to horses could be seen as the daily care they require, involving feeding and watering, fence maintenance, hoof care, occasional veterinary attention, and regular exercise, whether or not you need their help. In addition, horses need hay, the making of which either requires the use of a tractor or the labour-intensive process of mowing with a scythe and tedding (tossing and turning the grass to air-dry it) with a pitchfork. Compared with a rotavator or tractor, horses are potentially harder work, time-consuming and do not necessarily save on fossil-fuel use. However, the rewards gained in the enjoyment of having a positive relationship with a working animal more than compensate if you have a greater affinity with horses than with machinery, which can also demand hours of maintenance time.

A fossil-fuel-free option for horses is to use them to produce their own feed and manage their pasture. At La Borie Noble, a community in southern France, a horse-drawn finger mower is used to cut both hay and arable crops. The hay is then turned and put in windrows using a horse-drawn tedder and side-delivery rake. These latter two tools are now used for haymaking at Tinker's Bubble. I well remember the historic day when they were first introduced there, having been bought at a farm sale and painstakingly restored over the winter. They symbolised a significant reduction of hours spent in the hot sun, tedding the hay with pitchforks and hand-raking it into windrows, and the experience provided a vivid insight into the excitement with which such innovations would have been met in the past. Horses can also be employed for pasture-management tasks, such as chain-harrowing, which is required to rake out the dead grass, allowing space for new spring growth.

In recent times the most common use of draught-horses has been for entertainment, at rural shows and ploughing matches, pulling brewery drays or as a picturesque relic of the past at historical farms. With increased awareness of climate change, and the need to find alternative renewable sources of energy, horses and perhaps other draught animals, such as donkeys or oxen, could find a more practical role once again. Fortunately there are still some people alive who worked with horses prior to the age of the tractor, and it is important that we quickly learn from them the skills of farm-based horsemanship before they are lost.

As Philip Oyler, writing in the 1950s when horses were being super-seded by tractors, wrote, "I suspect many of the machines we use do not save us the time that we imagine, though they increase the cost of farming to a prodigious amount. Indeed, if our methods of farming were regulated solely on the basis of cost, we should use horses or oxen, not tractors, for all those who have compared these by keeping accurate accounts have found animals to be cheaper in the long run, even in the USA, where con-ditions favour the most economical use of the tractor." [13] Over the last 50 years the economics of farming have changed unrecognisably, distorted by subsidies, price-control mechanisms and enormous global differences in labour costs. Cheap and readily available oil have made machinery use eco-nomically more efficient than draught animals, but that could all change if oil prices continue to rise as a result of declining supply. If 'Peak Oil' pre-dictions are correct, Oyler's comments that draught animals are more effi-cient than tractors may be seen as more than an anachronistic quotation, and those who have made the effort to carry forwards the skills and knowl-edge of our horse-drawn forefathers will be the real heroes.

Fuel-powered machinery

"If a machine is useful then use it; if it becomes necessary then it is your urgent duty to throw it away. For it will inevitably catch you up in its wheels and enslave you."

– Gandhi, quoted in *Return to the Source* by Lanza Del Vasto [14]

When comparing the work capacity of a gallon of oil with that of a horse or a human being (oil 1 hour, horse 10 hours, human 97 hours) it is easy to understand why fossil-fuel-powered machinery has revolutionised so many aspects of society. [15] Machines have the ability to vastly magnify the amount of work a person can do per day and in an economy where the majority have access to machinery and the cost of labour (£5.35/hour min-imum wage) is currently valued more highly than a gallon of diesel (£1.59) (based on 35p per litre cost of red diesel, at the time of writing) it is hard to be commercially competitive unless you use machinery.

It thus comes as no surprise that nearly all the commercially active projects I visited were using machinery of one sort or another. 14 of the total of 28 projects were using a tractor for soil cultivation, cutting hay and cereal crops, topping weeds and moving materials around the farm. Other machines encountered regularly included rotavators, chainsaws for felling trees and cross cutting logs for firewood, lawnmowers and strimmers. Only two places, Tinker's Bubble and La Borie Noble eschewed the use of fossil-fuel-powered machinery altogether, and even La Borie Noble used a mains electricity-powered mill for grinding their grain into flour. A handful of projects used machines fuelled by non-animal, renewable energy. At Steward Wood and Brithdir Mawr, electric chainsaws powered by micro-hydro and wind power respectively were used for cutting firewood, whilst the steam-powered sawmill at Tinker's Bubble is fuelled with wood. Both Fivepenny Farm and Briggs Farm use biodiesel to power their tractors and Steward Wood was experimenting with bio-ethanol as a chainsaw fuel.

The cultural impact of machinery

The question of whether or not to use machinery, and if so how to power it, is central to any discussion about human energy in sustainable land use. The arguments for and against using machinery can be teased out into strands relating to the social impact of machines on individuals and society as a whole, their environmental sustainability and a practical comparison of the figures for fuel use, carbon emissions and time management when using machines and tools powered by other means. Today, machines perform so many of the tasks that were previously done by people that they are taken for granted, by many, as being an inevitable part of modern life. Before assuming that this is the case it is worth considering a couple of powerful movements which have challenged the assumption that machinery is generally beneficial to society – the Gandhi-inspired L'Arche Communities of Lanza del Vasto and the Amish communities in the United States.

Mahatma Gandhi is well known for his opposition to the sweeping industrialisation of crafts which could be undertaken by hand. He viewed the skilful use of hand tools as a means of personal and national empowerment, while machinery was a cause of enslavement and waste. Using the example of cotton, he observed the vast infrastructure of railway lines, ports, docks, warehouses, factories and banks involved in supporting its industrial processing into clothes, and compared it to the simplicity of farmers spinning home-grown cotton to meet the needs of their families and villages.[16] He observed the millions made unemployed and destitute by industrialisation, the waste of skill, the reduction in quality of workmanship when machines replaced craftspeople and the simmering discontent caused by underpaid workers who couldn't even afford to buy the stuff of their labours.

Influenced by the time he spent with Gandhi, Lanza del Vasto demolishes the arguments used by the supporters of industrialisation, as follows:

> "*Machines save time and labour* – If it is true (that they save time), how is it that in countries where the machine is master, one sees only people who are pressed for time? Whereas, in countries where men do everything with their hands they find time to do everything, as well as time to do nothing to their heart's content. If machinery saves labour, how is it that wherever it reigns people are busy, harnessed to unrewarding, fragmentary, boring tasks, hustled by the rhythm of the machine into doing jobs that wear a human being out, warp him, bewilder and weary him? Is this saving of trouble worth the trouble?

> *Machines produce abundance* – If it is true that machinery produces abundance, how is it that wherever it reigns, there reigns in some well-hidden slum the strangest, the most atrocious misery? How is it that if it produces abundance it cannot produce contentment? Overproduction and unemployment have been the logical accompaniment of the machine whenever it has been impossible to throw the surplus into some hole or devour it in some war.

> *Machinery multiplies exchanges between people and brings them into closer contact* – If machinery has done this, it is little wonder that the people in question feel unprecedented irritation with each other. There is nothing calculated to make me hate my neighbour and him hate me like forcing me upon him in spite of his will and mine. Forced contact does not engender union."[17]

According to Lanza del Vasto, work is as much a means of spiritual development as practical utility, a subject elaborated upon in Chapter Twelve, Siestas and Fiestas. In short, Gandhi's views are summed up by the quotation, "The machine enslaves, the hand sets free." [18] To this end, Gandhi encouraged Indians to empower themselves by making khadi, home-spun cloth, as part of the movement to achieve independence from the British Empire.[19] The international movement of L'Arche communities, started by Lanza del Vasto in 1948 to put Gandhi's principles of nonviolence into practice, is also characterised by its use of hand tools rather than machinery.

Members of the Amish community in the United States are highly selective in their use of machinery in their attempt to live a simple religious life, practising humility, lowliness, obedience and service to Christ. Their faith is central to their decisions about how to live, followed closely by their desire to care for their families and be good stewards of their land, and work is a concept that is embraced rather than avoided. Hence, Amish people evaluate technological inventions in terms of their impact on the family, their ability to care for the land and their faith, rather than whether it will save them time and work.[20]

An example of the impact of their faith on choice of technology is the decision that was made long ago to retain horses for agricultural work. The reason was to ensure that no individual family would expand to such a scale that they would push their neighbours off the land, resulting in the destruction of their community. As Stuart Pattison, a Devon-based farmer who uses horses, points out, the motivation to retain horses was well-founded.[21] In industrialised cultures, the introduction of ever more powerful tractors has contributed to the steady concentration of land into fewer and fewer hands. The social and environmental impacts of this trend have not been positive, as rural communities have been broken up and hedgerows removed to make fields ever larger. Pattison, who has discussed these matters in depth with Amish farmers who have travelled to England to take part in his courses on using horse-drawn tools, states that, "The Amish standpoint has nothing to do with efficiency as such, nor with energy conservation, nor indeed with economics as usually understood." Indeed, I have been interested to learn that the Amish philosophy does not altogether preclude the use of fossil-fuel-powered machinery. Modern horse-drawn equipment designed in Britain by Pintow Hitch Cart, involving a 25-horsepower petrol engine mounted on a hitch cart that can trail agricultural equipment requiring a PTO, is now being produced by an Amish firm for the American market.[22]

If an Amish man needs a technology, he will take a long time to decide, debate the matter with his brethren and maybe try using it, but if it gets in the way of his faith, family and stewardship of the land, then he'll stop thinking about it. This is beautifully illustrated by the story of an Amish man who, in the 1980s, kept a generator-run computer in his chicken coop, to explore its possible uses. "He quietly and thoughtfully agrees with many worldly writers that the computer – the cold, wired, electric-faced, non-organic computer – might be able to help a man stay at home with his family and with his community. He is testing the idea, without noise, without announcement. He just keeps the computer in his chicken coop and is teaching himself to understand its possible uses. He has thought most kindly about us non-Amish and hopes that the computer might help us stay at home and be with our families too."[23]

From an agricultural perspective, a technology must help to care for the land to be used by the Amish, since they are faithful stewards who see the land as being in trust to them for their lifetime. "The Amish man treats the land sensitively – he nourishes it with horse and cow manure; he treads on it lightly – with teams of animals instead of machinery that packs it down. He works it often by hand. The Amish man's fields flourish because he pays close attention to them, because he is sensitive to the earth, because he lets it guide him."[24]

The biofuel debate

Alongside these practical, spiritual and philosophical arguments, there are now compelling environmental reasons for minimising our use of fossil-fuel-powered machinery to reduce carbon emissions. Biofuels are now being heralded by politicians, industrial-scale farmers and the transport industry as a solution to the need to cut fossil-fuel use and carbon emissions, without reducing agricultural productivity and the convenience of car transport. It is argued that biofuels are carbon-neutral because the carbon they emit is reabsorbed by the next generation of plants destined to be used as biofuels.

Throughout the UK small enterprises are converting used chip oil into biodiesel, which local people can use to run road vehicles and agricultural machinery. The recycling of chip oil into fuel represents the re-use of a resource that is often seen as a waste product, but can only meet a small fraction ($\frac{1}{380}$) of our national demand for road transport fuel.[25] To meet the demands of the UK's road fleet would require crops to be grown specifically for biofuels and would entail between 40 and 70 million hectares of arable land.[26] When it is considered that there are only 6.3 million hectares of arable land in the United Kingdom, it becomes clear that imports would be necessary to meet the UK's needs. Tropical forest is already being cleared to make room for biofuel crops, destroying these valuable carbon sinks and threatening biodiversity, whilst food prices are inflated beyond the reach of the poorest people on Earth as land is diverted to biofuel production.[27]

Although powering cars with biofuels is morally questionable, Fairlie argues that there is a better case for using biofuels to drive agricultural machinery. He cites figures from Elsayed (2003) to show that "a hectare of land producing 8 tonnes of grain will produce bioethanol equivalent to 1,000 litres of diesel. It takes 100 litres of fuel to cultivate a hectare of wheat, and if we allow another 10 litres for the embodied energy cost of the machinery, that means that a hectare of bioethanol will power a tractor to cultivate that hectare and a further nine hectares. A hectare of biodiesel will provide power to cultivate only a further five hectares."[28, 29]

Interestingly, Fairlie compares the efficiency of fuelling tractors with biofuels with that of a more traditional form of biomass energy for farm traction, the draught-horse. He calculates that "eight tonnes of grain, grown on a hectare of prime land, will provide enough calories annually (72,000 per day) to keep two horses working at a moderate pace. Two horses are normally said to be capable of cultivating 10 hectares. So a pair of horses therefore appears to require the same amount of land as a tractor running on bioethanol – one hectare of grade 1 land out of every 10 cultivated is needed to supply fuel."[30] Moreover he points out that the cultivations required necessary to grow 10 hectares of grain shouldn't take a team of horses more than 100 days, and allowing two rest days per week, the horses would be available to do other work on 160 days at no extra fuel cost, whereas any additional work with a tractor would require extra fuel.

In weighing up the advantages of using horses and biofuel tractors, the labour input into each must be considered. Horses and other draught animals require daily care whether or not they are being used, whereas a tractor can be left in its shed. Conversely, old machinery or that which has been out of use for a while often needs attention from a mechanic before it will work properly. This can be expensive and can cause frustrating delays in cultivation. The choice of whether to use horses or machines often comes down to personal preference and the skills one already has. If one is mechanically minded, engines still offer attractions over horses, whilst someone who is confident with animals is more likely to choose the horse-drawn route. However, with the imperative to cut fossil-fuel use and maximise efficiency of production, the time has arrived when draught animals should be considered by everyone as a serious alternative to combustion engines.

Who uses which machinery?

At most of the commercial market gardens I visited (Longmeadow Organics, Little Farm, Tamarisk Farm, Galingale, Meadow Farm, Keveral Farm, Stroud Community Agriculture, EarthShares, Briggs Farm and Fivepenny Farm) tractors were used regularly for a range of field-scale cultivations, including ploughing, harrowing, rotavation, weed control and muck spreading. Two of the smaller-scale market gardens used a petrol-powered rotavator to cultivate beds, and many used a garden lawn mower to keep grass under control. On two out of the three farms where arable cultivation took place, tractors and a combine harvester were employed. In addition tractors were used around many of the farms and three of the communities for haymaking, topping thistles, mowing grass around the garden edges, banging in fence posts, and hauling heavy loads such as logs, manure or hay.

Among those who were working with wood, either for timber production or more detailed furniture making, chainsaws were frequently used for felling and in one place a petrol-powered mobile sawmill processed logs into planks. Whilst several of those who were using fossil-fuel-powered machinery expressed regrets that this aspect of their business was less sustainable than it could be, most believed that they would be unable to remain commercially competitive without machinery.

Seeking a sustainable compromise

Committed environmentalists are faced with a dilemma when choosing which technologies to use. Whilst the need to reduce greenhouse-gas emissions coupled with knowledge of impending oil price rises cause them to favour human and renewable sources of energy, current economics still make it hard to earn a living without using machinery. To a certain extent it is possible to subsidise the business by working harder and lowering living costs, by living a low-impact, subsistence lifestyle, but it is when these measures are taken too far that people become exhausted. How realistic a proposition is it for people seeking to earn their livelihood from the land in industrialised countries to avoid the use of fossil-fuel-powered machinery? What compromises is it reasonable to make when trying to run a financially viable, ecologically sound business without driving oneself to the point of collapse? A pragmatic approach is to find a compromise which combines selective use of machinery with hand and horse-drawn tools wherever possible.

It is interesting to compare the different combinations of technology adopted at the 19 places where commercial market gardens were in operation. Only four growers were cultivating solely by hand and they tended to be small-scale (less than an acre) and following a 'no-dig' system involving permanent beds and mulch. These systems tended to be producing a higher yield per area compared with less labour-intensive systems, but involved an extremely high input of work and attention to detail. For example at Tinker's Bubble, one man grows vegetables using only hand tools on fixed beds outside and in two polytunnels, the total area of which is about one sixth of an acre. Due to communal commitments it is only possible for him to spend three to four days per week on horticultural activities (including harvesting, marketing and paperwork), and hence on average only two days per week actually cultivating vegetables. Yet his small garden is now generating about £4,000 worth of produce per year, and he estimates that productivity could increase significantly were he able to spend a larger proportion of his time working there.

At Mulberry Tree Farm, in 2007 an acre of hand-cultivated land was providing enough produce to fill 20 weekly vegetable boxes (feeding 30-35 people) all year round, generating an annual turnover of £7,300. Typically the garden has two nearly full-time growers, supported by regular volunteers. Again there is significant potential to intensify and hence increase production from that area as the experience levels of the growers increase and their other commitments decrease. They did once try using a rotavator to speed up cultivation, but have found their current system of fixed beds, mulched with black plastic when not in use, to be a more efficient method of cultivation at their scale.

Another four enterprises used a minimal amount of engine power alongside very high inputs of labour or intensive use of plastic mulch and irrigation equipment. The power tools used by all four were rotavators, one of which was tractor-mounted and three were push-along 'walking-tractor'-style machines. These examples are interesting because they demonstrate the interaction between the economic strategy of the enterprise, the personal circumstances of the grower and the choice of technology. Tamarisk Farm has sufficient accommodation to enable it to host three or four WWOOFers on a regular basis in its two-acre market garden (working between four and six hours, five days per week). Hence, although a tractor-mounted rotavator is used for incorporating weeds and crop residues in some parts of the garden, all of the weed control, ridging up and much smaller-scale ground preparation are done by hand. Likewise, the very active farm shop at the Trading Post (which retails a wide range of goods alongside those produced in the garden) brings in sufficient income to enable the market garden to employ two full-time workers (in addition to the proprietor) to cultivate five acres. Mechanical tools used regularly include a lawnmower and a 'walking tractor', onto which various tools, including a rotavator can be attached, but the majority of the weed control is done by hand. As its proprietor said, when asked whether he'd recommend his set-up to others or suggest changes to it, "Either invest in machinery or go with people. You don't really need the machines. I've gone betwixt and between and not quite got there. Machines can cost as much as the people."

At Sea Spring Farm, instead of reducing machine use by increasing human labour, good design and investment in 'passive' tools such as black plastic mulch and irrigation equipment enable a series of intensively cropped polytunnels to be managed part-time by just one couple with occasional help from casual labour. Once a year the ground in the polytunnels is rotavated, before being covered with plastic mulch to control weed growth and conserve water. Drip irrigation pipes running under the mulch mean that whole polytunnels can be watered just by turning a tap. Arguably, the oil used and carbon emitted in producing horticultural aids such as plastic mulch, netting and irrigation pipes mean that from an environmental perspective such a system is no better than one dependent on machinery. However, at Sea Spring Farm the black plastic mulch is re-used and tends to last for about ten years, while the irrigation pipes were bought second-hand in 1989 and are still going strong. The longer these plastic tools are used, the lower their environmental impact, as their embodied energy is spread over more years. An interesting and much needed avenue of research would be to compare the carbon inputs of highly mechanised and plastic-dependent horticultural systems.

One grower who had previously been using a 'walking-tractor'-style rotavator had recently upgraded to using one drawn by a tractor. Whilst this was partly due to the fact that the opportunity arose to share a tractor with his neighbour, a significant factor motivating this change was the back problems which he had experienced from using the rotavator.

A third group of growers were using tractors on a regular basis not only for soil cultivation, but also for weed control, planting seedlings and harvesting root crops such as potatoes and carrots. Even in these systems, however, many jobs such as picking, fine weeding and erection of support for climbing crops still needed to be done by hand, and extra labour was employed seasonally. The main advantage of such machinery use was that it enabled one or two people to cultivate larger areas of land (between 2.5 and 11 acres) and produce sufficient vegetables to supply a large customer base at affordable prices.

The final group of horticulturalists I encountered were three who were combining the use of hand labour, horse-drawn tools and tractors. Those who were regularly employing horse-drawn tools tended to have used tractors to open up the pasture when the garden was established. Ed Ravel from Jade Gate Organic Produce, whilst using a horse for weed control, maintained that certain jobs such as ploughing, setting up the fixed ridges and muckspreading are more efficiently done with a tractor. Hence it was possible to keep only one modestly sized cob rather than a team of stronger draught-horses, who would eat more. The main use for the tractor at La Fermette, besides ploughing when the grassland was opened up, was to rotavate a five-metre strip around the cultivated area to deter slugs. At EarthShare, a tractor is used alongside two draught-horses throughout the year and does 90% of the ground cultivation, while the horses do the remaining 10%. Weed control, ridging up and thinning crops tend to be undertaken half by machine, and half by hand and horse-drawn tools.

Another area I was particularly interested in exploring was the different options for haymaking, since wherever horses are to be employed instead of machinery they will need to have forage prepared for the winter. There is still an element of fossil-fuel dependence if hay is made using conventional farm machinery, yet making hay by hand is time-consuming and in today's economy, economically inefficient. All three commercial market gardens using horse-drawn tools were feeding hay made using a tractor. The other two places where draught-horses were used regularly were both communities. At both places hay was made using hand tools (scythes and pitchforks) or horse-drawn tools (finger mowers, tedders and side-delivery rakes) or a combination of both. However, the availability of a pool of labour from the community and visiting volunteers was a significant factor in making such traditional hay-making techniques viable. Even then there is an awkward labour bottleneck, since haymaking time coincides with the busiest months in the garden.

In most of the places where forestry work was being undertaken, machinery was being used. David Blair at Dun Beag was using a petrol-powered mobile sawmill to turn a problem (low-value sitka spruce being cleared from an oak forest) into a valuable resource (planks which were to be used for building affordable homes). As he said, "while there are other options, it's about using what is appropriate." Alongside his chainsaw and sawmill, he was reducing human labour and fossil-fuel use by using a plastic chute to enable the planks to slide down hill by gravity and harnessing hydropower to provide a 240v electricity supply with which he could use mainstream power tools for building and joinery work. He made the point that even with power tools, such as chainsaws, human energy as well as petrol can be saved by keeping them very sharp.

The relationship between choice of technology, the number of people involved in a project, and the way they are organised became very clear during my research, and is summed up succinctly by the following quote from a community resident:

> "Farming can be done by one person, but you need machines and to employ people. It is much better in a group and that is how it always used to be done – mixed farming, anyway."

As we shall discover when different kinds of social structure and livelihood strategies are discussed, working in a group, which seems to be necessary in order to eliminate the use of fossil fuels entirely, brings its own set of challenges. The truth is that the best combination of technologies for working the land in a sustainable way (ecologically, economically and in human energy terms) is dynamic and will change as resource prices escalate, skills develop and attitudes change. What is most needed is more information about the relative carbon emissions of different tools and technologies, so that the environmental costs of each option can be quantified and accurately weighed up against the social and economic costs of choosing alternatives. At present the environmental credentials of different land-management tools are based on crude assumptions, which are wide open to critique from anyone who cares to challenge them, including many who would prefer to ignore the imminence of climate change.

Choice of tools and technology can make the difference between a thriving business, enjoyable self-sufficiency and a project that struggles both financially and in terms of the health and enthusiasm of those running it. In ending on a note of compromise I do not intend to be defeatist, but merely to point out how difficult it is at present to totally withdraw from a society and economy which is still wedded to fossil-fuel use.

There are, however, projects which have taken a purist stance by rejecting fossil-fuel use or machinery altogether. The three that I came across in this study were all communities, which I believe is no random coincidence and is discussed in the concluding chapter. Their technology choices extend beyond land management and livelihood into the domestic realm, so a comparison of the three is left until the end of the next chapter on domestic-energy use. Everyone's lives straddle both work and domestic realms to some degree, and how energy is used in the home is as important an ingredient in the human-energy equation as how it is used on the land.

A few final thoughts on tools

Sometimes the successful accomplishment of a task results not from the correct choice of tool, but from the adaptation of the task to fit the tools, people and skills available. For example, it may be that it is sensible to use a machine for a particular job, but not worthwhile to purchase that machine. The decision to hire in machinery or specialist help when required is just as important a contribution to the success of a project as knuckling down to doing the job yourself. This is particularly true when establishing a smallholding from scratch, when considerable development of infrastructure is necessary. Fields may need to be fenced to keep stock in or rabbits and deer out; tools stores, animal shelters, packing sheds and perhaps a home for the smallholder built; polytunnels erected and access tracks laid. Whether these jobs are done by you alone, with help from friends or with bought-in help from a contractor will depend not only on your skills and choice of tools, but also how much capital you have available and the time-scale on which you are operating.

Erecting fencing by hand is a skilled and time-consuming activity, but may be an appropriate way to spend time on the land if you are not in a hurry. During the first year after buying their land, the group at Mulberry Tree Farm spent one day a week together on the land building a fence. This not only saved them money and taught them how to build fencing, but gave them a purpose beyond observing the land when they visited and helped build the group into the strong community it is today. On the other hand, if it is necessary for you to live on the land to run your business and planning pressures require you to start earning a living from the land straight away, it may be wise to pay for contractors to erect fencing. They are likely to have specialist equipment which will speed up the process of banging in fence posts, and save your energy for other jobs.

The establishment of a smallholding is an expensive business. Cost is likely to be a major factor in choosing which tools and machinery to buy. Often savings can be made by searching for equipment at farm auctions and garage sales, in friends' sheds and in the advertisements in local newspapers or farming magazines. However, it can be time-consuming going to sales speculatively, in the hope you will find what you need, and buying equipment new has the advantage of certainty in getting what you want when you want it. There is such a vast choice of farm equipment available now for the smallholder that choosing good quality, well-designed tools can seem daunting to the beginner. It is worth asking the advice of a trusted friend or neighbour before investing in expensive tools. It might be that the cheap version is just as good, whereas in another situation quality is accurately reflected by price. How often are you going to use the tool? If the answer is occasionally, then perhaps it doesn't matter if the tool is not built to last. How easy is it likely to be to mend the tool or find spare parts if it breaks? If you or a friend have the skills it might be possible to adapt an existing tool for the purpose, rather than investing in another. Is it worth bodging together a tool, or is the inconvenience and wasted time of trying to making do with what you've got counter-productive? Building local networks of contacts who can help out with welding, mechanical problems and carpentry jobs, in return for some vegetables or a joint of meat, can sometimes help money to go a little further.

Finally, having somewhere dry and well-organised to store your tools is vital both for their longevity and your sanity. It is demoralising to see valuable equipment deteriorating because it is kept outside or in a leaky shed. It is equally frustrating not to be able to find a tool, and to waste time rummaging through a cluttered shed trying to find it when the weather is perfect for that particular operation. Creating an adequate tool-shed should be a priority for the new smallholder, and keeping it relatively tidy and organised is a first step to success. It is well worth stopping work five or ten minutes early to give you time to put tools away clean and in their right places, especially if you are not the only person who uses them. In the same way that, 'good fences make good neighbours', I think it could be said that well-cared-for tools make for communal harmony. Even if you work alone, your enjoyment and serenity will be greatly enhanced by knowing that your tools are ready and waiting to be used when you need them.

Chapter Seven

Domestic Energy

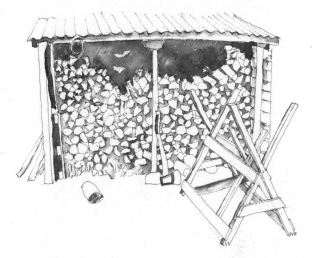

A smallholder's domestic and working lives are usually inextricably inter-twined, and it is almost impossible to isolate one from the other. To remain healthy and have enough energy to work effectively, it is important to have a warm, dry and comfortable home in which to relax, prepare and eat meals, sleep, look after children and do paperwork. Furthermore, where renewable energy is being used for heating, cooking and light, an efficient system is required, to prevent large amounts of time being absorbed by fire-wood management or maintenance of off-grid electrical equipment. This may sound obvious, but I have encountered situations where cramped, damp, cold or dark accommodation is having a negative impact on the health and ability of inhabitants to carry out their business. Whilst inade-quate housing may be a necessary temporary measure, while more perma-nent accommodation is built or planning permission sought, a well-designed, warm and comfortable home is a vital ingredient for the long-term sustenance of human energy.

House design

I was inspired by some beautifully designed homes, which were easy to heat with renewable resources and provided spaces conducive to both work and relaxation. This section draws on such examples and describes key building design principles which can affect human energy.

When the energy of the people who are to live in the house is considered, the efficiency of fuel use for heating and the choice of fuel for cooking are of tantamount importance. An ecological home should be easy to heat and exploit natural light. The principles enlarged upon below, provide a useful check-list in designing accommodation for a person or family who will be living in a low-impact way on the land:

- Roof and foundations

- Insulation

- Passive solar gain

- Thermal mass

- Surface area to volume ratio

- Scale.

Roof and foundations

An old saying used by cob builders is, "a house should have a good hat and boots." Both the roof and the foundations can make the difference between a warm, dry house and a damp and draughty one. Considerable energy can be wasted trying to keep a damp house dry, so it is a better idea to avoid damp in the first place. Numerous options are available for providing water-tightness, low embodied energy and aesthetically pleasing roofs. Two of those that particularly struck me were the hand-made shingle roof covering a reconstructed Pyrenean shepherd's hut, and the straw-bale-insulated turf roof which keeps Tony Wrench's roundhouse in Wales toasty warm, whilst making the house invisible from any distance.[1]

As for foundations, the options will depend on planning permission and the predicted lifespan of the building. The lowest-impact accommodation I saw were the benders at Steward Wood, which are constructed on platforms on the hillside. As well as creating a level building surface on a steep slope, these platforms have the advantage of lifting the dwelling above the soil, which can be a source of rising damp. It is important, however, to insulate the floor to protect against heat loss and draughts caused by air movement under the platform. This principle of lifting buildings off the ground can also be applied to more permanent buildings, by resting the entire structure on pad stones or wooden 'stilts'.

Insulation

Insulation of walls, roof and floor are fundamental in increasing the length of time a house will stay warm and the amount of fuel that is needed to keep it so. The building material may be a good insulator in itself, as in the case of straw bales which were used at Fivepenny Farm to create a low-cost, but cosy, house for one family. A turf roof adds a little further insulation and reduces the visual impact of the house, although adding extra insulation inside the roofing material will be more effective in retaining warmth. I was struck by the ingenuity of a floor I saw in another low-impact house, that was made with cross-cut discs of wood laid into subsoil. Apparently the insulating properties of the wood made the floor significantly warmer than an earth floor with rugs.

More conventional in appearance is the wood-framed house, modelled on a highly energy-efficient Swedish design, at Longmeadow market garden, built 20 years ago by Hugh and Patsy Chapman. Insulated all over (roof, walls and floors) with 6-inch-thick rock wool, with double glazed windows, the house is heated by a wood/coal stove and two night storage heaters powered by off-peak electricity. Solar water-heating is supplemented in the winter by an off-peak electrical immersion heater. The ease of living in such a comfortable, yet energy-efficient, house has enabled the Chapmans to channel their energy into running the most productive, economically viable and long-lived market garden I came across.

Passive solar design

When light energy from the sun enters a building and falls on internal surfaces it is converted into heat energy and is radiated from them. If these surfaces have a good heat storage capacity, some of the sun's energy is stored in them and slowly released into the house throughout the day and night.[2] Even in fairly northerly latitudes, such passive solar gain can provide significant amounts of heat to a building. Whilst the cooler, cloudier climate of Britain means that it is difficult to meet all of a house's heating needs from passive solar alone, its contribution to the overall energy budget of the house should not be underestimated. When a new building is being planned it is worth considering its orientation and the heat storage capacity of building materials to maximise the potential contribution of passive solar gain. Orientating the house so it faces south and placing large windows on the south rather than the north side of the house will enhance the potential for significant passive solar gain.

The most inspiring example of passive solar gain I came across was David Blair's beautiful house in Scotland. This tall, timber round-house (built by David with Sitka Spruce from his own plantation) was built on top of a 6,000-litre water tank surrounded by concrete and stone. As well as giving the house abundant natural light during the day, the numerous south-, south-east- and south-west-facing windows provided ample opportunity for passive solar gain. The water and high thermal mass stone/concrete water tank stored the sun's heat during the summer and slowly released it during the winter. The reservoir also provided under-floor heating in winter. I was impressed at how warm the house was on a cool November day without the wood stove being lit – a valuable lesson in the power of passive solar gain even in northern latitudes. Tragically, David Blair's beautiful house burnt down shortly after my visit, following a suspected arson attack. Six months later he had built a smaller, simpler version of his original house, but says that it took considerable energy to pick up his tools and start again.

Thermal mass

Thermal mass goes hand in hand with passive solar gain, since this is the term that describes bulk materials that are good at absorbing and re-radiating heat. Such materials include stone, cob, concrete and brick, but not wood. As well as being good at absorbing solar heat, thermal mass is useful for storing the heat radiated by fires. Incorporating a stone/cob wall or even just a chimney into an otherwise wooden house can create a valuable heat-storage unit. However, it is worth considering the pattern of time one spends in the house before planning to build entirely with materials which have high heat-storage capacity. Whilst high thermal mass will help a house to stay warm, it also takes longer to heat the house up in the first place, because the building materials absorb much of the available heat. Such a 'slow response' house is more suitable for people who are likely to spend longer indoors during the day, for example looking after children or doing paperwork. For people who are outside for most of the day and require instant heat in the evening, a well insulated 'fast response' house may be more appropriate.

Examples of high-thermal-mass houses were the renovated stone houses in which I found people living in France. In a continental climate like the south of France, the thermal mass has the dual benefits of keeping houses cooler during hot summers, as well as warmer during cold winters. In contrast, at Fivepenny Farm and Ourganics in Dorset, low-thermal-mass, insulated stud-work, wooden houses enabled people leading outdoor lives to heat their houses quickly at the end of the day.

Scale

A small house will obviously be easier to keep warm than a large one with equivalent insulation. However, a human energy consideration is the amount of personal space you need to stay sane. Fuel efficiency may be increased by using the same room for cooking and eating, sleeping, doing paperwork and as a children's play-room. However, if it means that it is hard to relax or you have to stay up late regularly doing paperwork, it could be a false economy. For a family, or even a couple, I would say it is important to have at least two rooms so that people can have personal space when they need it.

Domestic energy

Firewood management and the maintenance of renewable-electricity systems can be time-consuming compared to the convenience of fossil-fuel-powered heating and mains electricity. In the Western world we have lived for so long detached from the reality of the energy that supports our lifestyles, that learning to live independently of fossil fuels requires a radical change in mindset. My purpose in writing about domestic-energy use is to outline some of the options for making low-impact domestic life easier, thus releasing more time for land-based work and leisure. Low-impact living need not involve total rejection of fossil-fuel energy, and it is worth weighing up the amount of petrol or carbon emissions saved against the time and personal energy it would take to do the job by hand when choosing domestic equipment.

The main decisions that will need to be made when setting up an energy-efficient household will be how to heat space and water, what fuel will be used for cooking and how electricity will be supplied and what appliances it will power.

Firewood management

"Wood warms you thrice", so the saying goes, "when you cut it down, when you cut it up and when you burn it." The transportation of wood to where it will be used could be included as a fourth point of heating. In order to reduce the workload, the aim should be to minimise the amount of wood that is necessary to provide the desired amount of heat. It is important therefore to choose a stove that burns wood efficiently and directs the heat to where it is needed. A large firebox will enable longer logs to be burnt, and thus reduce the amount of time and energy it is necessary to spend sawing wood. Within a community, another factor which affects the amount of wood which will be used is the system for firewood management and use – whether heated space is shared or each person/family has their own place to heat. The methods by which wood is harvested, transported and cut to size will also affect the amount of time and energy invested in heating.

At Laurieston Hall, firewood management is a communal task to which each adult has to commit half a day per week. It was thus that I found myself going out 'wooding' with a group of about 15 people on the first morning of my visit. At that time wood was being harvested from a neighbouring forestry commission softwood plantation, where they had permission to fell and remove standing dead wood. The morning's work involved a couple of people with chainsaws felling the trees, while the rest of us removed side branches and cut logs to a manageable length with hand tools. They were then loaded onto a tractor-drawn trailer and taken back to the Hall, where a future morning would be spent cross-cutting, splitting and stacking them. The four large wood-sheds systematically filled with firewood at different stages of seasoning were an impressive sight, and a Lauriestonian's reward for their weekly wooding contribution is unlimited access to this valuable resource.

The downside to this system, in my view, is that it does not encourage efficient use of the wood. The combination of living in separate units in and around a large country house, and being obliged to prepare firewood each week however much you burn, results in about 80 tonnes of wood being used for a community of 24 adults, plus children and about 600-800 guests per year. Whilst some families were using wood for their heating as well as cooking, in many units gas cookers were also being used. Coming from a community that uses about 10 tonnes of wood per year for all space and water heating, as well as cooking for ten residents plus guests, I was struck by the comparison. Tinker's Bubble is no longer as communal as it used to be, in terms of fire use. However, the fact that meals are shared every evening, and breakfast and lunch are prepared using a central fire or kitchen range, contributes to less wood being used. Such communality used to be a feature of Laurieston Hall, but after 16 years the intensity of communal life led to people wanting their own, private spaces within the large central building and outlying dwellings.

Another explanation for so much less wood being used at Tinker's Bubble is that, whilst coppicing (done by hand, during a single social weekend each year) is a communal activity, it is up to individuals to transport and cut up wood for their personal use. When this is being done by hand it makes you more thrifty about firewood use, by thinking carefully about whether you need to light the stove in your house if you are going to spend the evening in the communal kitchen. Wood used for cooking communal meals and to heat the roundhouse is transported uphill by horse and cart and cut up during communal workday time.

The comparison between the wood systems at Laurieston Hall and Tinker's Bubble illustrates several interesting points. Firstly, the cost in terms of wood fuel of heating a large old hall and outlying homes is significantly higher than for small, low-impact dwellings despite their sometimes inadequate insulation. Secondly, the primary business at Laurieston Hall is the People Centre which requires significant quantities of wood, to heat water and maintain a comfortable temperature for guests on its various residential courses. Thirdly, the communal system of wood-cutting, transport and storage at Laurieston Hall which is more supportive for people who lack the physical strength or capacity (for example parents of small children) to cut wood, has to be balanced against the fuel-efficiency benefits of the system of private wood collection at Tinker's Bubble. In contrast, domestic facilities at Laurieston Hall were less communal than at Tinker's Bubble. It is important to remember the value of having a warm, comfortable space to be alone, or with just your family. While the shared kitchen and roundhouse at Tinker's Bubble reduce fuel need, the more communal life there is not to everyone's taste.

I like the compromise that has been struck at Brithdir Mawr, where people live in units in the main farmhouse and buildings around a courtyard. On four nights per week meals are cooked and shared in the communal kitchen, whilst other meals are prepared by individuals in their own kitchens. Whilst the harvesting (using mainly hand tools) and transport (by horse and cart) of one third of the wood used is done in communal workday time, people cut it for personal use in their own time. This is done using an electric chainsaw powered by the community's 1kw-rated wind generator (which produces 250 watts at average wind speeds), saving considerable time compared to cross-cutting with a bow-saw. A second source of firewood is straight, seasoned deciduous logs which are the by-product of a local conifer forest, bought by the truckload twice a year.

Residents at Steward Community Woodland were also using an electric chainsaw, this time powered by a small hydro-turbine, until a couple of dry winters rendered their stream too feeble to provide electricity (see Electricity section below). During the winter prior to my visit they were cutting firewood by hand, but a family who moved in during that winter struggled to keep up with cutting the amount of firewood they needed. As one of the family members said,

> "When I turned up there was no firewood apart from large larch logs, because it had all been used. In the winter I was spending four to five hours per day on wood. We nearly left because I couldn't use a chainsaw. Two gallons of petrol will do my firewood for one year. People use that just driving to the shops."

Like Tinker's Bubble, Steward Wood has a policy of not using fossil-fuel-powered machinery on site. It was agreed after much discussion to allow the temporary use of a petrol-powered chainsaw until a biofuel option was available or the electric chainsaw could be used again.

This example interests me for two reasons. Firstly, that two gallons of petrol could cut the amount of firewood that it would take many weeks for a person to cut. This is a graphic illustration of the comparative power of unskilled-people versus petrol. I should add, however, that where firewood is cut by hand, it tends to be collected and cut little and often throughout the winter, rather than all at once to create 'this winter's log pile' as tends to happen when a chainsaw is used. Nevertheless, in trying to reduce carbon emissions and dependence on fossil fuels it is important to consider the relative quantities of fuel that different appliances use and extra time/human labour that doing the same job by hand will involve. In this case, it makes more sense to curb car use than to abandon the use of fossil fuels altogether.

The second point I found interesting about this situation was the balance that had to be found between principles and pragmatism. It is more beneficial to the environment for people to make reasonable compromises in trying to minimise carbon emissions and hence maintain a quality of life that they can sustain, than to stick so rigidly to absolute principles that one gives up entirely due to burn-out. Of course, each person's threshold of the amount of work they are willing to live with in relation to their environmental impact varies. What I found refreshing about the chainsaw issue at Steward Wood was the dynamically flexible attitude they were willing to take to one of their core principles. Relaxing the fossil-fuel policy temporarily kept one family in the community, while other options for wood cutting were sought. For a period the community experimented with a chainsaw powered by a 50/50 mixture of wheat-derived ethanol and petrol, but found that this clogged up the saw. They now use Aspenfuel, which is a by-product of natural gas, and therefore a fossil fuel. It is, however, cleaner than petrol (no fumes) and works better, but costs twice as much. Although recently the stream-flow has been more reliable and they now have a better turbine, they find the electric chainsaw awkward since it can't be used in the rain and the power cable gets in the way. Trees are still felled using hand tools, unless they are particularly dangerous, but they are cross-cut using the chainsaw and occasionally planked using a guiding bar attachment on the chainsaw.

Space and water heating

Having harvested, transported and chopped your firewood, the next decision is how to burn it. Wood-burning stoves come in all shapes, sizes and designs, and each situation will have its own needs. For example, a family house which is occupied for much of the day will require a stove that gives off a constant heat over a long period for minimal attendance. By contrast, a farm worker who spends most of the time outside will want a stove that quickly heats up their house after dark.

The efficiency of a conventional steel or cast-iron wood-burning stove is typically 45-60%, since logs burn at a relatively low temperature and combustion is often incomplete, with unburnt volatiles re-condensing in the chimney as tar or blowing away as smoke.[3] These stoves heat mainly by convection, warming up the air as the fire burns. Masonry, or ceramic stoves, achieve 70-90% efficiency and are virtually pollution-free. This is because they burn for a short time at a very high temperature and the masonry fabric of the stove stores the heat, steadily releasing it as radiant heat over the following hours. Each burn lasts 45 minutes to an hour, and only in very cold weather would two burns per day be necessary. It is important to shut down the air intake after the wood has burnt to prevent cold air being drawn in and cooling down the system. A Forestry Commission paper published in 1980 stated that seven tonnes of air-dried wood are required to heat a typical three-bedroomed house for a year; three tonnes of wood were used to heat the reasonably well-insulated Oxford Eco House with a masonry stove.[4]

Whilst being highly efficient, masonry stoves have the down side that it takes longer to heat a room with them, since the heat stored in the fabric of the stove is released only slowly. So while these would be the ideal stove for a constantly occupied family house or workplace, they are less conve- nient for someone who spends most of the day outside. Measures such as keeping a long section of the chimney pipe inside, so as much heat as pos- sible is harvested before it leaves the house, or using a rocket stove (see Box 7.1) may be more appropriate for such people.

In an ideal world, water heating will go hand in hand with space heat- ing during the winter, so as to make maximum use of a single fire. For this reason, wood stoves which incorporate back-boilers are a common choice amongst those I interviewed. These water tanks, which are fitted to the back of solid-fuel stoves, are a common feature of cooking ranges, such as Rayburns, and are worth seeking out if this is the cooking option you choose. I encountered another design of wood-fuelled water-heating sys- tem, which was being manufactured by Romanian gypsies. It consisted of a wood-burning stove with a water tank that surrounded the straight, seven-foot-high chimney immediately above the firebox. Its efficiency was such that within half an hour of lighting it could heat enough water for six people to take a shower, making it a desirable option for communities and other places where a back-boiler would struggle to keep up with the need for hot water. In the summer, and the winter too, if they are well-designed, solar water-heating systems dispense with the need for an alternative energy source to heat water. These can range from the simplicity of a hose- pipe laid in a polytunnel for a few hours to more sophisticated systems which utilise solar radiation even on cloudy days. Hence, a well-designed solar hot-water system is the ultimate in human energy efficiency and qual- ity of life, since hot water can be obtained passively, providing the pleasure of a hot shower at the end of a long day's work!

Cooking

The aim in choosing cooking equipment is to combine ease of use with efficient use of energy. The most elementary way of cooking is over an open
fire and this is done on a regular basis at Tinker's Bubble and Steward
Wood. Although not perhaps the most efficient use of heat, when small
firewood is readily available this can be a surprisingly quick way of boil-
ing a kettle or preparing a hot meal at lunchtime, when waiting for a stove
to heat up would take too long. However, constant attention is needed to
keep the fire fed with wood. When catering for larger numbers of people,
where several pots of food are being prepared, considerable skill is required
to keep food warm and ensure it is all ready at the same time.

It is more common to find wood being used as a fuel for cooking ranges
with ovens, such as Rayburns or Stanleys. These take longer to get up to
heat than an open fire, since there is more thermal mass to heat, but once
fired up give a steady heat over a long period. They are hungry for wood,
however, and typically will require 10kg wood for an evening or 3 tonnes
in a year. In many cases, as well as being used for cooking, the range will
provide space and water heating. In the winter particularly, its hunger for
wood is therefore justified by its multiple functions.

Apart from Tinker's Bubble and Steward Wood, all the places I visited
were using gas or electricity instead of, or alongside, biomass (wood) for
cooking. This reflects the convenience of cooking with gas compared with
wood, especially during the summer when the space-heating warmth generated by a cooking stove is not as useful. Cooking on gas is undoubtedly
much quicker than on a wood-fuelled fire, since the heat is instant and
doesn't require the collection and cutting of fuel, as one community member, who was new to cooking with wood, observed:

> "The biggest change is cooking on an open fire/wood burner. We used to have
> bottled gas. You have to allow time to cook."

In countries such as India, where firewood is in short supply because the
majority of the rural population are dependent on biomass for cooking, the
production of methane from biomass or cow dung is being pioneered.
Biogas, which is composed of methane (60%) and carbon dioxide, is generated by the anaerobic degradation of organic matter by bacteria. Natural
microbial activity results in 600-900 million tons of methane being
released into the atmosphere worldwide, with devastating results since, as
a greenhouse gas, methane is 20 times more potent than carbon dioxide.
Collecting methane and burning it instead of kerosene or firewood for
cooking, lighting and heating therefore has multiple environmental benefits in that is saves forests from being cut for firewood and turns methane
into the less potent greenhouse gas, carbon dioxide. Furthermore, the

Box 7.1 – Rocket Stoves

A recent addition to the range of wood-fuelled cooking options is the rocket stove, designed by the Aprovecho Research Centre in Oregon, USA. The aim of the scientists at this appropriate technology centre was to invent a stove that would reduce the amount of wood and other biomass required by the three billion people on Earth who rely on these fuels.[5] Such an achievement is urgent, due to the fact that in many poorer countries wood is being cut and burned faster than it can be replanted and grown. The other much needed feature of the rocket stove is that its efficient burning of wood gases results in a much cleaner burn. More than 1.6 million women and children die every year from respiratory illnesses resulting from breathing in the microscopic particulates found in wood smoke.

Whilst most Westerners trying to live on the land are currently not so desperately dependent on the diminishing resource of firewood, the application of rocket-stove technology is still appropriate. The high population density of Britain means that there is limited space available for growing firewood, were significant numbers to transfer to using this renewable resource. Furthermore, from a human-energy perspective, a cleaner, more efficient burn means less time needs to be spent cutting and transporting firewood.

The principle of rocket-stove design is to ensure that wood is burnt as thoroughly as possible and the heat it produces is directed precisely to where it is needed. This is achieved by ensuring that enough air is available for combustion (the air/fuel inlet should have the same area as the chimney) and by insulating the fire area and short chimney above the fire to burn up the smoke and speed the draught. Finally, the resulting heat is forced against the cooking pot or griddle, by using properly sized channels around them.

The exact dimensions and specifications of the rocket stove are the result of twenty-five years of research and development. However, the principles can be applied to many different materials and they are simple enough that they can be manufactured with basic metal-working equipment. As well as being used for cooking, rocket stoves can be used for water- and space-heating, and adaptations have been created to cater for the cooking needs of widely varying cultures. Aprovecho Research Centre publish books and manuals on how to design and build many different kinds of stove, as well as offering training and consultancy services.[6]

residual organic matter which is left after bio-digestion has a higher nitrogen content than the best compost made through open-air digestion, making it a valuable fertiliser. This is because the nitrogen present in manure is conserved in the enclosed biogas digester, whereas during open-air composting the same nitrogen evaporates away as ammonia. If the residue from a biogas plant is used immediately, each daily kilogram of compost can yield 0.5kg extra nitrogen.[7]

Biogas production also has social benefits, in that it reduces the amount

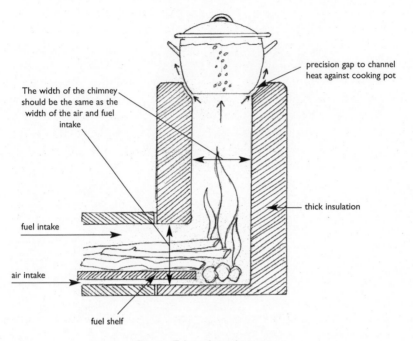

precision gap to channel
heat against cooking pot

The width of the chimney
should be the same as the
width of the air and fuel
intake

thick insulation

fuel intake

air intake

fuel shelf

Figure 7.1 – A rocket stove.

of time spent searching for firewood, treats potentially hazardous dung and does not produce smoke when it is burning. For example, in Sri Lanka the charity Practical Action has helped commercialise on-farm biogas schemes which feed gas directly into the farmer's household for cooking, laundry and lighting. Over 60 new schemes, which meet 75% of cooking needs, have resulted in household incomes rising as women and girls are freed from up to two and a half hours domestic labour which they can use instead for income generation.[8] The health benefits of biogas plants are two-fold. Firstly, pathogens and organisms present in cow dung, such as typhoid, cholera and tapeworm, are killed in the bio-digestion process. Secondly, the respiratory problems caused by working in the smoky environment created by indoor fires are reduced by cooking with biogas.

Whilst attention is being focused on its many benefits in developing countries, in the wealthier, northern nations methane produced through anaerobic digestion is rarely used domestically. Yet, considerable amounts of potentially valuable methane are released into the atmosphere by careless management of animal manure or are burnt off from ducts draining landfill sites. Any holding which keeps animals indoors for a period of time each day, so that manure can easily be collected, has the potential to produce its own biogas. A simple digester design is outlined by John Seymour, in *The Complete Book of Self-Sufficiency*.[9] It consists of a series of insulated barrels and pipes leading to a gas-collector, and eventually to a stove. Using this design, Seymour estimates that the daily manure production of a single cow or pig would be sufficient to boil five kettles full of water. To build a larger and more efficient biogas digester is a skilled and potentially dangerous operation, due to the explosive nature of the biogas, and should be undertaken only after considerable research into possible designs. However, considering the environmental benefits (renewable cooking gas, nitrogen-enriched compost, firewood conservation and utilisation of a potent greenhouse gas) and social benefits (a quick, clean and easy source of energy for cooking), it is surprising that more attention has not been focused on developing bio-digesters for farm and domestic use in the so-called developed world.

Electricity

Mains electricity is a form of energy which most people in the modern world take for granted, and miss greatly when they are deprived of it by a power cut. At the flick of a switch lights will come on, washing-machines operate and music will play. All we need to do to maintain its supply is to keep paying the bills. By contrast, building and maintaining a system to generate your own electricity requires knowledge, skill and frequent attention. Although it is possible to employ someone to install an off-grid system, in terms of mental energy, as well as financial investment, it is a costly alternative to being connected to the grid since it requires constant monitoring and regular maintenance. Yet, the replacement of mains electricity with an off-grid system of renewable energy is a powerful way to curb demand so that it matches the supply, usually resulting in less wasteful patterns of energy use.

Another option is to do without electricity altogether and depend entirely on traditional forms of lighting and human energy instead. Only one of the places I visited, Vallée de Mérens, didn't use electricity on a regular basis. Smallholders there tailor their work and leisure to fit in with daylight hours, using candles if they need light, and wash all their clothes by hand. It means that domestic tasks take longer, but since their mainly subsistence lifestyle fully integrates domestic work, food preparation and preservation and land work, the balance seems to work. It was noticeable, however, that in the household where I stayed, traditional gender divisions of labour were clearly evident, with outdoor work for the women only being possible when domestic duties were complete. Likewise, at La Borie Noble, where very little electricity is used, men seemed to be in charge of agricultural activities, while women were more engaged with food processing and administration roles. It would be unwise to draw generalisations from such a small sample. However, it is interesting to contemplate whether it is the time-consuming nature of domestic work without electricity, the strength required for agricultural work without machinery, the practicalities of combining work with child-care or some ideological consideration which resulted in such traditional gender roles.

When generating your own electricity, irregularity of supply means it is necessary to be thoughtful about how electricity is used. For example, on still, cloudy days a system dependent on wind and solar power may be short of power, while windy and sunny days produce more electricity than the batteries can hold. The scale and style of electricity systems selected by the off-grid case studies relate to human energy in two ways. Firstly, they determine the kind of labour-saving appliances people can use, and secondly the amount of time and expertise that is required to maintain the system.

Of the 28 case studies, 11 were entirely off-grid, but varied greatly in terms of the source of energy and the scale of equipment they were using. The most common systems I encountered were simple, small-scale 12v or 24v circuits powered by wind generators, solar panels or both, and involving batteries to store excess energy for low periods. In contrast to these small-scale systems one community, Brithdir Mawr, has invested in a one kilowatt rated wind turbine which, alongside a micro hydro system (constant 100 watt) and four solar panels, generated enough electricity for the community to run a 240v circuit and use conventional appliances. Hence, community members regularly use a full range of domestic appliances, including TVs, DVD and CD players, laptop computers and broadband in individual households and a communal washing-machine and food-processor. In addition, the renewable system is sufficient to power wood- and metal-working tools such as angle grinders, a circular saw and bench press drill in the communal workshop, and an electric chainsaw, which is used for cutting firewood. The only omission to the appliances you'd find in a conventional household is a refrigerator, which they estimate would add another 35% onto the community's daily power use. This is considered to be superfluous to their needs, since their goats provide fresh dairy produce daily and leftover food is usually consumed within a day. Despite having access to all these appliances, individual community members only use ⅕₅ of the UK per capita electricity use. This is achieved mainly by not leaving things on standby when not in use and choosing efficient appliances, such as laptop rather than desktop computers.

A significant difference between the 240v off-grid renewables system at Brithdir Mawr and a mains power supply is that it is the responsibility of the community to carry out maintenance work, rather than an 'outside expert'. They estimated that they spend 20 minutes per week on routine maintenance jobs, such as removing leaves from the hydro intake, as well as one or two days per year repairing worn parts of the system. The total cost of operating the Brithdir system is £1,000 per year, which covers a rolling ten-year fund for both repairs and complete replacement of all components as required.

Hydroelectricity is used in at least three other places, in addition to those that employed a hydraulic ram pump to mechanically harness hydropower to move water uphill. Again scale varied greatly, ranging from the 100-watt generator at Brithdir Mawr to the hydro-turbine at Dun Beag, which produces 500 watts at peak river flow. Usually photovoltaic solar panels complement the hydro system, since the summer is when the river flow is at its lowest. At Dun Beag, the panels have the capacity to produce 1 kw in midday summer sun. Power from the hydro-generator and solar panels feeds a 48 volt battery, and is then passed through an inverter which converts it to 240v alternating current. This enables David Blair to use conventional electric appliances, including power tools in a woodwork shop. He estimates that he spends two hours per week maintaining the battery store and hydro-generator and occasionally has to devote several days to repairing a part of the system when it goes wrong. The system was set up to maximise the efficient use of the power. For example, surplus electricity was 'dumped' first into domestic hot-water tanks, and then the 6,000-litre reservoir underneath David Blair's house, to supplement passive solar heating and provide winter under-floor heating.

These systems involved a high degree of supervision to balance demand with supply, and where they were used by more than one person, the role of electrician was usually delegated to the person who knew most about renewable energy technology. In community situations this sometimes led to an interesting power balance, in which everyone was dependent on that one person for maintaining electricity supply. At Brithdir Mawr this issue had been addressed by educating and informing the rest of the community about the renewable system, so they could take responsibility for their personal use of electricity. This was achieved by investing in monitoring equipment to show the rates at which electricity is entering the system and being used, and the power status of the batteries. The monitor was mounted on an interpretation panel just inside the front door, where everyone would notice it on a regular basis. Hence, whilst those who were most knowledgeable about electricity still carried out the routine maintenance, the rest of the community could play a more active role in regulating their use of electricity to match supply. At the time of my visit a clothes washing-machine had recently been acquired and members of the community, who had been travelling to the local laundrette or doing their washing by hand, were appreciative of the time saved. A system involving cardboard numbers being placed on piles of washing, meant that when a resident noticed the monitor showing that enough electricity was being generated they could start the washing-machine for whoever was next in the queue.

Whilst renewable electricity generation is highly desirable from the perspective of reducing carbon emissions and fossil-fuel dependence, being off-grid is not necessarily a panacea. Unless the supply of power is constant, which is rare in the case of sun and wind, batteries are needed to store electricity and the chemicals involved in batteries are far from benign. The energy involved in manufacturing batteries and other renewable equipment might be more efficiently invested in larger installations, which spread the embodied energy 'cost' between more people, than by replication of small-scale systems by neighbouring smallholders. Although it is sometimes possible to re-use batteries cast off by industry, where a group are looking at investing in a renewable energy system, it might be worth considering whether to connect to the national grid. In this way, the grid can be used as a battery, by absorbing electricity when it is in surplus and providing power during periods of deficit.

At Laurieston Hall, a significant proportion of the electricity for the main house and a couple of dwellings is produced by a hydro-generator, but the entire community also remains connected to mains. This means that as demand and supply fluctuate according to the number of people resident and the weather, there is enough electricity to meet everyone's needs. The fluctuation in demand is exacerbated by the temporary increase in the Hall's population during the summer, when the 'People Centre' is hosting courses, which coincides with the time of year when the river flow is at its lowest. Catering for large numbers increases electricity use, meaning that in the summer only 15-25% of power is provided by the hydro generator and the rest is supplied by mains. In the winter, however, this is reversed, with the main house using 85% hydro and 15% mains electricity. On average, about 40% of the power produced by the hydro-generator is used as electricity in the house, whilst the remaining 60% is 'dumped' into hot-water heating, significantly reducing the community's use of gas.

Currently there is little financial inducement to invest in costly renewable-energy equipment for connection to the national grid because of the volatility of prices received for energy compared with those charged by the Grid. By contrast, in Germany a feed-in tariff policy requires electricity companies to buy power generated on a small scale from renewable sources over a 20-year period. This provides a strong incentive for people to invest in small-scale solar electricity-generation projects, since an annual return on investment of 3-4% is guaranteed and the costs for photovoltaic equipment can be recouped more quickly than in the UK.[10]

A *holistic system*

True sustainability requires a holistic approach. The artificial barriers that divide home life from work in conventional society tend to dissolve when people live and work on their land. A typical day will consist of the integration of land-based work and domestic activities, such as child-care and wood-cutting, and will usually be governed by the weather. If the domestic set-up is too labour-intensive, then there may be insufficient time to invest in the managing the land or earning a livelihood. Conversely, it is important to reserve enough energy within the working day to attend to jobs like wood-cutting or monitoring the renewable energy system. It is demoralising to arrive home at night, exhausted, to a cold house and have to cut firewood, carry and heat water and sort out problems with the electricity.

As I have shown in Chapters Five to Seven, it is worth investing careful thought at an early stage in the choice of tools and holistic design of the home and surrounding land, so as to conserve human energy. Each smallholder will have their own objectives, but whether these are to be self-sufficient or commercial, to minimise fossil-fuel dependence or to use whatever machinery is necessary to run a viable business, quality of life is likely to be a major consideration. It is sometimes necessary to compromise on ideological beliefs in order to achieve a sufficient quality of life. Nowhere is this more apparent than in the three communities which are endeavouring to exist without using fossil-fuel-powered machinery.

Three low-carbon communities

Tinker's Bubble and Steward Wood, both in the south-west of England, and La Borie Noble, in the south of France, all illustrate how land-based communities can function using minimal fossil-fuel-based technologies. It is interesting to compare their reasons for avoiding combustion engines and where they compromise in their use of fossil fuels.

Tinker's Bubble

The policy of not using internal combustion engines on the land is one of the defining features of Tinker's Bubble. The aim of the community's 16 residents is to derive their livelihoods from the sustainable management of the land and its resources. The motivation for the fossil-fuel policy came partly from a desire to minimise carbon emissions, but also, as one of the founders states, "because working with hand tools is a saner way to work land. Machinery leads to only one person per 1,000 acres being needed." Since 1994, the community has succeeded in not only avoiding the use of combustion engines on the land, but also limiting the domestic use of fossil fuels to the occasional use of paraffin and candles for lighting when no electricity is available. Wood provides the fuel for all cooking, space and water-heating, and a wind-generator and solar panels provide enough electricity for lighting, stereos and laptop computers.

A forestry enterprise operates using hand tools to fell trees, which are then extracted by horse and sawn into planks with a wood-fuelled, steam-engine-powered saw bench. Both domestic and commercial gardens are cultivated by hand, and occasionally with horse-drawn tools, and goods are moved around the site by horse and cart. The horse also helps manage the grassland for himself and the house cows by pulling a chain-harrow and a hay-turner, to dry the hay which has been hand-cut with scythes. The internal combustion engine policy only extends as far as the boundaries of the land, enabling the community to operate two cars. These are run on biodiesel, are shared between members and used for transporting produce to farmers' markets, as well as personal trips. A mileage charge, that incorporates a proportion of the costs of maintaining and replacing the car, encourages car-sharing and the use of alternative forms of transport.

Steward Wood

The development and demonstration of affordable, home-made ways of generating renewable energy are central aims of Steward Community Woodland. The community was established in a Devon woodland in 2000 to be a living example of integrated woodland conservation, permaculture and low-impact sustainable living.

Dwellings are heated with wood-burning stoves and cooking is done either on an open fire or the wood fuelled Rayburn. Electricity is generated with a combination of micro-hydro-power and solar panels. The first micro hydro system was built using reclaimed materials and powered by a small stream. This has now been replaced by a more efficient Turga Turbine, which produces 300 watts for the community's 240v a/c circuit. In the summer, the flow is insufficient to provide power, but the long light evenings mean electricity is less in demand than in the winter.

The firewood used for cooking and heating is a by-product of managing the woodland. Whilst trees are felled using hand tools, until winter 2005/06 an electric chainsaw was being used to cross-cut large logs into lengths which could be easily split. However, the perpetual shortages of electricity resulting from insufficient stream-flow during a succession of dry winters, and low battery capacity, resulted in the decision being made to allow minimal use of a petrol chainsaw (see pp.135-6). A natural gas derivative, Aspenfuel, is now used to power the chainsaw – creating one exception to the community's policy of avoiding the use of fossil fuels. The community's vegan ethos and the high percentage of wooded land mean that, compared with the other communities, a smaller proportion of their food is produced on site and more imported produce is consumed. For example, dairy protein is substituted with soya products produced overseas, adding carbon emissions from food miles. Recently, however, some of the vegan principles have been relaxed for health reasons, making it possible for organic eggs, cheese and locally caught fish to be consumed by individuals. Some vegetables are produced in a garden at the edge of the wood. All vehicles on site are run on biodiesel, but individuals are encouraged to minimise car use and whenever possible use public transport, walk or go by bicycle.

Steward Wood is less strict than Tinker's Bubble and La Borie Noble about avoiding fossil-fuel-powered machinery. In trying to accommodate the needs of individuals (e.g. parents with small children, people with jobs that can't be reached by public transport), they have made compromises in their environmental policies. Nevertheless, they have calculated their carbon footprint to be only 39% of the national average and by attracting residents who might otherwise be living more conventional lifestyles, these compromises are arguably bringing a net environmental benefit.

La Borie Noble

La Borie Noble was the first of the L'Arche communities formed in 1948 by the Italian, Lanza del Vasto, following his encounter with Gandhi. The communities, of which there were 11 at one time, engender the Gandhian principles of nonviolence, service and manual work. Gandhi's vision saw manual work not only as a means of achieving high-quality craftsmanship and political autonomy, but as a way of developing the worker more holistically than is possible in the fragmented work of industrialisation. The L'Arche communities have therefore been managing their land, processing the harvest and meeting many of their other needs for clothing, crockery and furniture through manual labour for 60 years. At La Borie Noble, where I stayed for a week in October 2006, 120 acres of land are cultivated to produce wheat, vegetables, eggs and dairy produce, using hand tools and horsepower in a community consisting of 20 full-time residents and various working visitors. The community is entirely income-sharing, and all residents take on two or more areas of responsibility for providing for the needs of the rest of the community. At the time of my visit, six cows were being milked by hand twice daily and the milk was being processed into cheese, butter and yoghurt. A barn at a neighbouring community stores an impressive array of horse-drawn tools and carriages, including mowers, hay-turners, cultivators and even a hearse!

Haymaking is a time of great joy and hard work which goes on for about a month each summer, and involves ten to fifteen adults on a daily basis. The vast loaves of sourdough bread, which are baked in a wood-fired oven, provide enough for La Borie Noble and a neighbouring community, and are one source of communal income. Others are surplus pottery, woven garments, hand-printed cards and other handicrafts, which are sold to visitors from an informal shop.

In contrast to Tinker's Bubble and Steward Wood, with machinery rather than carbon emissions being the defining issue, the use of fossil fuels was permitted. Gas cookers are used for communal meals, and while most of the community used candles for lighting, one or two of the older women (in their eighties) were using mains electricity.

It is no coincidence that three out of the four places I visited which were avoiding the use of fossil fuels or machinery were communities. There is a close connection between the kind of tools and external energy employed, and the degree of communality. Social structure therefore goes hand in hand with choice of technology as an important variable in the human-energy equation, and it is to this that I turn my attention in Chapters Nine and Ten.

Chapter Eight

Livelihood Strategies

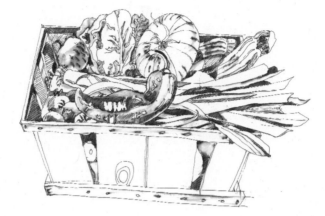

A common reason why people get burnt out is that they subsidise their business with too much of their own energy to make it economically viable. There are many ways to keep you fed, clothed and with a roof over your head whilst living on the land. Far from being the dull subject that many who've chosen this lifestyle wish to flee from, economics when applied to the day-to-day practicalities of how to earn a living from the land can be fascinating and exciting. After all, what is real economics but the wise use of resources? The projects I visited demonstrated a wide range of economic strategies. This chapter can be seen as a menu, outlining some of the options for successfully managing to make ends meet financially without driving yourself into the ground with hard work.

I will look at the subject of livelihood strategies from two different angles. Firstly, there is the question of whether you are going to meet your needs directly from the land or trade your produce and buy that which you can't produce yourself. Included in this discussion will be the option of combining an income earned from non-land-based work with subsistence or commercial activities and some examples of how the land can also be used indirectly to generate an income. Secondly, there is the question of who owns the land itself and how rent, mortgage or loan repayments influence the balance of enterprises you may wish to operate. Among many environmentalists the subject of land ownership is approached awkwardly, since it implies that the Earth, which nurtures life itself, is being reduced to a mere commodity. Yet many land-based projects stumble through lack of clear delineation of ownership. Communicating openly about people's individual and collective needs to own or share land improves the likelihood of achieving harmony when people work together.

A menu of livelihood options

Pure subsistence

For those who are more interested in providing for themselves from the land than producing commercial crops there is a spectrum of degrees of self-sufficiency. As Patrick Rivers points out in his excellent book, *Living on a Little Land*, at one extreme you may attempt to meet every possible need from the land and reduce your need for money to the barest minimum. At the other end of the scale you will have a job and a vegetable garden and grow as much of your food as you have time for. "Each of us will place ourselves somewhere between the two, depending on a host of considerations: age, money, aims and aptitude." [1]

It is virtually impossible in today's world to live without any money at all, but there are many ways to work the land so as to provide for the majority of your needs for food, fuel, shelter, light, clothing and craft materials and so significantly reduce the monetary income you need to survive. I was impressed by the level of self-sufficiency I encountered whilst staying in Vallée de Mérens, in the French Pyrenees. Hidden away in this forested valley, high in the mountains, about 20 families have created smallholdings and are spinning out meagre incomes by growing and preserving most of their own food, making clothes, furniture and their own entertainment, and are enjoying a quality of life enviable to most. A typical household in this valley would be growing vegetables in their own garden and collecting wild berries and mushrooms from the surrounding mountains and forest. To ensure year-round supply of fruit and vegetables, they have become skilled at preserving and their larder shelves groan with colourful jars filled with green beans, sweetcorn, tomatoes and blueberries. Most families keep hens and goats, which roam the mountains collecting the varied grasses and herbs to provide milk, which is preserved as delicious cheeses. The goats and chickens also provide occasional meat for special occasions. The surrounding beech woods provide an ample supply of firewood, as well as timber for building; and the stream that gushes its way down the valley, feeds into numerous large stone sinks, or *lavoirs*, where dishes and clothes are washed and people cool down on hot days.

A little produce (vegetables, cheese and honey) is sold at market stalls in the local village and town – but the emphasis is on providing enough food to enjoy a varied diet throughout the year, without needing to buy much in. Most people in the valley have some form of outside work to bring in a small income, and for many this is concentrated into two or three months of seasonal work each year. Several of the younger folk travel to the foothills of the Alps to pick apples in large commercial orchards, and one young man has an annual winter job as a shepherd in south-east France. Others earn money from building work, nursing and carving the wooden handles of pocket knives to sell in tourist shops. However, their level of self-sufficiency means that most people require only a little money for buying goods such as olive oil, flour and luxuries such as coffee and chocolate.

A year later I returned to France and had the opportunity to visit a very different, but equally striking, example of self-sufficiency at the community of La Borie Noble. Self-reliance is at the heart of this Gandhi-inspired community (Chapter Two, p.41) whose motto is, "It is in making things that human beings are themselves made." To this end, community members are personally responsible for acquiring the skills to meet their own basic needs for bread, a roof over their heads and clothing. They consciously aim to limit their needs and thereby free people in all parts of the world from the tyrannical economic systems which underpin global consumerism. In practice residents are collectively involved in farming the land, processing its produce, constructing and maintaining the buildings and making furniture, crockery, clothes and metal work for daily use. Magnificent cheeses, great loaves of sourdough bread, beautifully crafted candlesticks, bowls, wheelbarrows and buildings were a testimony to what human beings can do without machinery when they collaborate for a common cause. The community's income, which is generated from selling bread, cheese, crafts and books, is shared, meaning that when a resident has the occasional need for money they must request it from the treasurer. Their degree of self-sufficiency means that the average living costs of each community member are little more than £2,500 per year.

Whilst I found nowhere in the UK that matched up to these two examples of French self-sufficiency, I did observe that the other communities tended to focus on subsistence rather than commercial activities compared to individual or family projects. This may be because with more people it is easier to engage in a wider range of activities, therefore meeting a more diverse spectrum of subsistence needs. Conversely, the lack of land-based commercial enterprises operating in communities could reflect the challenging nature of working in a group, or the shortage of time left over for personal projects after community obligations have been met. It is often easier to earn any money you might need from a part-time job outside the community than to shoe-horn the time-consuming business of running an agricultural or horticultural enterprise into three or four days per week.

Certainly the subsistence element of community life in several of the UK communities contributed to the much lower than average living costs enjoyed by residents. At Laurieston Hall, Brithdir Mawr and Brockhurst, a large part of the 2-3 days per week workday commitment is communally farming the land to produce food and fuel for residents and visitors. People take responsibility for different parts of the vegetable garden, milking the cows or goats, processing the milk into cheese, butter and yoghurt, tending the chickens or pigs and collecting and cutting firewood. The rest of the time they are free to earn a living however they choose and most tend to have outside jobs. However, many commented on the quality of fresh, organic food that community life gave them access to on a low income, as well as the freedom from having to work five days per week at a less fulfilling occupation. At Tinker's Bubble a high level of subsistence is integrated with small-scale commercial activities, with the community benefiting additionally from produce that returns unsold from markets.

A land-based income

Earning a living from selling goods that I have grown, raised or processed is one of the most satisfying experiences I have ever had. Not only is there a basic honesty about working to produce a high-quality product which people actually need, but the appreciation expressed by customers seems to magnify the monetary value of the produce several fold. That said, it is hard work and takes considerable skill, in both efficient production and marketing, to translate that hard work into a reasonable living. Very few of the projects I visited were 100% dependent on the income from their land-based business.

In some cases farming was the sole occupation, and was being supported by either agricultural subsidies or working tax credit while the business was in its infancy. Horticulture is one agricultural sector which has had to manage without agricultural subsidies, and new growers are faced with either having to retain another job until the business becomes profitable or take advantage of government schemes designed to help young enterprises through the first few years. The problem is that with the abundance of cheap food resulting from industrial agriculture and imports, the prices people are willing to pay for local and organic food sometimes barely cover the real costs of production. One interviewee had a sad tale to tell about how the aggressive pricing practices of a new supermarket in town had eventually driven her organic market stall out of business. Others have fared better during the rises and falls in popularity of organic food that have occurred during the past two decades. At present people spend an average of 10% of their income on food[2] and until they are forced to

Type of Marketing	Holding	No. of holdings selling this way
Market Stall	La Fermette Fivepenny Farm Galingale Land of Roots Les Jardins de Mondoux Little Farm Meadows Farm Ourganics Tinker's Bubble Vallée de Bernède Wood White Tony Wrench	12
Box scheme	Briggs Farm La Fermette Mulberry Tree Farm Ourganics Trading Post *Used to:* Little Farm Longmeadow Tamarisk Farm	5 now; 3 in past
Farm shop/ farm gate	La Borie Noble Les Jardins de Mondoux Longmeadow Sea Spring Tamarisk Farm Trading Post	6
Wholesale to local shops and the catering trade	Fivepenny Farm Galingale Keveral Farm Ourganics Tamarisk Farm Tony Wrench Vallée de Mérens Woodwhite	8
Mail order	Real Seed Catalogue Sea Spring	2
Courses and camps	La Borie Noble Brithdir Mawr Dun Beag Keveral Farm Laurieston Hall Ourganics Pentiddy Woods Sea Spring Farm Steward Wood	9

Table 8.1 – Types of marketing practised by the holdings.

pay more realistic prices, through the increased cost of conventional production and long-distance transport, the market for food that is sustainably produced and local will be limited to a committed minority who are
prepared to pay for its wider benefits. However, the market for local and
organic food is growing rapidly and the rising cost of oil is likely to
improve further the financial viability of small-scale, local and organic production.

Mixed farms centred on market gardening, but producing fruit, eggs
and meat as sidelines, seem to be well-positioned now to generate a reasonable income for supporting a family. Vegetable box schemes are one
very effective way of building a loyal customer base and receiving a guaranteed weekly income for home produce. Several of the businesses were
operating successful box schemes, or had done so in the past. However,
with the increased availability of organic produce, the market has changed
and to be competitive it is often necessary for box schemes to offer exotic
fruits and vegetables alongside that which they can produce themselves.
Hence market gardeners may have to buy in produce and divert a significant amount of time to collecting, packing and doing the administration
for produce which is not their own.

At present it seems that retailing other produce alongside your own is a
pragmatic way of attracting a wider range of customers, whether you are
direct marketing via a box scheme, a market stall or a farm shop.
Alongside price, convenience is the other aspect of supermarkets that has
made them so popular and, apart from the most committed ethical consumers, most people don't have the time to shop at more than a handful of
outlets each week. One man, who was running a successful farm shop
alongside his market garden, said: "In other places they only sell what they
produce. If you buy in other things people need, then you create a good service for people – eggs, milk, bread and a few other things. Then they can
come for most of their supplies." In this case, the 'other things' means a
fairly full range of wholefood groceries as well as mouth-watering, locally
produced cakes, pies, meats and other high-quality foods.

Direct marketing

So, what are the human energy implications of the various options for
direct-marketing produce? The main forms of direct marketing I encountered were box schemes, market stalls, farm shops and mail order. For all
four methods it should be considered that there is a trade-off to be made
between the benefits of increased control over, and knowledge of, your
market and the extra time and hard work that is spent preparing produce
for selling, on advertising and administration. However, despite the fact
that direct marketing entails greater work, enthusiasm and commitment

	Box schemes	Market stalls	Farm shop	Mail order
Pros	• Guaranteed weekly income • Greater commitment from consumers. • Seller has choice over what produce harvested and sold each week.	• Low capital investment and overheads • Flexibility of what you need to produce each week.	• Possible to stock a wider range of goods and thereby offer greater convenience to customer. • Tending a small, informal farm shop can be integrated with other farm administration or household activities.	• A much larger market can be accessed because geographical restrictions are lifted. • Low capital investment and overheads
Cons	• Box packing is time-consuming and can be dull. • More time spent driving around the countryside delivering boxes. • Increased stress from ensuring that there is enough produce to fill boxes each week (Can be alleviated by careful crop planning).	• Risk of produce not being sold and wasted. • Highly weather-dependent (i.e. customers less likely to come out when raining or very cold).	• High capital investment required to start. • Staffing costs and overheads if open full-time • Time spent managing staff, stock control and administration.	• Greater 'food miles' involved, yet takes advantage of existing distribution services (often Royal Mail) so still quite green! • Success relies on promoting the product nationwide. Often this depends on advertising, which is expensive.
Time away from production (per week)	• collecting bought-in produce • packing boxes • delivery (half day to whole day)	• Market preparation (half to one day) • Market stall attendance (half to one day)	• Full-time job for one or more people if open full-time. • If open part-time (tending shop whenever open) • Self-service (daily restocking and regular removal of cash from honesty box)	• Packing many small retail orders. • Administration and deliveries to post office (daily)

Table 8.2 – A comparison of the advantages and disadvantages of various direct-marketing methods.

than selling wholesale, most producers are unequivocal about the rewards they reap from having a closer and more secure relationship with the consumer. Table 8.2 (on the previous page) outlines some of the pros and cons of these four methods of direct marketing, although it should be remembered that differences in scale and the detail of how each individual business is run make each point below open to debate.

For example, while a farm shop that is open six or seven full days per week will need to be staffed by at least one full-time member of the family or an employee, to allow the producer to carry on producing, other more informal options exist. At Tamarisk Farm, the shop opens only twice a week, on Tuesday afternoons and Friday mornings, and sells only produce from the market garden and farm (vegetables, fruit, lamb, beef and flour). Another option is to operate a self-service farm shop, where goods are displayed on a market cart or in an open room, and customers place money in an honesty box. Whilst such farm gate sales are more common when only one or two products are for sale, such as vegetables, honey or eggs, one farm I know sells a wide range of locally produced preserves, ice-creams, juices, vegetables and cheeses alongside their own meat, Jersey milk and cream via a self-service/honesty box system.

The marketing systems at some of the farms had evolved through several different types of direct selling, and most continued to combine elements of direct and wholesale marketing to find homes for all of their produce. Box schemes and market stalls are a good precursor to the financial commitment of opening a farm shop (see Box 8.2 on Longmeadow, p.161), whilst mail order is a way of reaching distant customers with more specialised products. However, if future fuel shortages result in increased transport costs, mail order companies may find themselves having to seek more local customers. Mail order should perhaps be seen as a temporary marketing solution, enabling businesses to develop until a large enough proportion of the local population is willing to support local producers.

Markets are the oldest and most direct way of selling produce, and can be found operating all over the world. Vendor and customer face each other over a table, on which the items for sale are displayed for all to see, and often the price is agreed through a process of negotiation. Until recently, street markets in Britain were a pale shadow of their former selves, having become the province of cheap, low-quality, imported goods. Over the last decade, produce markets have experienced a revival, with farmers' markets creating venues where people can find fresh, locally produced food and meet the people that have produced it. However, most farmers' markets operate monthly, or at most fortnightly, meaning that consumers need to find other places to buy their food in between times and often forget or are unable to attend the market when it operates.

Box 8.1 – Send it by Post: The Tale of Two Mail Order Companies

Peppers by Post and The Real Seed Catalogue are two thriving, horticulture-based mail order companies being run in very different circumstances.

Peppers by Post specialises in growing chilli peppers in polytunnels. During the six month harvest season chillies are picked and posted first-class on the same day, so they reach customers the day after harvest, much fresher than chillies available in any shop. The business started in 1996, when the husband and wife team decided that in order to earn a living from their market garden they needed to specialise. Until then they had been growing a range of vegetables and selling them at markets, to shops and to restaurants, but it was a struggle to generate enough income to raise a family and pay off a mortgage. Peppers suited them because they are a high-value product and require relatively little labour to produce, yet there is a limit to the number of chilli peppers it is possible to sell locally. The idea of selling them mail order took off from the outset and the company has gone from strength to strength. Publicised by numerous articles in magazines and national newspapers, the advent of the company coincided with growing public interest in exotic ingredients and they now run courses on growing chilli peppers and cooking with them in different cuisines.

The Real Seed Catalogue is a seed club that provides members with access to a selection of open pollinated seeds and heirloom vegetable varieties, tailored for home gardeners to grow fine-tasting produce. It is part of a movement to protect valuable heritage seeds from disappearing forever, due to legislation that prohibits them from being sold unless they have passed through a very costly registration process. Like 'Peppers by Post', the business is family-run, but differs in that the couple live in a community rather than on their own holding. The work of the seed business is spread throughout the year (growing seeds in spring and summer; harvesting, sorting, packing in the autumn; and the busiest selling season in late winter and early spring) enabling it to mesh with the demands of parenting and community duties of shared cooking, land management and administration. Many of the seeds sold in the catalogue have been collected and grown by the couple in their garden at Brithdir Mawr, but to ensure that customers are offered a full range of vegetable varieties they also buy-in seed, which they rigorously test for germination before putting it in the catalogue. The annual catalogue is the main point of communication with the members and it includes fascinating snippets of history and personal recommendations about vegetables with particularly good flavours. A shift towards internet sales has resulted in significant increases in efficiency, meaning that expansion of the business has been able to take place within the time limits of community life.

At towns which still have a regular street market there is nothing to stop producers setting up shop alongside the cheap clothes and pet-food stalls. Fivepenny Farm established a weekly market stall in Bridport, Dorset soon after they had bought land in the area. At first they sold fruit and vegetables bought from an organic wholesaler, meaning that when their own produce came on stream they already had a loyal customer base and could sell whatever they could grow. It was decided from the outset to continue buying-in produce that could not be grown at the farm, such as avocado pears and lemons, to provide a convenient one-stop shop for fresh produce. The two couples who own the farm take turns at running the stall on alternate weeks, and use the profits generated from bought-in produce to pay market costs, thus maximising income from their own produce. Their regularity of attendance at the market, rain or shine, has brought them quite a following and many of their customers buy a significant proportion of their fresh produce from the stall. Alongside fruit and vegetables, eggs, home-made preserves, hand-made herbal cosmetics and occasionally their own pork or lamb are sold, and the market stall has also become a place where the farm can seek help for labour-intensive activities such as tree-planting or strawberry-picking.

Another alternative is to take your stall to the customers. At La Fermette in France, a couple were doing just this, by loading up their horse-drawn market cart with vegetables and eggs and driving it half a mile to the local town. There they would wend their way through the suburbs, ringing a bell to bring people out of their houses, before stopping outside the supermarket for a couple of hours to catch some more custom.

The benefits of wholesale

There are other options, however, besides the time-consuming requirements of direct marketing and the large, regular quantities, rigorous cosmetic demands and financial uncertainty of selling to supermarkets. Selling wholesale to local shops, caterers and producer marketing co-operatives cuts out the need to stand and wait for individual customers to come and buy your produce, and the administration and delivery involved in running a box scheme or mail order company.

Several producers in the survey sell produce wholesale, including flour, charcoal, eggs and vegetables to local shops and garages. Ourganics, a small permaculture garden in Dorset, sells about 15 kilograms of salad leaves per week from March through until November to local shops, box schemes and private caterers, to supplement direct-marketing outlets. Independent shops and chefs at restaurants, pubs and hotels are often keen to promote local produce and will buy it in significant quantities. One man was struggling to keep up with caterers' demands for eggs and vegetables from his 300 hens and growing horticultural enterprise. He was able to combine food deliveries with selling £2,500 worth of his own charcoal to garages and shops each year.

In recent years 'middlemen' have received a bad press, being accused of taking too high a proportion of the price paid by the consumer and thereby depriving producers of their fair share. However, where middlemen can enable producers to get on with what they are really good at, be it growing vegetables, making cheese or raising animals, I believe they have a valuable role and deserve their cut of the product price. I became acutely aware of this when I visited Keveral Farm in Cornwall, where individual producers are now selling a high proportion of their salad crops and other vegetables to a popular Cornish restaurant. The relationship between multiple small-scale producers and a restaurant, that in the summer was buying £1,000 worth of fresh produce per week, was made possible by Shaun, a community member, working in partnership with another man as a marketing agent. Thus, the restaurant could interact with a single business, Buttervilla, who would place orders with individual producers both at Keveral and other local farms, ensure they were of a suitable quality and deliver them to the restaurant.

Not only is this relationship more efficient in terms of transport, removing the need for each individual producer to deliver, but it frees up their time so they can produce more vegetables, knowing they have a guaranteed market for them. The only problem was that in the winter period orders dropped off to £300 per week, and by acting as a middleman, Shaun has less time to earn his own living by growing vegetables. Whilst remaining passionate about supporting small-scale producers by helping them sell their produce, he is now reducing the number of suppliers he sources from so he can spend less time on the telephone and more time in the garden.

Meeting local needs

If you are producing food, a good starting point is to remember that everyone needs to eat. Whilst the people who are most commonly attracted to organic food are those with an awareness of environmental issues and people on higher incomes, there are ways of broadening access to fresh, local produce, which are welcomed by people on lower incomes. Inspired by schemes first set up in Cumbria, Somerset Community Food have been developing fresh food co-ops in towns throughout the county. Each week a bulk order of local, and often organic, produce is delivered to central drop-off points (village halls and community centres) where it is shared out, and sometimes delivered, by volunteers. Local residents, who have pre-ordered the bags, come later in the day to collect them and can pay as little as £3–£5 for a bag full of mixed vegetables. The fruit and vegetables are supplied by a combination of conventional wholesalers and Somerset Organic Link, a local producer co-op and marketing company.

A more direct link between villagers and a grower came about in 2001, when foot-and-mouth disease stopped customers being able to collect their vegetable boxes from Galingale Farm, in Somerset. Instead, the farm started to sell their vegetables from a stall outside the vicarage on a Saturday morning and people from all walks of life started to buy their produce. Seven years later the stall is a regular village fixture and production is only limited by the amount of time the couple are able to spend working on the farm.

Inspired by this example, I experimented with selling vegetables outside the village school near Tinker's Bubble, reasoning that child-collection time would be a good focus for bringing people in the village to the same place at one time. Unfortunately, the perception of organic produce being an expensive luxury put most parents off coming to even look at the stall, even though our produce was very reasonably priced. The following summer we were invited to set up the stall outside the village shop, and were heartened to find that many more people became regular customers. Timing was crucial, and we chose Thursday afternoons from 3.00pm to 6.30pm to coincide with school collection time and enable people to pick up vegetables on their way back from work.

Your imagination is an invaluable tool in finding local markets for your produce. By thinking carefully about what people need and how to offer a service that best meets that need, you may hit upon a successful formula for selling your produce. It then takes time to refine your chosen marketing method, and over the years it will adapt both to changing public tastes and trends, as well as to your own needs (see Box 8.2 on Longmeadow, p.161). However, if you are willing to embark on meeting the growing demand for fresh, local and organic food, you will experience a sometimes challenging, but nevertheless rewarding adventure.

Land-based diversification

Selling produce is only one way to generate an income from your holding. The land may provide the materials or the context for the enterprise, but translating them into a livelihood can involve a diverse range of skills and processes.

'Adding value' is a term that is frequently used in the context of farm diversification, and several smallholders were successfully earning a living from adding value to the primary products of their land. A classic example is green-woodworking, a traditional skill by which the products of woodland management can be transformed into high-value furniture. Over the

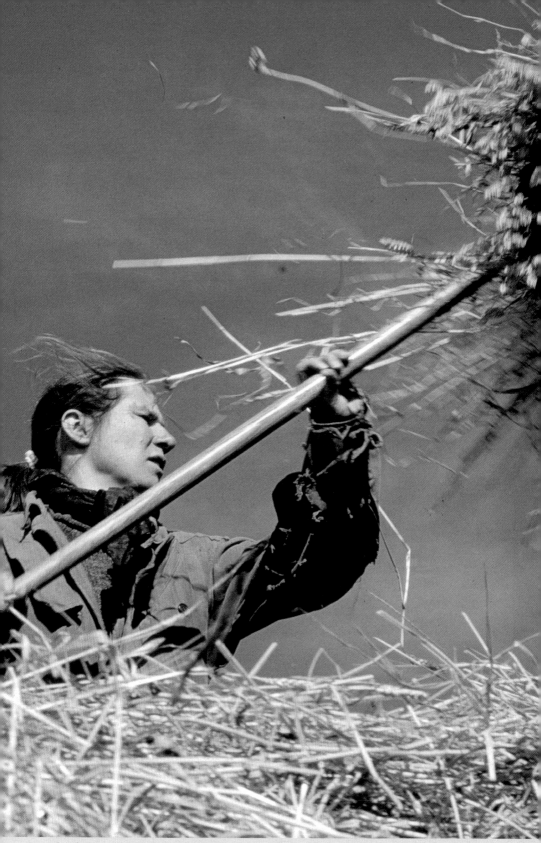

Threshing at Tamarisk Farm requires sustained physical effort from everyone in the team.
Photo by Michael Michaud/Sea Spring Photos

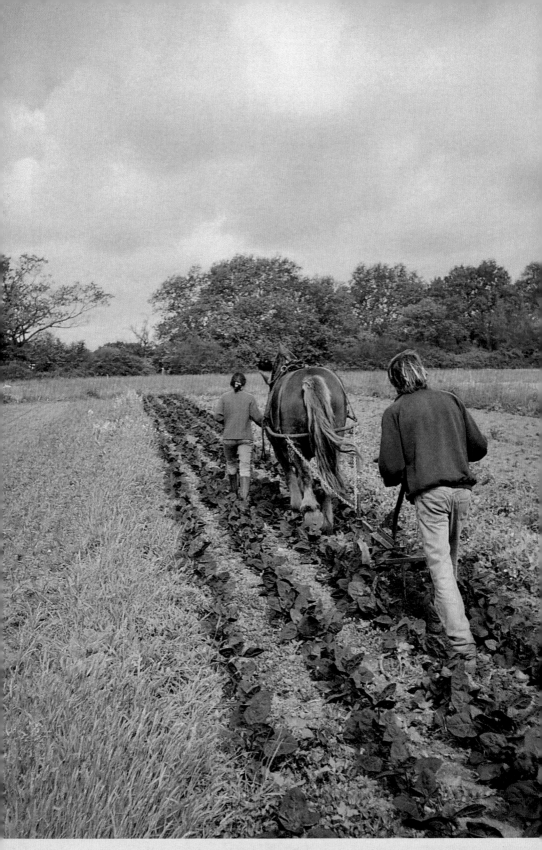
Hoeing amaranth, an early spinach substitute, with a PROMMATA Kassine (see p.112) at La Fermette.

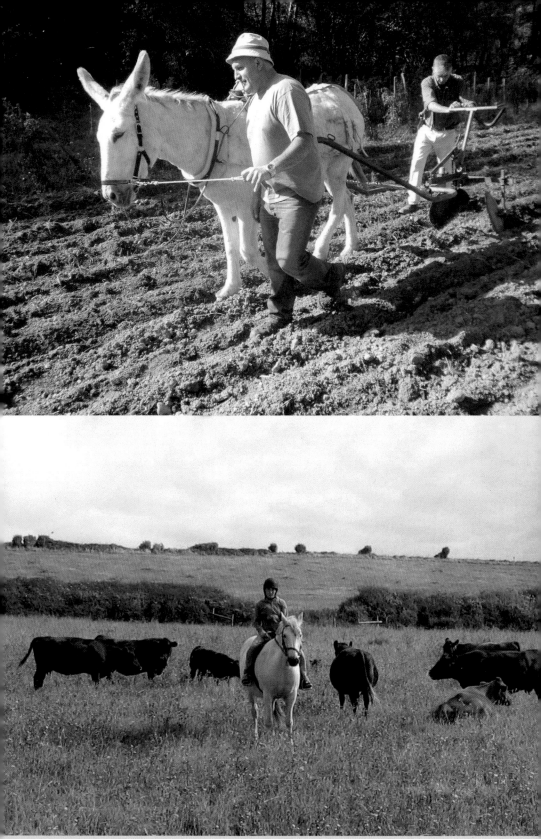

Above: A variety of tools, such as these ridging discs, can be fixed onto the Kassine frame. *Photo by Jo Ballad*
Below: Stock-checking on horseback – Devon Red cattle at Tamarisk Farm. *Photo by Adam Simon*

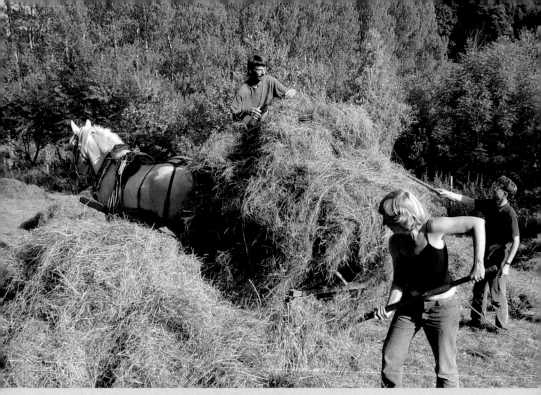

Above: Bringing in the hay at Tinker's Bubble – a mixture of hard work and celebration.

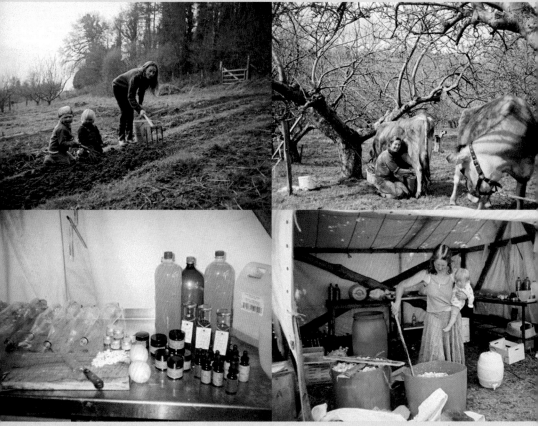

Middle left: Children are keen to help in the garden. *Middle right:* Hand-milking creates a rewarding relationship with your cow. *Below left and right:* Elderflower cordial and other herbal products produced at Tinker's Bubble

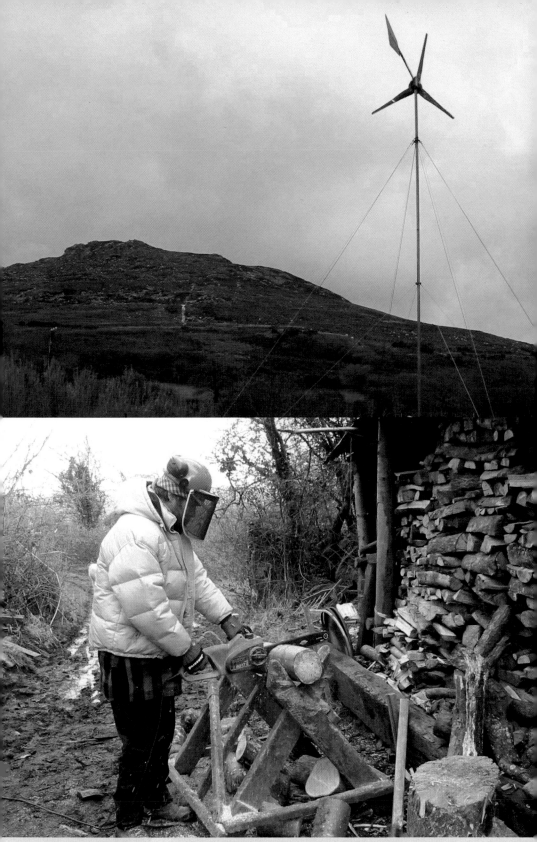

The renewable energy system at Brithdir Mawr *(above)* powers a range of labour-saving appliances, including a washing-machine and an electric chainsaw *(below)*. *Photos by Ben Gabel*

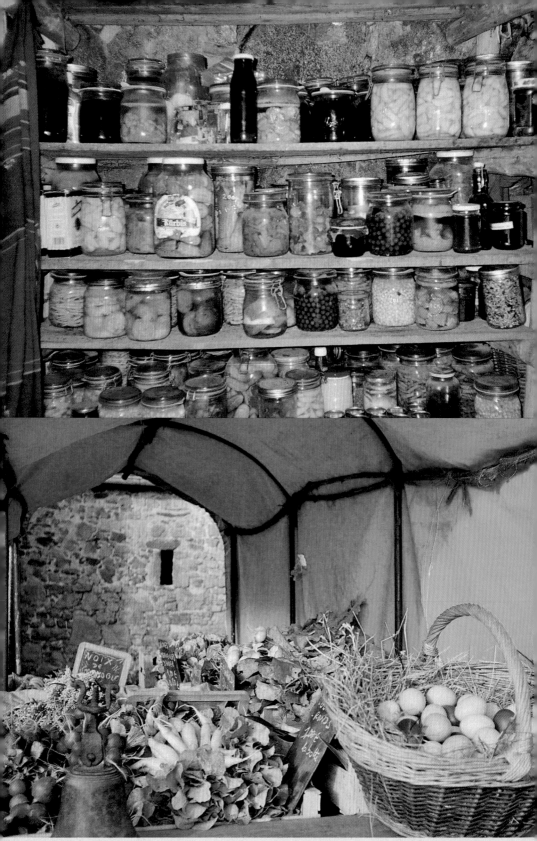

Above: All set for winter. A store cupboard like this represents many hours of hard work.
Below: Fresh, green and convenient – door-to-door sales of organic vegetables from a horse-drawn cart.

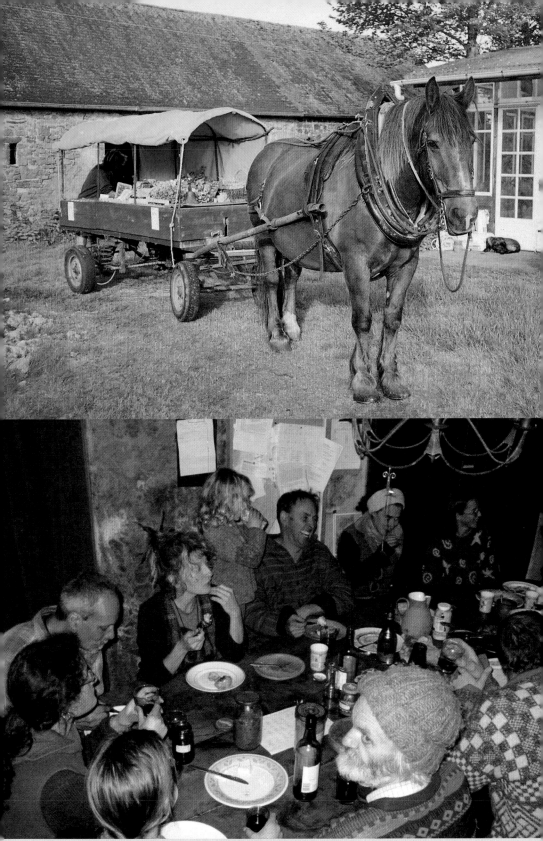

Above: Ready to go! The market cart at La Fermette, Loire Atlantique.
Below: Regular shared meals and cameraderie are a major attraction of communal life. *Photo by Ben Gabel*

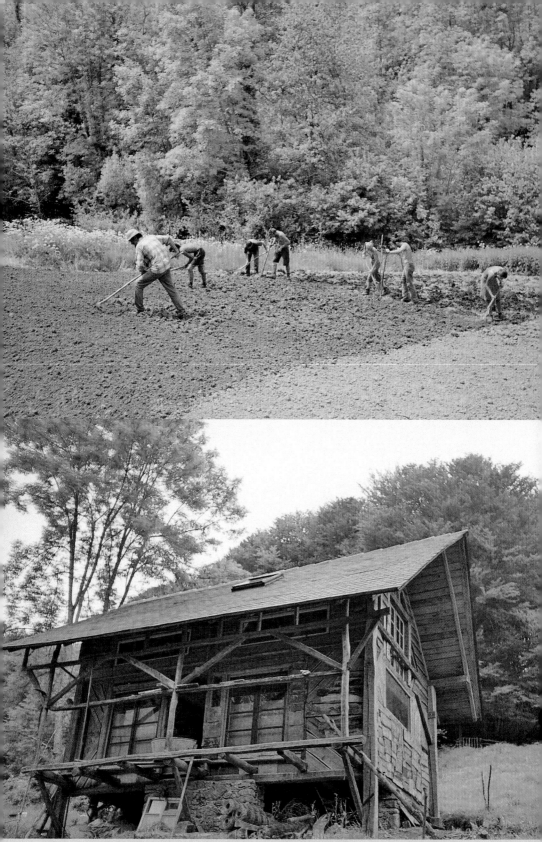

Above: Many hands make light work – a family work party in the Pyrenees.
Below: A new generation of smallholders are building their homes in Vallée de Mérens.

Box 8.2 – The Evolution of a Market Garden: Longmeadow Organics

Hugh and Patsy Chapman bought their nine acres in Dorset in 1987, and started growing field-scale vegetables and sharefarming sheep with their neighbours. In the early years they sold most of their vegetables wholesale via the first organic marketing co-op in the country, Somerset Organic Producers. They also sold a few via a self-service vegetable stand outside the house. Hugh did a small amount of extra part-time work in the beginning to supplement their income. When the co-op folded in 1993, due to the recession, a downturn in organic sales and dissatisfaction with supplying supermarkets, the Chapmans were forced to develop more local outlets. In 1994 they started a box scheme, and also supplied a restaurant and a wholefood shop in nearby Dorchester. At its peak the box scheme was an outlet for most of the vegetables from 6.5 acres under cultivation. Each week 140 boxes were sold to families who picked them up from collection points in local towns and villages within a 15-mile radius. Most of the produce in the boxes was their own, but they did buy-in certain vegetables, especially at the beginning and end of the season. Even with the help of mechanical cultivation, running the box scheme was extremely hard work, involving heavy and repetitive manual work whilst preparing literally tonnes of carrots, leeks and other vegetables for the boxes. However, the Chapmans found it to be a reliable outlet and by taking a seasonal break for the 'hungry gap', between March and July, they were able to sustain their energy from year to year. Also, the positive feedback they received gave them the sense that customers were supportive and sympathetic to their needs.

As they have grown older Hugh and Patsy have started looking for easier ways to sell their produce. A recent development has been the establishment of a farm shop in a converted outbuilding. The farm shop business is actually owned and run by a couple of their friends, and sells a wide range of other organic products alongside the vegetables and fruit grown or sourced by the Chapmans. In the future they plan to scale down the market garden, so that they are just growing a few high-value vegetables to supply the farm shop.

years one man has honed his skills with the pole lathe and now makes beautifully finished Windsor and American ladder-back chairs. Another uses offcuts from softwood saw logs to make rustic garden furniture on commission. Heartwood Creations, part of the Pentiddy Woodlands Project in Cornwall, makes a mixture of stylish indoor furniture and rustic outdoor benches, tables and chairs using a combination of coppice wood and sawn timber. Using an electric lathe, one smallholder contributes to his income by making bowls and plates out of interesting, knotty pieces of wood.

Herbal products are another form of adding value, and four women were using both herbs they had cultivated themselves and ones they had gathered from the wild. In France and Italy I have come across beautiful herbal tea mixtures, which combine colourful, dried flower petals and leaves to create 'tisanes' with various medicinal properties. A friend with a deep knowledge of herbs infuses alcohol with herbs such as elderflowers, mullein and hyssop to make tinctures which can help with various minor ailments. She also processes large quantities of elderflowers and berries into cordial and syrup each year, and makes a fine elderflower champagne which she sells at festivals. Another friend infuses oil with comfrey and calendula petals which she uses as the base for a variety of soaps, salves and hand creams.

Another approach to diversification is to see the land itself as a product, offering both a resource for education and a venue for leisure. Several projects ran or hosted courses and camps. For many years Laurieston Hall has offered dormitory accommodation, catering and facilitation services to courses run by outside organisations, through its workers' co-op, the People Centre. The People Centre is run by community residents, pays rent to the community for the facilities and buys vegetables, eggs and dairy products from the housing co-op to use in catering for the courses. In their spare time, course participants can enjoy walking in the extensive woods around the hall, swimming in the loch or sweating in the lakeside sauna.

Going slightly more upmarket, as they have grown older the couple running Tamarisk Farm have diversified into holiday cottages, which are marketed on the basis of being located on an organic farm next to the sea in Dorset. People staying in the cottages, one of which is fitted with facilities for disabled people, can pre-order vegetables, meat and flour from the farm shop and are provided with breadmaking machines. Guests can explore Tamarisk Farm via a network of public footpaths, and thus can enjoy the flora and fauna which result from the farm's conservation grazing programme.

Pentiddy Woodland Project uses its land as an educational resource for courses in bushcraft, as well as providing a venue for a monthly forest school for local children. Thus, the integrity and biodiversity of the mature mixed woodland can be conserved, whilst generating a small income as both children and adults build shelters, forage for wild food and make fire with bow drills. Adults can also take part in green-woodworking and rustic furniture-making courses, which will increasingly draw from the woodland resources of Pentiddy as the hazel and chestnut coppice they have planted comes to maturity. The couple at Pentiddy are also seeking permission to operate a woodland burial site. This will enable more people access to the beauty and tranquillity of this evolving permaculture project. Several other farms run permaculture courses, using their own sites and other nearby projects as examples of permaculture in action. Ragmans Lane Farm in Gloucestershire, where I took a permaculture design course, is a prime example of this. It combines diverse enterprises such as apple juice making, shiitake mushroom cultivation and willow production with a camping barn where several permaculture courses take place annually.

Keeping the day job

Tempting though it might be to quit all previous employment and throw yourself wholeheartedly into your land-based livelihood, it is important to weigh up the pros and cons of spending all your time working solely on your own project. Generating enough money to live on from the land is tough and requires long working hours, efficient systems and creative marketing skills. Working part-time off-site or at another, more lucrative, occupation can remove a considerable amount of the financial pressure to make your land project work and make the difference between enjoyment and endurance. However, there are more than just financial reasons for keeping another job. Many people coming into organic or local production are moving from other occupations, and are often highly skilled at, or passionate about, what they were doing previously. Combining a land-based project with another job that fulfils different aspects of a person's interests and work needs may be important in maintaining their happiness, motivation and a holistic sense of meaning in life.

A few people I spoke to cautioned against being entirely financially dependent on your land-based project. Having tried several combinations of income generation, the couple who run 'Peppers by Post' strongly recommended 'keeping the day job'. Alongside running their very successful mail order business, Joy works as an editor and runs a library of horticultural and agricultural photographs. Her husband Michael is developing a career as a freelance writer and runs courses on growing and cooking with chillies. Previously, before they had specialised in chilli peppers and while they had a young family, he worked as an inspector for the Soil Association, which brought in a reliable supplementary income.

The downside of having another job is that it reduces the amount of time you have available to work on your own land. One couple were on the brink of having to give up, or at least scale down, their successful market gardening business because they were finding it too exhausting meeting the growing demand for vegetables on top of holding down a full-time and a part-time job. It was necessary for them to keep their other jobs to cover the expenses of living in a conventional house (mortgage and bills) and they hankered after the chance to build a more energy-efficient, low-cost house on their land so that they could afford to focus entirely on running the smallholding. Another couple were in a similarly frustrating position, being forced to continue tree surgery work and teaching to cover their conventional living costs, when being able to live on their land would have enabled them to develop their horticultural, egg and charcoal enterprises to their full potential.

Not only does keeping another job increase the ability to pay the bills and invest in a fledgling business, it can also be a valuable way of getting out into the community and having a change of activity. One woman I interviewed was deeply ambivalent towards the child-care work she had to do alongside managing her smallholding. On the one hand she hated having to tear herself away from the long list of jobs that always needed doing on the smallholding, and having to keep clothes clean and ironed for work. However, she recognised that her outside work was a link into a valuable network of customers for her produce, and in some ways enjoyed the contrast of working with people after being alone on her holding. Several other people retained a part-time job off the farm due to a personal interest or skill, rather than out of financial necessity. Two women take time out from their farms to undertake jobs in land-rights campaigning and training counsellors on breast-feeding.

Although a truly sustainable model of food production requires a radical increase in the number of people working on the land, it is unlikely that most people in today's society would be happy spending all their time labouring on the land. The modern education system has emphasised the development of mental abilities at the expense of manual skills to such an extent that insufficient numbers of people are willing or able to undertake full-time many of the jobs that underpin society (e.g. farming, building, plumbing and electrical work). Yet, I am aware of many people in the UK who are keen to live a simpler, more land-based lifestyle. Not only do they lack the confidence in their ability to earn their entire living from the land, but many would like to combine partial self-sufficiency with a part-time version of their current employment. For those with sufficient capital to buy land with housing on it, such a dual-income model is possible. However, it is hard for people without significant capital to buy properties with land at the same time as scaling down to a part-time income so they can practice self-sufficiency.

Balancing 'head' work, with 'hand' work is a vital ingredient in creating healthy, happy and fulfilled members of society and is a key to sustaining human energy. Yet without radical action being taken to address the issue of affordable rural housing, society will continue to be polarised between those who are working too hard at white-collar jobs to enjoy life, and those who are doing land-based work they enjoy, but are scraping along on a minimal wage and lack a secure home.

Land ownership

One decision which must be made at the outset of any land-based project is whether to buy or rent land. The subject of land ownership is riddled with emotional and spiritual issues, as well as the practicalities of finance and legal documentation. Land is, after all, a portion of the Earth's surface and is the fundamental means to our survival, so it is not surprising that throughout history, and all over the world, land rights have been fought for and valued, sometimes more than life itself.

Whilst the concept of private land ownership may be distasteful to some, who see land as a resource that should be held in common, the reality is that in most parts of the world private land ownership is the system that holds sway and in order to secure access to land it is necessary to engage with that system. Owning land does not have to preclude holding the view of land being a common treasury for all, it just re-frames it in a longer-term perspective. The Amish people of North America have sovereignty over their holdings, yet take the view that they are stewards of the land rather than owning it. For an Amish man, "it is his privilege to live on it; the land is in trust during his lifetime. He is so serious about being a faithful steward that he nurtures his earth, he brings forth the harvest of its own disposing, he tends the land until it glows with contentment." [3]

The following quote, from a wonderful book about peasant farming in the 1930s in the Dordogne valley of south-west France, sums up how issues of land ownership and personal sovereignty can affect motivation and ability to tend the land:

> "The peasants own their houses, fields, vineyards, plots of woodland, whether they are farmers, carpenters, wheelwrights, masons, cobblers and so on. No-one is a complete specialist, even when he has a handicraft. Everyone is his own master, does his own work in his own way in his own time. Ownership is the very basis of freedom and independence and, as far as the land is concerned full production from it is possible only under individual ownership. A paid agricultural worker or a tenant for that matter cannot be expected to do as well by the land as he would if he owned it. Everyone has the right to sunshine and air and should have a right to as much of the earth as he and his family can cultivate – but no more. In a Christian community – Christian, in fact – no-one would be denied this right and no-one would want to possess more than he could cultivate well." [4]

Whatever your beliefs about land ownership, it seems that security of tenure is key not only to ecological sustainability but also to the sustaining of human energy. Whether you are working alone or with other people it is important for motivation to know that the labour investment you make in the land in terms of soil improvement, biodiversity conservation, infrastructure (fencing, water, buildings) and tree-planting will be valued and not destroyed by whomever inhabits the land after you. Many people also feel the need to experience the short- to medium-term benefits of labour and capital investment themselves, and will be reluctant to invest significant amounts of energy and money into land to which they might at any moment lose access. It is therefore a vital precondition to any successful land project that access is secure, whether it be through ownership or tenancy, private or collective.

As is all too often the case, it is the cost of property that is at the root of many people's problems in gaining secure access to land. Despite the downturn in agricultural fortunes in recent decades, land in the densely populated UK is expensive relative to neighbouring European countries, such as France where there is more land per head of population. The perceived attractions of rural life – quiet, crime-free, wholesome and healthy – combined with increased mobility and, more recently, the internet allowing more people to work from home, have resulted in rural property prices escalating well beyond the reach of those earning their living from the land. Estate agents quickly realised that there was a demand for houses with small amounts of land, and as farms have gone out of business and been sold, farmhouses have been parcelled up in small acreages to maximise their value, whilst the rest of the farmland has been sold off at agricultural prices. Unless you are fortunate enough to have access to large amounts of capital, a house with enough land from which to earn a living or even land with planning permission to build a residential building, is too expensive to buy outright. Increasing numbers of people are buying bare land holdings at agricultural land prices, hoping to gain residential planning permission in the future; but even these prices have risen sharply in recent years. This leaves the options of borrowing money, renting land or joining with others to share the costs of land purchase.

Borrowing money

Trying to run an economically viable land-based business is demanding, but not impossible. Having to earn enough to cover mortgage or loan repayments, or pay rent to retain your right to the land and any buildings, adds an extra degree of pressure. Some producers stated categorically that they would not have attempted to set up their project had they had to borrow money to buy their property. Others have gone down the mortgage route, but have had to retain a significant outside income to supplement their land-based livelihood in covering repayments. As far as I know, only two of the farms had taken out loans to buy their property. One project had borrowed money from an ethical investment bank, while the other had arranged loans directly with a series of private investors, many of whom were friends and family, by issuing loan stock when they needed to raise money to purchase their land.

Loan stock is a system which enables housing co-operatives to borrow money from people outside the co-op, thus helping them raise finance. The term was coined by Catalyst Collective, an organisation that advises and helps to register newly forming co-operatives, to enable co-operatives to advertise publicly that they are seeking financial support.[5] The system involves people lending money to the co-op for a set period, usually five years, as a fixed-term loan. The co-op pays interest to the investor ('loan stock' holder) either directly at the end of each year or in the form of an extra loan-stock certificate which covers the interest. At the end of the set period the investor is paid back in full. When issuing loan stock, an opening and a closing date are advertised, and investors are invited to send a cheque for the sum they wish to invest between these two dates and in return are issued with a certificate stating the terms of their loan and its interest. Loan stock is a valuable way of formalising loans from friends, family and associates who want to support a particular co-operative project. It makes administration of the loans easier by standardising timescales of repayment, interest and paperwork.

Renting land

If borrowing money to buy land doesn't appeal, renting land is another option, although not one chosen by any of the projects I visited. I didn't question interviewees about why they had chosen to buy rather than rent, but I can imagine the following reasons might have applied. Firstly, like a mortgage or loan repayment, paying rent to secure the right to use land is a significant regular financial commitment and, for fledgling enterprises, creates additional pressure at a time when outgoings are usually greater than income. In conventional agricultural economics, to demonstrate financial viability 'rent' is supposed to be included in any calculation of business expenditure, whether the enterprise is a tenant or an owner occupier. However, few small-scale producers adhere to this practice. This is because they tend to view sustainable stewardship of their land, and providing fresh, good-quality food to local people, as more important than applying an accounting convention that would condemn their business as non-viable.

The other unattractive aspect of renting land, rather than owning it, is that the effort you put into improving it (adding organic matter to the soil, building infrastructure, planting trees) will not be rewarded if you have to leave the land. That is not to say that what one person sees as improvements will necessarily be reflected in the selling price if land is owned, but at least there is an opportunity to benefit from your financial and labour investments in the land if you sell it. All that having been said, I have heard of instances where tenants have been offered first refusal to buy land when the landlord wanted to sell up. They have been offered affordable terms of purchase and even the chance to pay for the land in labour (for example by planting a hedge for the vendor). Renting land might just put you in the right place at the right time, by demonstrating to the seller how well you will care for their land and make it work.

On the other hand, renting land from an existing farm and offering to produce a complementary product create benefits for both the landlord and the tenant. For example, a meat or dairy farmer might be willing to rent land to a vegetable grower, who could use manure from the animals and provide vegetables to sell alongside meat or milk in a farm shop or on a farmer's market stall. Likewise, a poultry business on an existing cereal farm, or a pig enterprise alongside a cheese-making operation, enables a two-way flow of useful products – grain for feed in return for manure, or the utilisation of a 'waste' product, whey, for fattening pigs. Integrated, mixed farms make economic and ecological sense, but to manage the land and market the products of all the different elements of a mixed farm are too much for a single person, especially if they are trying to minimise machinery use. The traditional buildings present on many farms, considered too small for modern machinery, are ideal for small-scale packing and processing of vegetables, cheeses and other hand-made products. Where they have not yet been converted into luxury homes or holiday cottages, a farmer might be keen to rent them for a function closer to that for which they were designed.

From a business perspective, renting rather than buying land could also be a wise move if you have a limited amount of capital available. It is generally considered wise not to spend more than a half of your capital on land anyway, due to the many other investment costs that are incurred in establishing a smallholding, farm or forestry project. This principle can be taken one step further by renting, which transfers the cost of the land from being a capital cost to a running cost, and liberates capital to be spent on developing the business. Being able to invest in good-quality tools, netting, to protect crops, and irrigation equipment could make the difference between an enterprise which struggles and one which quickly becomes profitable and is sustainable in terms of human energy.

Community Land Trusts

In the current economic climate, once land has been purchased, it is likely to increase in value, especially if residential planning permission has been acquired. One option for creating permanently affordable access to land and housing is the establishment of a Community Land Trust (CLT). The CLT movement originated in the United States, to address the issue of lack of affordable housing and to protect small farms from subdivision by developers in north-eastern states.[6,7] Community Land Trusts are a legal mechanism devised to enable the democratic ownership of land by the local community, represented by three complementary sets of stakeholders – leaseholders on the land, representatives of the wider community and professionals (conscious architects, finance experts, builders). The land is initially purchased by or gifted to a Community Land Trust, which will hold it in perpetuity. Houses on the land are sold to individual home-owners, who lease the underlying land from the CLT, but are able to sell their homes when they want to move on. Alternatively, the housing stock might be owned and managed by a separate housing co-operative. The idea is that land is taken out of the market and separated from its productive use, so that the impact of land appreciation is removed, therefore enabling long-term affordability and sustainable development.[8]

The application of the CLT model to agricultural projects is still in its early days in the UK, with the most noteworthy examples of successful rural CLTs being the Scottish community buyouts of Gigha, South Uist and the Amhuinnsuidhe estate.[9] In 2006, Fordhall Farm in Shropshire was saved from development when 8,000 members of the public bought shares of £50 each in a CLT which would own the organic farm. Thus, Charlotte and Ben Hollins, the latest of several generations of tenants, have secured the land in community ownership. They are now tenants of the Fordhall Farm Community Land Initiative, an Industrial and Provident Society with charitable status. They live in the farmhouse, manage the land, its livestock and wildlife, run a farm shop to pay their rent and are developing Fordhall Farm to be an educational resource to build the connections between people, organic food and wildlife. Through disconnecting land from its market value and thereby maintaining its affordability, CLTs may offer new opportunities for community groups to access land and affordable housing.

Collective ownership

Buying property collectively is an approach that has been taken by others searching for ways to find affordable access to land. Whilst many of the issues surrounding living communally and working collectively have already been discussed, it is worth emphasising here the importance of clear communication about property ownership when it is being shared. One of the most common causes of conflict in communities is the question of land-ownership, and spending time at the beginning agreeing a legal structure that sets out members' rights to the land is a valuable way of investing in future communal harmony. When people know what is expected of them and feel that their contributions of both labour and money will secure them a fair stake in the land, they are more likely to be motivated to co-operate than if they don't trust the group and feel insecure about their place in the community.

Paradoxically, agreeing a 'get-out clause' for community members at an early stage in a group's formation can be a good way of making people feel secure and confident about a land-sharing arrangement. Although it might seem like a pessimistic thing to do when a new group is in its first flush of enthusiasm, knowing that there is an arrangement for fair distribution of resources if things go wrong can actually increase the chances of a group staying together. Without such 'worst case scenarios' having been considered, the fear of what might happen if the project folds can undermine trust and motivation.

I encountered a variety of communal land ownership models, which illustrate the strengths and weaknesses of different approaches. The land and buildings at the two oldest communities, Laurieston Hall and La Borie Noble, were owned outright and collectively by residents and exuded a sense of stability. Laurieston Hall is a housing co-operative, and residents pay a low rent, in addition to their work commitments, which gives them the right to accommodation, collective access to the land and a democratic role in decision-making. Several other communities are in the process of paying back long-term loans to private individuals who were major capital investors when the land was purchased (see Box 8.3 opposite). In this situation clear legal structures, good record-keeping and written agreements are the foundations to the transparency and trust necessary for communal harmony.

In my opinion, informal arrangements, especially where one person owns the land and allows other people to live on it for nothing or a very low rent, are a time-bomb waiting to go off. This is illustrated by the farm (house, outbuildings and land) where another community were living, which is still owned by the founder of the community, who was no longer a resident. For many years an informal arrangement existed whereby the residents paid a very low rent and had been left pretty much to their own devices. The landlord is now keen to sell the farm and at the time of my visit the community were going through a period of change, consolidation and debate about their future. The changes included the establishment of a housing co-operative to which community members had to pay a much higher rent, which covered the costs of maintaining the property more realistically (including its renewable energy system), as well as paying the landlord for the property in monthly instalments. The increase in rent had changed the nature of the community from being a relaxed place where people could live without pressure to earn much money to one where people were hard-pressed to meet their three-day per week communal work commitment and then earn enough to pay rent.

During my visit I encountered differing opinions about the changes. Some

Box 8.3 – A Tale of Two Communities

To demonstrate the value of formal procedures and clear communication it is informative to compare two communities where loans were being paid back to private investors. At one, a housing co-operative had been set up to own the land and buildings, and was the vehicle for repaying the landowner as well as for maintaining and developing the property. Residents pay a rent of £195 per month which gives them access to an equal stake in decision-making, collective ownership and management responsibility for the land and the right to accommodation in the main farmhouse, its outbuildings or a self-built low-impact dwelling. The culture of the community emphasises clear communication and, despite differences in individuals' aspirations, there seemed to be a high degree of trust and harmony. The quality of self-built dwellings is high, since, being owned by the housing co-operative, it is in the interests of the whole community to support individuals who are building their own homes by giving them practical help and time-off communal tasks while they are building.

In contrast, the informal arrangements and confusing legal set-up of another community are at the root of recurring conflict and a low level of trust. When it was bought, the property had been paid for by a combination of 'shareholders' who paid £3,000 each and one individual who invested enough capital to pay the balance. These people are tied together by an arrangement of trust, and the deeds of the land state that two individuals, the major shareholder and one other shareholder, hold the land on behalf of the trust. A limited company was set up some years ago to own the land when it has been bought from the major shareholder, and very slowly shares are being bought by the community, who each contribute £5 per week to a land fund. In addition, when new members join the community they buy shares from the major shareholder. For some people the arrangement works well, since they are able to live very cheaply, there is little pressure to repay the loan, and community members respect the decision-making process of the regular, minuted meetings. However, record-keeping about who holds shares is very slack and the lack of a formal legal structure leaves the community vulnerable to both internal power struggles and external attack should things to wrong (e.g. somebody tries to sue the community).

found the drive to earn money stressful and felt the community was losing its alternative edge (home education, vegetarianism, leading a simple, spiritual life), whilst others felt that the changes were necessary and reflected more realistically the cost of living in the community. One man said, "It feels a bit like animal farm. We've been dragged kicking and screaming into relating with the outside world and all the things we were trying to get away from." Others expressed profound worries about whether they would be able to stay on the farm and believed that the changes were necessary to secure their tenure. As one person said, "Sometimes it feels as though we're working backwards because it was set up by people who had different objectives. We're here with the land, accommodation, animals etc., yet we're still trying to get our structures, principles and core values sorted out. Its better to do your visioning before you start, so you know that everyone subscribes to your core values. Trying to do it now, in amongst everyone's work commitments, is like trying to push jelly uphill!"

For some people, however, there are a number of inherent weaknesses in collective ownership of land that no amount of communication and well-recorded agreements can overcome. Probably the most significant is that when you share land it is very difficult to gain a financial return on any improvements you might make to the land. This may not matter if you intend to stay in the community for the rest of your life. However, if you decide to leave for some reason, you may need capital to establish yourself in another situation, either to buy more land, for a deposit on a house or to set up a business. Some communities have provisions in place for giving people who are leaving a capital grant, as a form of 'golden handshake', to thank them for the work they have put in. However, young communities rarely have the resources to do this, especially if they themselves are still repaying loans to secure their land. Another weakness of communal land ownership is that parents are less able to pass on property to their children, who may well not want to live in the community.

These sentiments were expressed by several people I spoke to. A young man, who had grown up in a community and returned to live there with his young family didn't want to stay there longer than five more years, despite enjoying the lifestyle it offered him. "We want a bit of financial security. Many people will get parental inheritance. If I stay here I won't get a chance to provide that for my children. But it's hard because if we do move, our standard of living will drop. I don't really know what I want to do if I do move." A woman who had recently left a community with her husband and young family to establish a farm of their own, gave their reasons for doing so as, "We definitely wanted to build a house. We decided we wanted to own land so that work we did was there for our children (e.g. capital gain or ideally a farm)". She went on to state later in the interview, that "with communally owned land you don't benefit in the long run from work you've put into the land because you don't own it."

Some people attach less importance to personal ownership and inheritance, and view labour and capital investments as a gift to whatever land they may be living on at the time. However, whether or not individuals feel inclined to invest personal capital into long-term improvements of collectively owned land (for example, planting fruit trees or building a barn) usually relates closely to their sense of security about staying at the community and their trust in its long-term future. Living and together working harmoniously is a skill which will be considered in the next chapter.

Chapter Nine

Living and Working Together

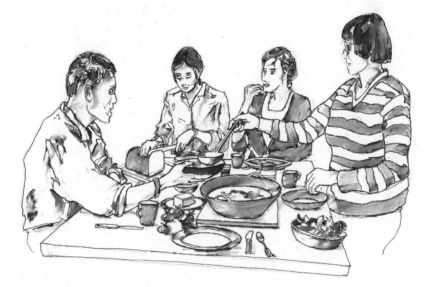

Living together

All aspects of life feed into the human-energy equation, and the details of community organisation are no exception. The nine communities that I visited varied greatly in size and the degree to which people shared their lives. Where people live, how often they eat together, how work is organised and which resources are shared are all variations on the theme of living and working collectively. In the rest of this chapter I will look at the following aspects of those communities:

- Physical infrastructure
- Eating patterns
- Servicing the community's needs
- Meetings
- Working together

Physical infrastructure

The most obvious difference between communities' infrastructure was whether their buildings pre-dated the establishment of the community, or the community had started from scratch on a bare land holding. Five possessed buildings at their inception, ranging from a large country house with outlying cottages at Laurieston Hall to Brithdir Mawr, where residents live in the farmhouse and converted outbuildings surrounding the farmyard. Tinker's Bubble, Steward Wood, La Sorga and Mulberry Tree Farm all started with bare land holdings and over the years have built, or are in the process of building, communal facilities and accommodation for individuals as well as renewable electricity and water supplies. Dwellings at these communities range from simple canvas-covered benders to timber, strawbale and cob buildings.

Inheriting buildings is a mixed blessing. The advantages are that the basic domestic infrastructure already exists, and it is possible to get on with the business of managing the land more quickly. The disadvantages are firstly, that the property is likely to be significantly more expensive and secondly, that the buildings are not tailor-made to meet the community's needs. The buildings may be in poor repair, ill-suited to communal living and difficult to heat efficiently. The skills and cost involved in restoring and maintaining such buildings can be a drain on community resources (both financial and labour) unless adequately planned for.

The advantage of a bare land plot is that you have a clean slate to design the infrastructure that best suits the community's needs, including energy-efficient buildings made from sustainable materials. The downside is that implementing those designs is time-consuming and requires a wide range of skills and financial resources. Above all, gaining planning permission to build on a bare land plot is very difficult and can involve a long and emotionally draining process of planning applications and appeals. It is with good reason that new developments in the open countryside must justify why they are necessary and that they are going to provide net benefits to the environment and local community. However, whilst there is a strong case for re-using old buildings rather than leaving them empty, if new developments are needed anyway, it is better that new developments have high-sustainability credentials. The environmental and visual impact of an ecological, land-based community is likely to be significantly lower than that of a conventional, energy-consuming housing estate of the kind that is spreading out all over Britain to meet projected housing needs.

For communities that start from scratch, money is usually in short supply and development is incremental, starting simply and becoming more elaborate with time, as skills develop. The advantage of such gradual development is that buildings and infrastructure are more likely to meet the exact

needs of the community, rather than being planned ahead to meet antici-
pated needs which may be different in reality. Conversely, the situation often
arises where a temporary and unsatisfactory structure, such as a kitchen or
guest accommodation, becomes permanent because it is functional and
other more urgent tasks mean that it takes a long time before the final
improved version is worked upon. More than once I witnessed frustration
due to the discomfort and inefficiency of using inadequate (dark, damp,
scruffy and hard to clean) facilities which had been erected to fulfil a temporary function and had become permanent due to lack of time to replace
them.

In all four 'built from scratch' communities, individuals or families live
in separate, self-built structures, but share facilities such as a kitchen, compost loos and bathing facilities. At Steward Wood, individual dwellings
also contain cooking facilities. At the communities that use pre-existing
buildings, residents typically live in flats in either the main house or outbuildings. The flats tend to have their own kitchens, whilst some share
bathrooms. Laurieston Hall offers a variety of accommodation, ranging
from self-contained cottages to bedrooms along a corridor, which share a
kitchen. In this sense they resemble ecovillages rather than communes,
since self-contained accommodation for families, couples and single people
mean that it is the work rather than the domestic sphere that brings people together.

Eating patterns

A Zimbabwean visitor to Tinker's Bubble once commented, "The reason
your community stays together is because you all eat out of one pot." I
would agree that sharing the cooking and eating of meals is one of the pleasures and practical advantages of communal life. Everyone has to eat, and
coming together for mealtimes creates a regular informal social gathering
where information can be exchanged, jokes shared and a sense of unity created. Some of my happiest times, both at my own and other communities
have been spent over food, around a fire or a kitchen table. It is a different
experience from a supper party, since there is greater equality between
those present and a sense of continuity, due to the frequency of being
together, which creates depth and substance to the conversations. Hence,
communal mealtimes feed one emotionally as well as physically, and can
be a time when energy is created through social interaction.

The disadvantage of eating communally on a regular basis is that an
intimate part of daily life is made public. This is more of an issue for families and couples than for single people, who benefit most from the companionship of communal meals. Parents in particular reported finding

mealtimes challenging, since their parenting skills are on display. I witnessed children playing up or refusing to eat the food that was available more often when in the company of other children than when they were at table with just their family. This created situations where parents needed to exert discipline, but felt they were being watched and possibly judged. For a seasoned community member, or in a supportive community, this need not be a problem, and the combined efforts of several adults can be helpful in teaching table manners. However, some parents prefer to eat at least some meals in the privacy of their own homes. Even for couples without children, regularly sharing a meal separately from the community is an important part of building and nurturing their relationship.

The frequency with which meals are shared varies among the communities, and is reflected by the degree to which kitchens are communal or private. At Tinker's Bubble and La Borie Noble a hot meal is shared daily. This is lunch at La Borie Noble, whilst breakfast and a communally prepared light supper are eaten in individuals' apartments. At Tinker's Bubble, residents help themselves to breakfast and lunch in the communal kitchen and an evening meal is prepared by different people in rotation.

At Laurieston Hall, no regular meals are eaten communally except during maintenance weeks, when residents and working visitors are all engaged in the same work. Throughout the summer, meals are prepared centrally for people attending courses, which some residents may choose to attend, especially if they are involved in hosting the course. However, most individuals and families eat separately in their own apartments or houses especially throughout the winter. A few, who live along the same corridor in the main house and share a kitchen, have a regular arrangement for sharing meals in smaller groups. Most of the residents at Brithdir Mawr have the facilities to cook meals in their own apartments, but choose to eat an evening meal together four times per week (Monday to Thursday) and cater for themselves at weekends. I liked this arrangement, which combined the best of both worlds and meant that at the end of a day's work people could look forward to a good meal in a convivial environment, whilst having more flexibility and privacy at week-ends.

Communal meals are eaten only once or twice per week at Steward Wood, a situation which has arisen partly as a result of the different diets (vegan, raw food, eggs and fish) and also because of eating times preferred by residents. At some places children are fed earlier, whilst at La Sorga an older woman prefers to eat earlier than her younger fellow residents and thus eats separately in her own house, but comes and joins the others when they eat later for the companionship.

As well as feeding people physically and emotionally, sharing meals is also an efficient way of organising time and fuel use. Rather than five or ten families/individuals cooking each day in their own homes, taking turns to cook for everyone means that for, say, six days out of seven people can get on with other jobs, knowing that a meal will have been cooked for them. When cooking less often, the incentive to cook something really good is greater than when cooking every day, and the diversity of different cooks means that the variety and quality of catering is usually quite high.

Servicing the community's needs

Living communally by definition entails some degree of sharing of the work that is necessary for daily survival. Cooking, washing up, cleaning, food production, infrastructure building and maintenance are all activities that are typically shared between adults and older children living in a community. Usually it is required that all residents spend a certain amount of time each week doing communal jobs, and table 9.1 shows the work commitments each community asks of its members.

Community	Number of communal work days per week	Work done together / at different times by individuals
Brockhurst	1 and cook one evening	Same days
Brithdir Mawr	3	When convenient
Tinker's Bubble	2 (inc. one domestic day/fortnight)	Same days
Laurieston Hall	2.5	When convenient
Steward Wood	1.5	Same days
Mulberry Tree Farm	1	Same days
La Borie Noble	5	
Keveral Farm	none (some paid work done for community by community members)	Same days -

Table 9.1 – Comparison of communal work commitments.

Communal work is sometimes performed as a group activity on the same day/s each week or workdays may be done separately, when it is convenient to individuals to get on with their particular communal jobs. Often when it is done together, one of the main purposes of workdays is to do large jobs that require many people, such as constructing a communal facility or doing something tedious like ragwort-pulling or dung-collecting, which benefits from many hands. Even if everyone is doing communal work on the same day, they may be scattered all over the site. For example, on a workday at Tinker's Bubble there might be four people working in the communal garden, three people on the sawmill, one person building the guest house, a couple repairing some steps and a person on domestic. I experienced a great sense of pleasure and solidarity from knowing that all over the site we were contributing to the goals of managing the land and its infrastructure and producing food.

The kind of work that is included as 'communal' varies. Cooking, washing up and firewood management for communal spaces are the most common communal tasks. At Laurieston Hall, every adult spends half a day per week (part of their workday allocation) on firewood duty with a group of others, either felling and cutting up timber, transporting it or splitting and stacking logs to fill woodsheds with logs which can be used by all community members for their personal use. At Brithdir Mawr firewood is carted up to the woodshed from outlying parts of the site on work days, but sawing and splitting for personal use is done by individuals in their own time.

Certain communal jobs will be taken on by people who have a special interest or aptitude for them. For example, milking goats or cows is best done by the same two or three people so as to give the animals continuity. It is also better for people who have the skills and are familiar with the procedures to process milk into cheese, yoghurt or butter. Communal vegetable gardens are often divided into sections with people taking responsibility for different crops or parts of the rotation. Skilled jobs, such as managing renewable-energy systems tend to be the responsibility of one or two individuals who have specialist knowledge.

At Brockhurst, child-care is also included as a communal responsibility, even though at the time of my visit only one couple had children. This meant that on work days, any community member, rather than just the parent, might entertain the children and this work would be considered just as valuable as milking a goat, mending a fence or cooking a meal.

Another area of shared responsibility at communities is administration and the hosting of visitors. Regular, time-consuming domestic jobs, like collecting money for food, rent and phone bills alongside dealing with outside agencies such as Companies House, site insurance companies and DEFRA are usually allocated to one or two members. Likewise, one person often takes on the role of responding to enquiries from potential visitors and hosting them when they arrive. Alternatively, different people may volunteer to 'sponsor' each visitor to spread the load, since hosting visitors on a daily basis can be disruptive of other work. Whichever way it is done, having a particular person allocated to ensure that visitors or WWOOFers are shown around and generally looked after is important, since at communities it is all too easy for everyone to think that someone else is doing the hosting.

Meetings

Any group of people who are trying to organise themselves to live or work together need to communicate formally as well as informally. Hence, meetings are an inevitable part of community life. The pattern of meetings will relate to the legal set-up of the community, with different levels of decisions being made either at full community meetings or delegated to specialist subgroups. The other distinction that can be made is between meetings for deciding on practical matters and those which are to facilitate emotional communication and harmonious relationships amongst community members.

Formal meetings are at the heart of any community, since these are where decisions are made that affect the lives of all residents. It is therefore well worth investing time and effort into ensuring that they are managed fairly and don't run on for too long. Whilst important decisions take time, people may become alienated if they are forced to sit through hours of discussion about a subject that they feel bears little relevance to them, or if they don't feel they are being listened to. Meetings are often the times when opposing personalities come face-to-face most directly, which is why some communities choose to focus on feelings and emotions either in separate meetings or as a regular part of business meetings (see Chapter Ten). Creating a space where feelings can be aired is a valuable tradition to establish from an early stage, since without it there is a greater likelihood that they will be regularly vented during general management meetings, distracting people from objective discussion of the issues on the agenda.

Community	Frequency	Subjects
La Borie Noble	Weekly	General community business
	Twice daily	Prayer and meditation
Brithdir Mawr	Weekly	Land-management work
	Irregular	Feelings meeting
Brockhurst	Weekly	Emotional sharing followed by housing co-op business
Keveral Farm	Monthly	Housing co-op business
Laurieston Hall	Weekly	Housing co-op business
Mulberry Tree Farm	Weekly	Land management and domestic
	Irregular	Feelings
Steward Wood	Monthly and weekly	General community business
	Irregular	Feelings meetings
La Sorga	Irregular but frequent	General community decisions
Tinker's Bubble	Monthly; fortnightly	Land and community management, specific work allocation

Table 9.2 – Comparison of meeting types and frequency at the nine communities.

All the communities stated that they operated as non-hierarchical groups and used the consensus process to make decisions, rather than relying on a voting system. Consensus decision-making aims to find solutions that everyone in the group can live with, rather than just the majority, in the belief that more effective, long-lasting decisions will be made. It is a process of finding common ground through dialogue between equals, and although it may take longer to arrive at agreement, the likelihood of the final decision being implemented is greater since all concerned will be committed to that outcome.

Whilst consensus decision-making may be the stated aim of a group, its true and effective practice is less common. Improperly used it can cause frustration, when people misuse the ultimate tools of blocking or vetoing a decision or feel that in reality their voice is still being sidelined. Correct use of the consensus decision-making process requires training, practice, time and patience and is best embarked upon when a group is in its early stages of formation. The eleven steps recommended by 'Seeds for Change', a small co-operative that offers training in consensus decision making (see Appendix 2: Resources section), are as follows:

1. The problem, or decision needing to be made, is defined and named. It helps to do this in a way that separates the problems/questions from personalities.

2. Brainstorm possible solutions. Write them all down, even the crazy ones. Keep the energy up for quick, top-of-the-head suggestions.

3. Create space for questions or clarification of the situation.

4. Discuss the options written down. Modify some, eliminate others, and develop a short list. Which are the favourites?

5. State the proposal or choice of proposals so that everyone is clear.

6. Discuss the pros and cons of each proposal – make sure everyone has a chance to contribute.

7. If there is a major objection return to step 6 (this is the time-consuming bit). Sometimes you may need to return to step 4.

8. If there are no major objections, state the decisions and test for agreement.

9   Acknowledge minor objections and incorporate friendly amendments.

10. Discuss.

11. Check for consensus.

It is often helpful, especially when a group is new to the consensus process, to have a facilitator to guide the group and keep them focused on the decision in hand. Whilst appearing straightforward on paper, the process of actually finding agreement through these steps can be difficult, due to differences of opinion. These are natural and to be expected. At the heart of the consensus process, which is dealt with in more depth in the publications of 'Seeds for Change', are a series of tools for exploring and incorporating varying opinions. There are also various 'levels' of disagreement which can be registered, leading to different responses from the group:

- *Non-Support:* "I don't see the need for this, but I'll go along with it."

- *Standing aside:* "I personally can't do this, but I won't stop others from doing it." The person standing aside is not responsible for the consequences. This should be recorded in the minutes.

- *Veto/major objection:* A single veto/major objection blocks the proposal from passing. If you have a major objection it means that you cannot live with the proposal if it passes. The group can either accept the veto or discuss the issue further and draw up new proposals. The veto is a powerful tool and should be used with caution. Some groups even avoid the position where someone can veto a decision, by putting an issue to the vote if consensus has not been reached after three meetings.

- *Agree to disagree:* The group decides that no agreement can be reached on this issue. This position can be alleviated with a variety of possible strategies.

- *Leaving the group:* If one person continually finds themselves at odds with the rest of the group it may be that this is not the right group for them. They may volunteer to leave themselves or the group may ask them to leave.

Other tools I encountered being used to help make meetings more effective included the publication of the agenda at least a day or two before the meeting; starting the meeting with a 'go-round' and the use of talking-sticks or facilitators. Publicising the agenda ahead of time gives residents the chance to prepare themselves for the meeting by thinking about issues and discussing them with other community members. This can save lengthy discussions occurring in the meeting that don't need to involve the whole community. A 'go-round' is the term used for giving each person at the meeting a brief chance to say something in the order of where they are sitting. This can be used to find out how each member of the community is feeling at the beginning or end of each meeting or to rapidly canvas opinion about a particular issue. A talking-stick, or any other object (ball, hat etc.), is a way of ensuring that only one person speaks at a time and is listened to by all the others. Only the person who is holding the talking-stick is permitted to talk, and those people who wish to speak must wait until the speaker has finished and then indicate their desire to be passed the talking-stick.

Working together

Earning a living from the land requires skill and hard work at the best of times, and when it is combined with the demands of living in a community it is not surprising that few of the community members I met were entirely dependent on land-based livelihoods.

As a result of sharing resources and the subsistence contribution of land-based community work, living costs at communities are generally lower than for a similar standard of life in mainstream society. It is usually necessary, however, for community members to have some income with which to pay for community expenses, such as rent, communal food and equipment, as well as to cover personal needs such as travel, clothes and entertainment. Table 9.3 shows a range of monthly financial contributions which members of some communities are expected to pay and the resources that this payment gives them access to. At the two income-sharing communities – La Borie Noble and Mulberry Tree Farm, all income is pooled in a communal pot. Whilst at La Borie Noble the only money paid to individual community members is when they have a specific need for something that cannot be provided by the community, at Mulberry Tree Farm each of the adults receives an equal weekly wage of £50 no matter what work they perform.

Community	Contribution per adult	Pays for
Brithdir Mawr	£200/month	Rent, electricity generation (food?)
Brockhurst	£195/month	Rent, building insurance
	£115/month	Food, wood, vehicle running costs
Laurieston Hall	£80/month	Rent, electricity, wood
Steward Wood	£132/month	Rent, food, car running costs
Tinker's Bubble	£92/month	Food, equipment, timber, insurance, loan repayment
La Sorga	At least one third of personal income or a minimum of £70/month	Food, equipment, bills and maintenance etc.

Table 9.3 – Comparison of financial contributions and what they cover.

At all the communities I witnessed a great diversity of income-generating activities. I was interested in the degree to which community members were economically dependent on the land, and whether these land-based enterprises were being run collectively or by private individuals. The relative level of each community's economic dependence on the land is shown in Figure 9.1 below, which reflects the number of residents earning a land-based livelihood and the proportion of their income derived from the land.

At La Borie Noble collective self-sufficiency is a primary aim. As an income sharing community incorporating all the basic food production activities (vegetables, fruit, dairy, bread) as well as skills such as joinery, pottery and textiles production, the 30 residents are able to survive on an annual income of £77,500, or £2,580 per person.

A high proportion of residents at Tinker's Bubble (50%), and Mulberry Tree Farm and Keveral Farm (75%), derive their income directly or indirectly from the land, compared with the other communities in the study. By indirectly, I mean either that they process produce into goods that also contain bought-in ingredients, or they use produce from the land in off-site activities (for example willow for sculptures, charcoal for blacksmith workshops). At Laurieston Hall and Brithdir Mawr, the land-based nature of commercial activity is also indirect. The central enterprise at Laurieston Hall is the People Centre, a workers' co-operative that hosts camps and courses run by outside organisations. A significant proportion of the food (vegetables, eggs and dairy produce) for the catering is produced on the land by community members, as is the wood which is used to heat the hall where visitors sleep. Other residents generate a livelihood through off-site employment (e.g. gardening in the village, nursing and youth work) or on-site self-employment (e.g. shiatsu treatments). Most people at Brithdir Mawr earn their livelihood from outside work or on-site grant-aided conservation work, while one couple run the heritage seed mail order business,

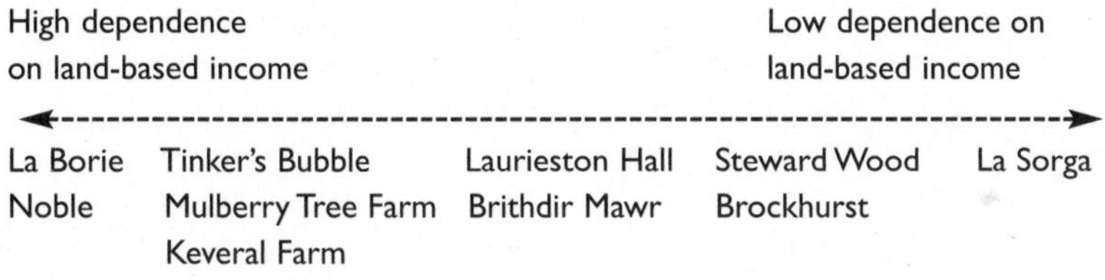

High dependence on land-based income

Low dependence on land-based income

◄--►

La Borie Noble	Tinker's Bubble	Laurieston Hall	Steward Wood	La Sorga
	Mulberry Tree Farm	Brithdir Mawr	Brockhurst	
	Keveral Farm			

Figure 9.1 – The spectrum of land-based economic dependence at communities.

'The Real Seed Catalogue', described in Chapter Eight on p.158 (Box 8.1). Land-based enterprise is less common at the remaining three communities. Steward Wood sells a small amount of hand-felled timber. They also host one or two 'Introduction to Permaculture' courses each year, which use the land-based infrastructure as a demonstration. During the spring prior to my visit two community members had completed a six-week forest school for local children, and were looking forward to further developing this aspect of their work. Educational work is the only land-based commercial activity at Brockhurst, where Tamsin, helped by her partner, grows willow which they use in rustic craft workshops for children at fairs and adults at 'special needs' learning centres. Both are involved in a local environmental education workers' co-op and have recently built a visitor centre, to enable groups to use the community's land for field trips.

Working collectively in groups, where responsibility for generating an income and managing the land sustainably is shared between individuals, is challenging. The main reasons that I have been able to identify for collective working being so difficult are:

- Decision-making involves finding consensus between multiple opinions and can be slow and inefficient.

- Mutual economic dependence relies on a high level of trust in fellow co-op members to pull their weight.

However, workers' co-ops can and do work and it is instructive to examine in some detail the varied examples of workers' co-ops that I discovered on my journey. Some were working well, whilst others had evolved towards looser forms of co-operation. The successful workers' co-ops included businesses run by two large, long-established communities, La Borie Noble and Laurieston Hall and one small, relatively new community, Mulberry Tree Farm. In contrast, the co-operative experiences at Tinker's Bubble and Keveral Farm provide useful insights into the difficulties of trying to generate a land-based income collectively.

Successful workers' co-operatives

La Borie Noble in south-west France has been running for almost 60 years and achieved a high degree of stability and skill at farming and various crafts. Whilst predominantly concerned with self-sufficiency, the sale of produce from a number of activities provides a modest shared income. Sourdough bread and cheese are sold to a neighbouring Buddhist community, whilst pottery, felt, hand-spun and woven garments and cards printed on the printing press are sold at a small on-site shop. In addition, the community earns some money from hosting annual retreats and camps for groups involved in promoting nonviolence. Key to its success and longevity is the commonly held philosophy of Gandhian truth, simplicity and nonviolence that binds the community and guides its members in their daily work. "We try to live a coherent unified life under the guidance of the one Spirit of Truth which animates our prayers, our work, our family life, our view of economics, education, authority, farming, medicine and even of national defence." [1] The adherence to truth means a high level of honesty, and therefore trust, exists between members, whilst emphasis is placed on finding agreement nonviolently when important decisions are made. Decisions about the running of particular aspects of the community, such as the farm, the garden, the bakery and the dairy, are delegated to the individuals whose responsibility it is to manage them. Other community members defer to them when working in that area. Such clear delineation of roles aids efficient decision-making, as well as reducing the potential for conflict when two people have different ideas about how something should be done.

Laurieston Hall, whilst not a religious community, has also achieved a noteworthy track record of stability for working co-operatively. Whilst the community used to share income, the People Centre now offers paid work opportunities to those community members who wish to work for it. Income from the People Centre, paid to the Laurieston Hall Housing Co-op, is significant and reliable, and makes a valuable contribution to keeping rents low for individual community members. A core group of six adults do the main administration and housekeeping for the centre, whilst other members of the community commit themselves to catering for or facilitating particular camps. As at La Borie Noble, the specific roles taken on by individuals in the People Centre mean that smaller decisions can be taken in sub-groups or unilaterally, increasing efficiency and reducing the risk of conflict. Systems have been established that enable the high standards of catering, cleanliness and organisation to be combined with a relaxed and welcoming atmosphere for visitors.

Many community members have lived at Laurieston Hall since its early days, so there has been time for a high level of trust and knowledge of each other's working patterns to develop. As one man told me, "The community feels rock solid. I worry about us rusting together rather than falling apart." This comment reflects an interesting strand of discontent that emerged in other interviews at Laurieston. The high standards, efficiency, and scale of the People Centre operation, whilst providing a reliable income for the community and a valued service to some organisations in Scotland, left little room for innovation and creativity among newer members of the community who felt bound by having to maintain the status quo. "The People Centre is like a big machine that swings into action. It has to happen and the (housing) co-op work gets left behind. Its hard graft

– can't stop once its started." There was a sense among a few members that the People Centre was running the community rather than the community running the People Centre, and younger members struggled to combine their work and community duties with child-care. Likewise, senior members of the community wondered how they would manage to sustain the intensity of work during the six-month summer visitor season as they grew older.

Mulberry Tree Farm is a much smaller and more recently established community than La Borie Noble and Laurieston, consisting of two families who have been living on their jointly owned land since 2003. The development of the community, however, started many years before this. Meetings to discuss a shared vision of a permaculture project began in 1997, and the group enlarged and shrank a couple of times before a core of five people, who had been working together regularly on gardening, eco-building and festival catering projects, started seriously searching for land. Their 15-acre holding was purchased in 2001 and three more years were spent commuting to the land from the families' existing homes for weekly communal workdays before they finally started to live there. As financial and time commitments of the project increased, one of the five decided to leave the group. The remaining four, who each had off-site professions, set about developing land-based enterprises that used their skills and complemented their other work. For example, Nick started coppicing the woodland and using its products (hazel poles and charcoal) in the green-wood furniture and blacksmith workshops at community festivals, as he had been doing for many years. The two women, Kath and Anna, started growing vegetables and within a year had established a small box scheme. Bill took on the management of the community's small flock of sheep. All four continued to integrate some degree of off-site work with their land-based enterprises.

For the first year of living on-site all four adults were self-employed, and transactions between different enterprises on and off-site were complicated and bureaucratic. To overcome this problem, they decided to establish an umbrella workers' co-op. The co-op is a company limited by shares and has the four community members as directors, as well as employing them all. Members continue to work at their previous activities, but rather than being paid independently, their varied wages go into a common pot which pays an equal weekly wage to each employee, which has been calculated according to what they need to cover living expenses. The new set-up means that tax calculations are simplified and transfers of produce from one enterprise to another no longer have to be recorded. Effectively, Mulberry Tree Farm has become an income-sharing community, with the higher wages of the main off-site worker subsidising the lower-paid but environmentally beneficial land-management activities.

Successful income-sharing is the ultimate manifestation of a functional community, because it reflects a situation of genuine co-operative working, with everyone pulling their weight and contributing towards the overall aims of the project. Mulberry Tree Farm illustrates how the essential pre-requisites of working together – trust, common vision and clearly delin-eated roles – have contributed to harmonious co-operation. Having worked closely for so many years before they moved to the land, the four of them knew well each other's styles of working and had developed a deep level of trust. Furthermore, the long process of discussions and gradual evolution of the group meant those that were left were all in agreement about the project's objectives and underlying philosophy, and therefore motivated to work towards achieving them. Finally, by enabling each person to continue focusing on work they enjoy and are skilled at, clear roles were established at the outset and one potential area of conflict (agreeing who does what) was eliminated.

The challenges of land-based co-operation

The story of the evolution of the workers' co-op at Keveral Farm demonstrates the importance of clearly delineated roles in sustaining goodwill and motivation. The residents at Keveral Farm started running a vegetable box scheme in 1997, with the help of a rural development grant, which committed the community to continuing the enterprise for at least four years. During that time eight people developed a business with an annual turnover of £70,000, supplying local people with up to 200 boxes per week. Since no one had experience of commercial growing, one couple, who had visited another box scheme, took the lead in building the business. It was, however, a workers' co-op where everyone worked the same hours in return for a wage of £50 per week.

For the first four years enthusiasm generated by the success of the project motivated people to work long hours (40-50 hours per week), despite low wages, but it reached a point where some people started to have families and wanted to earn more money, while others did not want to work so commercially. The scale of the box scheme reached a natural ceiling as limited growing space at Keveral meant the co-op needed more land and had to buy in bulk vegetables, such as carrots and potatoes, to provide enough for the boxes. They rented land on an organic farm two miles away, but found it hard having to travel several times a week to work on someone else's windswept land, while their own, smaller, plots were getting neglected. In the fifth and sixth years discontent grew as people felt frustrated that, however hard they worked, they couldn't earn enough to live.

The couple who had initiated the box scheme found themselves in the difficult position of being expected to take responsibility for co-op management tasks, but experiencing resentment when they asked others to do certain things. This situation was profoundly stressful for both of them and resulted in health problems that caused first one, then the other to withdraw from the co-op.

After that the co-operatively-run box scheme continued for three years, until one member asked if they could rent land and start their own horticultural business rather that continue to work for the co-op. Within a year the rest of the community had followed suit, and now all individuals rent their plots from the co-op and sell their produce individually. The box scheme continues, but is run by one community member who buys produce from co-op plot-holders as well as other local producers. Another resident has established an organic wholesale business supplying a large restaurant and sources produce from individual Keveral gardeners, other local growers and his own plot. Community members appreciate the fact that there is now a more direct relationship between the work they put into growing and the returns it brings, as well as enjoying the choice of markets and freedom to choose what to grow. While the co-op box scheme always struggled financially, the person growing for the restaurant is now making a reasonable income, as is the person running the box scheme, now that these are run as individual enterprises.

Some community members have scaled down to grow purely for subsistence, whilst others have started to diversify their crops and markets. One man is growing gourds which he carves into lanterns, musical instruments and bird boxes to sell at a nearby tourist attraction, and he and a fellow resident appreciate being able to put more time into their other enterprise, producing liquid plant-feed. Managing the plots individually has also allowed a flourishing of diverse growing techniques, ranging from hand-cultivation and mixed cropping to tractor cultivation of single crops. In the 'workers' co-op days' every decision was a commercial one and there was little individual choice about how to cultivate.

I had the opportunity to talk in detail with most members of the community about the transition from running the box scheme co-operatively to the current set-up, and all seemed much happier with the latter arrangement. Some people expressed sadness that they were no longer working so closely together, but on the whole people felt that the new system was fairer and had improved relationships between people in the community, as these comments reflect:

> "I think it's worked really well. I take responsibility for what I want to do and am happy with it. There's a lot less resentment. Before, different people were putting different amounts of energy in and it was breeding discontent."

"(Now) People have more control over their own time and money. You don't have to ask anyone else before you do something. But I think there were quite a lot of advantages with the old system. Now there's quite a lot of overlap and competition. It's better if you can work together."

"The personal freedom is an advantage. I've started working loads more because I can get back what I put in. It felt fair before, but not the same. You feel more responsible for plants, tools etc. Before, you were not responsible for the whole life of the plant. It was nice, that feeling of sharing on the communal workdays, but it feels much better now."

"There's less conflict now, but people working together does break down barriers. They communicate when they might not choose to. Now I can be free to experiment and be more inventive. I don't need to convince everyone else before I do something."

"People have a level of autonomy because they are responsible for their own business. If something goes wrong they have to sort it out."

"(Now) There's a lot less conflict and people get paid better. People are reaping the rewards of their own labour, whereas before it was just disappearing into a big pot. It's a bit sad that people are not working as closely as before, but there's nothing to stop people co-operating and some people already are."

Equally interesting were people's reflections on why the co-op had failed, since some seemed to believe that under different conditions they could have continued working more closely.

"We'd got ourselves into the bizarre mentality of having to do the same things, rather than recognising different people's skills."

"Different people have different standards and expectations. There was no common vision. The result was disunity and dissatisfaction because we weren't achieving a common aim. There were a lot of financial pressures from the outside world because we weren't earning enough to live on. Maybe we could have been more inventive. You need to be imaginative to earn a living from the land and when you're busy doing daily chores you don't have time to be creative."

I asked, "Under what circumstances could a group business work?", and received the following reply:

"If there are clearly defined roles and responsibilities. People need to be respected for the roles/skills they play. With that structure there's no reason why it couldn't work, but we'd gone too far down the other route."

This pattern of collective effort evolving into privatised activity was familiar to me, since a similar situation had occurred at Tinker's Bubble. For the first five or so years most work at Tinker's Bubble was necessarily collective, since before anyone could start to earn their living from the land there was a huge amount of infrastructure development required. Building the round house and communal kitchen, laying water-pipes, fence construction and creation of a barn, animal shelters and the cider house were all priorities and took a long time, since timber for building and fence posts had to be felled, extracted and sawn without fossil fuels. On top of this, gaining planning permission to live on site involved a five-year bureaucratic struggle and public relations effort to win favour with local people. Some individuals earned a living off-site and developed subsistence activities – growing vegetables, keeping pigs, milking goats, but the only commercial activity was selling apples and a few vegetables at a collective stall at Glastonbury farmers' market. As at Keveral, one or two individuals took the lead in building infrastructure and planning how to manage the land.

Gradually three potential group enterprises emerged, based on the main resources of the land – the softwood plantation, the orchards and the grassland. The arrival of a steam engine and saw bench provided a means to add value to Larch and Douglas Fir saw logs, felled by hand and extracted with a horse, and occasional commercial orders for timber started to be met by the community. Likewise, a manual apple crusher and cider press made it possible to process the large quantities of Bramley, Russet and Cox apples into apple juice. A cheese-making micro-enterprise began, as a way to store large volumes of milk when the community's Jersey cow had her first calf. Not using fossil fuels, all three enterprises were labour-intensive, but aimed to generate a modest hourly wage to pay those who chose to work at them, and thereby provide a financial return for managing the land. Each, by its nature was too much work to be undertaken by a single individual and required co-operation by a sub-group of the community.

After five years a couple of individuals erected polytunnels and started growing vegetables to sell at farmers' markets as a way of increasing their land-based income. A slow movement towards private enterprise was joined by others who had skills at green-woodworking and making herbal products. These activities differed from the group enterprises in that they were very intensive, requiring only small areas of land to generate a better return on effort. It was also possible to work on them independently, rather than having to make arrangements to work with other people and spend time agreeing how to proceed. Above all, when living closely in community, having greater control over one aspect of your livelihood was so attractive that people began to devote more time to their private activities than to the group enterprises. For those who were still focused on the forestry, apples and grassland management, the burden of working with too few people and the frustration of slow progress, resulting from not getting more help from other community members, began to take their toll, resulting in resentment and conflict.

The balance between the extensive group activities and the intensive private enterprises has continued to be difficult to achieve. Of the three extensive activities, the apple group has probably been most successful, managing to pay community members for time spent pruning, harvesting, pressing, bottling and marketing, out of the income generated from wholesale and direct marketing of juice and cooking apples. The cheese-making ceased to be commercial due to lack of facilities approved by environmental health inspectors, and a different milking regime means that only enough milk for the community's consumption is now produced. The forestry enterprise operates when enough people with the right skills are available to work at its various stages, but most sawn timber is used for communal buildings or is bought by people closely associated with the community.

As at Keveral, financial remuneration from working collectively seems to be hard to achieve, whilst the stress of both working hard for a very low wage and finding agreement with co-workers makes private enterprise significantly more attractive. Whilst the apple and forestry enterprises continue to operate seasonally or at a low level at Tinker's Bubble, it is the vegetable growing, processing of herbal products and green-wood working that are the main income generating activities for community members. It is interesting to observe how the patterns at Keveral and Tinker's Bubble reflect the failure of communist work models, as the inefficiencies and loss of motivation resulting from collectivism give way to private enterprise which directly rewards people for their work.

Earning a living from the land is challenging, as is working in a group, and when the two are combined the challenges can result in overwork, stress and conflict. It is not surprising that there are so few examples of land-based workers' co-operatives. Yet the examples that do exist provide valuable clues about how to establish workers' co-ops that could stand the test of time. Above all, the following prerequisites are a necessary starting point for any group wishing to work collectively:

- A high level of trust
- Deeply shared common vision/philosophy
- Clearly delineated roles

The preceding examples demonstrate how demanding on human energy working in groups is, yet also indicate that there are significant advantages in collective economic activity. This paradox begs the question, is there a way of combining the efficiency of co-operation with the freedom and control of working alone? Two possible solutions to this conundrum are eco-hamlets and community-supported agriculture.

Eco-hamlets – a sustainable way of living and working together

Eco-hamlets are geographically clustered smallholdings or farms, at which environmentally sustainable land management, livelihoods and lifestyles are a primary aim. They may be designed intentionally or may have evolved naturally, due to a particular locality offering individuals and families affordable opportunities to set up land-based projects. They tend to be smaller than eco-villages and occur in rural areas, with the occupations of inhabitants being at least partially land-related.

The main difference between eco-hamlets and intentional communities is in the pattern of land-holding. In eco-hamlets individuals or families privately own their holdings and dwellings, whereas in communities land and accommodation are common property by law, even though individuals may rent or borrow portions of the land for their own, exclusive use. Whilst such separate ownership of land facilitates individual entrepreneurship, the proximity of holdings leads to informal co-operation between neighbours and sometimes the establishment of business partnerships. For example, neighbours can look after one another's animals if a person needs to go away or help each other with tasks such as building or hay-making, and may also choose to market produce together through a joint market stall or farm shop. In short, eco-hamlets enable people to have control over their own land projects and businesses, whilst enjoying many of the social and practical benefits of community in its broader sense.

Three projects in this book could be described as eco-hamlets. The first is the Vallée de Mérens in the Pyrenees, where about 20 couples and families have colonised abandoned stone buildings and their surrounding land, and have developed independent smallholdings over the last 30 years. Each household is an independent entity, with its members supplementing land-based subsistence with varied income-generating activities, but strong social ties exist between households and the transfer of gifts, bartered goods and financial interactions link them together. Some households co-operate regularly at working on tasks that are too big for one person or couple to undertake alone, whereas others prefer to work alone.

Another eco-hamlet evolved out of a fragmented community. Brithdir Mawr was, until recently, joined with two neighbouring holdings in a farm comprising 170 acres. Differing aims and lifestyle choices had led to three 'hubs' developing in different parts of the farm. One woman wanted to live a very low-impact lifestyle without electricity and at a greater distance from mainstream society. She withdrew to a cluster of cob roundhouses at the edge of the woodland of Tir Yspadrel, where she grows vegetables, keeps chickens and goats and makes baskets. Tony Wrench and his partner Jane Faith, also built their renowned turf-roofed roundhouse in a more remote part of the farm, but choose to generate modest amounts of electricity to power lights, a computer and stereo with their own renewable energy system. Their roundhouse is deeply integrated in their two-acre permaculture plot, which enables them to be self-sufficient in fruit, vegetables and eggs, but they also work part-time off the land. The community of Brithdir Mawr, comprising ten adults and five children, is based at the farmyard and is closest to the entrance to the farm, reflecting its links with wider society where some of the community work, do business or send their children to school. Their lifestyles are more environmentally focused than most people in mainstream society but combine labour-saving modern appliances with renewable energy sources. They produce their own vegetables, eggs and goats' milk, share equipment and generate enough electricity with their wind-generator to run a washing-machine and electric chainsaw, as well as lights, a computer and stereos.

The split into three separate holdings has enabled different members of the community to live the level of 'green lifestyle' that they personally feel most comfortable with, removing previous tensions caused by conflicting priorities. Yet, being located next to each other, the three holdings interact regularly, both socially and economically. Tony and Jane buy goats' milk from Tir Yspadrel and use the internet connection up at the farmhouse to manage their website. People from all three holdings belong to a band which plays for circle dances, and one or two people from Brithdir Mawr have moved to Tir Yspadrel on retreat, when they have found that they too want to live a simpler lifestyle.

The third eco-hamlet is Fivepenny Farm, which is in fact two farms. It is owned and run by two couples who co-operate as partners for marketing their produce, sharing machinery and registering their land as organic. The couples bought the 43-acre holding together, but immediately divided between them to enable each couple to pursue their vision of how the land would be developed. However, from the outset they have co-operated closely to ensure that their enterprises complement one another rather than competing, collectively planning crops to supply their joint market stall. The set-up combines the benefits of mutual support without the frustrations and inefficiencies of collective decision-making about the minutiae of land management and livelihoods. In fact, the eco-hamlet comprises more than just the two holdings of Fivepenny Farm, since another case study in this survey, Briggs Farm, is just ten minutes walk up the road, and further along the valley is another smallholding. Tractor tools are shared between the farms, and Jyoti from Fivepenny Farm sells salad and eggs to Briggs Farm for distribution in the box scheme. Olly, the other grower at Fivepenny Farm, now cultivates seedlings to sell to Briggs Farm, and throughout the autumn smallholders in the valley gather at each other's holdings to make cider. This eco-hamlet has evolved naturally, as people in a local area with a common interest in farming, self-sufficiency and low-impact living have identified each other and developed networks of co-operation.

In his revised book on self-sufficiency, John Seymour advocates developing local networks, just like the one described above, to improve quality of life for people trying to live self-sufficiently. He says that, "The thing I have learnt is that it was a mistake to try and live like this alone. We have tried to do too much, have worked too hard, have forgotten what it is to sit and listen to music in the evening, or read something for pleasure or to engage for hours in amusing and interesting conversation."[2] He recommends setting up 'Self-Sufficiency Groups', to bring local self-supporters together initially for monthly social gatherings at a pub or each other's houses. As the group get to know and trust each other, skills and produce can be bartered and joint projects undertaken, gradually forging the group into a community which offers mutual practical and emotional support, as well as social gatherings where music, poetry readings, walks, meals and visits to interesting places can be enjoyed.

An alternative approach is intentionally to establish an eco-hamlet by buying a large piece of land and dividing it into smallholdings. This is the approach being taken by Lammas, an innovative project in south-west Wales. Eventually Lammas may consist of 20 five-acre holdings, held by agricultural leasehold, which are conditionally tied to requirements set out in the eco-hamlet's management plan. Residents will be committed to deriving at least 75% of their basic household needs (food, fuel, clothing, water and council tax) from the land, minimising car-use and building genuinely low-impact dwellings. The project has arisen in response to the opportunity created by a new planning policy in Pembrokeshire (Policy 52, Joint Unitary Development Plan for Pembrokeshire),[3] which allows low-impact development to occur where other development would not normally be allowed. The conditions include:

- The proposal will make a positive environmental, social and/or economic contribution with public benefit.

- All activities and structures on site must be low-impact in terms of the environment and use of resources.

- The proposal requires a countryside location and is tied directly to the land on which it is located, and involves agriculture, forestry or horticulture.

- The proposal will provide sufficient livelihood for and substantially meet the needs of residents on the site.

- In the event of the development involving members of more than one family, the proposal will be managed and controlled by a trust, co-operative or other similar mechanism in which the occupiers have an interest. (Appendix 4, Pembrokeshire County Council)

The eco-hamlet project will be managed by Lammas Low-Impact Initiatives Ltd, a co-operative registered under the Industrial and Provident Society Act, and a community 'Hub' building will provide a base for various employed staff who will contribute to the smooth running of the project. As well as acting as an administrative centre for the project, the Hub will also be a social centre for the community and contain shared facilities such as a shop and a part-time café. By establishing this eco-hamlet, Lammas aims to demonstrate a thriving example of low-impact development which can be used as an educational resource pointing the way to future sustainable rural developments. It will provide affordable opportunities for people to live and work on the land in close proximity to others, without the sometimes stifling intensity of communal living or co-operative working.

At present Lammas is in the planning stage, with nine households having been accepted to buy plot leases in the first phase. The selection process included applicants submitting comprehensive proposals showing their land-based livelihood strategies, plans for their low-impact dwellings and farm buildings, permaculture designs for how they would manage the land and an indication of what they proposed to contribute to both the Lammas community and the wider locality. The organisers of the project anticipate that, whilst households will run their own individual enterprises, including growing nuts and fruit, breeding milking ewes and offering horticultural therapy to people with learning difficulties, co-operative arrangements between the holdings will evolve as the project matures. It is, of course, too early to know whether this model will prove successful. However, in theory it answers the need for a compromise between working together and working alone.

Community-supported agriculture

A very different model of working the land with other people, which also combines the efficiency of autonomous decision-making with the practical and social support of collective endeavour, is community-supported agriculture (CSA). There are various different forms of CSA, but all involve a partnership between farmers and consumers, where the responsibilities and rewards of farming are shared.[4] The support offered to the farmer by the community can take the form of practical help, committing in advance to buying produce for the whole season by paying a subscription, or investing capital to secure ownership of the farm by the CSA. In return, farmers are accountable to the consumers, providing them with fresh, high-quality food and opportunities to influence the running of the CSA.

CSA is thought to have evolved simultaneously in Japan and Europe in the 1960s, as a consumer response to the rapid post-war industrialisation of food production. It was introduced to North America in 1985 and by 2000 there were estimated to be 1,000 CSAs in the United States. In the UK, CSA was introduced in the early 1990s at a time when farming incomes were starting to decline and public interest in organic produce and local food was increasing. Development of the British CSA movement was slow during the late 1990s, due to competition from supermarkets selling organic produce, but as the farming crisis deepened and a series of food scares (BSE, salmonella, *E. coli* and foot-and-mouth disease) focused consumer attention on how their food is produced, CSA has become a tool for farm diversification and community development.

The classic form of CSA is the subscription vegetable box scheme, for which consumers pay at the beginning of the season, helping to cover the costs of seeds and equipment, and providing a guaranteed return for the work of producing the boxes. Unlike commercial box schemes, the quantity of produce may vary according to what is seasonally available and the success and failure of crops, and members are warned to expect times of scarcity which will be balanced by times of plenty. In this way, the risks (poor weather, pest attack, poor germination) inherent in farming are shared with the consumers, as are the rewards (bountiful harvests and job satisfaction). Other forms of CSA include customers paying for their produce by a monthly standing order, 'renting a tree' from a pick-your-own fruit farm, or buying a share in a pig rearing co-operative. The amount of customer involvement varies from a simple financial commitment, to joining in with weeding on monthly members' work days or taking part in a regular pig-feeding rota. Another model involves people becoming members of a community co-operative which actually owns the farm. Co-op members buy a share, which does not entitle them to produce from the farm, but gives them a vote and an opportunity to influence the co-operative's activities by participating in the management committee. A CSA may either be initiated by the farmer or by the consumers, who might either approach an existing farmer and ask him to produce food for them or rent land and employ a farmer to grow the produce. One feature of CSA schemes is the organisation of community events for members, often combining work with a social gathering such as a harvest supper or barn dance.

From a human-energy perspective, CSA has both advantages and disadvantages. Having followed its development through the 1990s, I was aware of a couple of schemes which had failed due to insufficient support from the community, resulting in the people running the CSA becoming burnt out and disillusioned. Whilst in theory, having practical help from customers could ease the workload significantly, the help sometimes fails to materialise, volunteers usually need close supervision which can be time-consuming and administration can be complicated by the need to communicate with members and allow them a say in the running of the farm. However, it seems that in recent years some models of CSA have overcome these problems, and provide vibrant, thriving examples of how groups can work together to produce food for large numbers of local people. Two projects that came to my attention in particular are EarthShare in Nairnshire and Stroud Community Agriculture in Gloucestershire. Although unable to visit them, I contacted a representative from each and sent my interview questionnaire to the farmers to find out how they fared in terms of human energy.

EarthShare CSA is a small, not-for-profit company run on co-operative principles that provides fruit and vegetable boxes for 175 local families all year round. It was established in 1994 and grows produce on 16 acres of their 23-acre farm in north-east Scotland. Subscribers sign up for a year at a time and are encouraged to part-pay for their box by working on the farm. These work contributions are organised in terms of work-shifts, to which subscribers just turn up to help. Vegetable work-shifts take place on Wednesdays and Saturdays, and CSA members can help with soft fruit picking on Thursdays and Fridays. Members are expected to do at least three work-shifts per subscription year, and in return receive a discount on their annual subscription. Over three-quarters of subscribers choose this option rather than paying the full rate for their box. The scheme employs two farmers full-time, plus another person who works three days per week with harvesting and box-packing and some extra casual help during the spring and summer when the workload is heavy. One of the farmers owns a team of draught-horses, Tommy and Morgan, and uses them for hoeing, ridging and some cultivation. Three tractors, one of which is run on LPG, perform much of the rest of the cultivation and weed-control in combination with hand weeding, thinning and harvesting.

Stroud Community Agriculture (SCA) started in 2001 when people in the local community took on the rental of a 23-acre biodynamic farm within one mile of the town of Stroud, in south-west England. The business is owned and controlled by its subscribers, who elect a core group of eight members to make management decisions, and employ two part-time farmers as well as some seasonal labour. The scheme has 175 member families, who pay an annual membership fee of £24 (£12 concession) and then £35 per month to pay for their share of vegetables. Of this, £10 contributes to the farm rent and wages for the farmers and £20 to pay for the actual produce, including staples such as potatoes that are bought in during poor seasons to supplement the farm's own vegetables. Subscribers are also encouraged to help out with farm work on monthly farm days, and a limited number of people have a written agreement with the farm to do a certain number of hours of work in return for their vegetable share. Vegetables are collected weekly by subscribers, who may have to pick part of their share, directed by noticeboards in the vegetable patch announcing what quantity to take of each item. Members also have the option of joining 'Hog Hands', a subgroup of SCA, in which they raise pigs for their own consumption. To receive half a pig (25kg meat) they pay £150 in either one or two instalments and commit to a pig-feeding rota, which entails feeding pigs daily for three weeks spread over a four-month period. At present most of the weeding and all of the harvesting is done by hand, with the farm's diesel tractor and contractors being used for cultivation and heavier work.

The most significant difference between EarthShare and Stroud Community Agriculture is that whilst the former is a company supported by its consumers, the latter is actually owned and run by its subscribers, being an Industrial and Provident Society Community Co-op. This means that every member has a vote, and should the organisation wish to raise capital, they could ask members to invest and become a profit-sharing organisation. Whilst in both cases the farmers who do the actual growing are employed rather than being self-employed, the management process for Stroud Community Agriculture is shared by the core group.

I was interested to find out how decision-making was split between the core group and the farmers, who have the technical knowledge and are doing the day-to-day work. I asked whether having so many people involved creates an unbearably complicated system of administration and accountability. It transpires that the farmers are free to farm in the way they think best, following an agreed strategy and reporting progress to the core group as they go. They attend the monthly core group meetings, which last 2-3 hours, where broad farm-work priorities are agreed and lists of administration jobs are agreed and shared between members of the committee to undertake between meetings. Although participation in the core group entails voluntary administration work (10 and 20 hours per month spread between six to eight members) on top of monthly meetings and helping on the farm, in the five years that SCA has been operating there have always been enough members willing to stand for election. There is a rolling system, whereby one third of the group are replaced each year, and nobody stays on the core group for more than four years. Wider participation in the decision-making process is facilitated by the quarterly planning meeting to which all subscribers are invited.

It appears that SCA generates a great deal of administration work (membership management, book-keeping etc.). The farmers end up by doing about 20 hours administrative work per month, much of which is on top of their paid work. This is in addition to the jobs which are shared between the core group members. Whilst the farmer who answered my questions appreciated sharing responsibility for the farm administration, compared with private enterprise, he said, "The decision-making process is much more involved and drawn out, involving lots of meetings and e-mails and differing opinions. We have the occasional clash (who doesn't), but we have always managed to make our decisions by consensus."

I was keen to find the answers to three main questions, the answers to which can be seen on Table 9.4 overleaf (p.200):

- In reality, how good are subscribers at contributing to farm work? Do they come forward readily to do their share or do they need a lot of chasing-up? Is the community really supportive, or does their involvement entail extra work?

- What is the farmers' experience of working for the CSAs and do they consider it sustainable in terms of human energy?

- What advice would you offer to others setting up a CSA?

One feature which characterises CSA schemes is the social events which build the connection between subscribers and the land. Working together on work-shifts and on farm days provides one valued form of social interaction for subscribers, but the schemes also organise specific events to celebrate various seasonal milestones, as described in Chapter Twelve, 'Siestas and Fiestas', p.270.

	EarthShare	**Stroud Community Agriculture**
1.	A small, hard-core group always rally when help is needed. Other people need quite a few reminders before they come to the field. Good weather helps! The involvement of subscribers affects the morale of the farmers hugely. When they come in the right numbers and at the right time, hoeing, thinning, fruit- and potato-harvesting are efficient and fun. Otherwise it's a struggle.	The number of subscribers coming to monthly farm days can vary between two and 20. Three or four members come most weeks to help for an hour or two. There is no shortage of labour, with about 5-10% of the work being done voluntarily
2.	Very positive. Whilst long hours are worked at certain times, contributing to occasional overwhelming tiredness, this is compensated for by shorter hours and more time off during winter. Farmer feels healthier and keen to continue working for Earth Share in the long term. He recommends CSA as, *"being really an answer to providing local food, treating farmers fairly and involving consumers."* He appreciates the shared work-load, flexibility and social/cultural aspects of the community support.	*"It gives me a good balance between working on my own, working with a team and working very socially with members and volunteers."* The variety of work, shared responsibility and social contact are cited as particular advantages to the CSA set-up. In mid-summer and on picking days the intensity of the work can become overwhelming, but, *"there are times, like September, when the work eases and I can enjoy the fruits of our labours. I have no plans to stop working like this and my health is good, although I'm a bit stiffer in my joints since working here."*
3.	*"I would suggest pricing the vegetables a bit higher at the outset. Sometimes it is a bit worrying wondering whether we will have enough subscribers to be viable."*	*"We started small and gradually expanded, which was great. If you have to start big then it would require much more fore-thought, planning and financing beforehand."*

Table 9.4 – A comparison of the experiences of two farmers working for CSA schemes, based on the questions outlined on p.199.

Chapter Ten

Together or Alone?

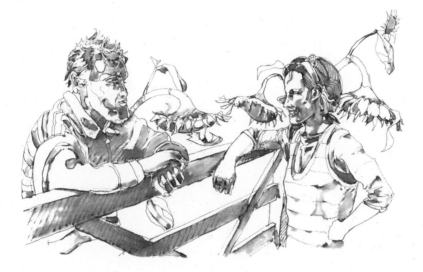

The choice of whether to live on and work the land with other people or remain independent may be straightforward for some people, but for others it is a difficult conundrum. The arguments on either side are fairly well matched and it is not uncommon to be pulled in two directions at once. Experiencing this dilemma first-hand was one of my motivations for undertaking this research, since I was keen to discover how people in different social set-ups were managing to sustain their human energy. Hence a central question in my interviews was: "What would you say are the main advantages and disadvantages of your social set-up compared with a family farm/community/cluster of smallholdings?". Responses to this question ranged from the social and practical implications of living and working collectively or independently, to more philosophical issues.

When contrasting the experience of living and working alone, in a family or as part of a community, a theme that crops up regularly is the simultaneous advantages and disadvantages of details of everyday life which make choosing between collective and more individual modes of life so difficult. Towards the end of the chapter I will address the issue of paradox, the tension between two seemingly mutually exclusive truths, which can lead to creative solutions as well as perplexing dilemmas.

The social experience

The most obvious difference between farming as an individual or family, and being part of a land-based community is the social situation. The former, especially as a single person, has the potential to be isolating, since home and work are the same place and social interactions depend either on visitors or employees coming to the farm or trips off-site. In contrast, at a community, you have a ready-made social life, being constantly surrounded by other people who can provide companionship and practical support. However, living in such close proximity can give rise to time-consuming social interactions and potential conflict. For single people and family farmers, the local community is usually an important source of social contact and support; whereas, the self-contained social nature of living in a community can potentially cut people off from the wider community.

The isolation of working alone is one of the main causes of stress and depression amongst conventional farmers, especially now that traditional meeting-places like livestock auctions are being replaced by marketing via supermarket contracts or big companies.[1] Forms of direct marketing, such as farmers' markets, farm shops and box schemes go some way towards re-creating social contact for individuals and family farmers, and are highly valued for this role. A few years ago, while researching the reasons why farmers choose to sell at farmers' markets, I found that the contact with the public and other stall-holders was a significant motivating factor for farmers continuing to attend, even though in the early days farmers' markets were not particularly profitable for some producers. Several of the smallholders I interviewed also mentioned their marketing system being a key link with the local community.

Since all of the single/family farmers in my sample were practising some form of direct marketing, isolation was not so much of an issue as it is for mainstream farmers. However, two single men cited loneliness and not having the strength of a support network as disadvantages of their set-ups. A woman, who had been happy to be living and working alone for the first six years of her project, admitted to me that during the past winter she had felt lonely and wished there were others with whom she could eat and socialise in the evenings. Although frustrated by the time absorbed by the part-time child-minding she needed to do to supplement her income from the land, she also recognised the importance of the regular social contact it gave her.

The long hours entailed in market gardening and other land-based activities mean that at the end of the day there is little time or energy left for going out. For family farmers and single people, this in itself can lead to a degree of isolation:

> "I get fed up not going to parties much on Saturday nights because I work on a Sunday."

"I do resent the tiredness – not having the energy to do cycling. We get nasty with each other and turn down invitations, when the other thinks we ought to be partying."

Another disadvantage of family farming is the pressure that it puts on a relationship. One woman, who had previously lived in a community, said:

"I felt I got more personal space in my relationship (in the community) because there were other people to work with besides each other, which takes the pressure off having to work with my husband. The children also had other adults to talk with, which took the pressure off."

On the whole, families and single people seemed to be well integrated with the local community, so could call on neighbours for practical support and had regular contact with friends for emotional support. WWOOF volunteers provide company as well as labour and were cited as a source of companionship by two of the single farmers.

For community members, the benefits of having other people around included companionship, emotional support and practical help. Sharing meals on a regular basis, or simply having people who share your ethos living nearby, reduces the need to travel to find companionship. Living in a community can thus significantly cut car use when compared with the needs of a single rural person desiring any semblance of a social life. A couple of community members also mentioned opportunities for enjoyment created by living in a community, ranging from spontaneous music sessions to large parties.

It's not just adults who benefit from the companionship brought by communal life. Children seem to thrive on the stimulation provided by other adults and the easy access to playmates when there are other children in the community. A charming book written by members of Old Hall Community in Suffolk to celebrate their twenty-fifth anniversary includes vivid accounts of growing up within a community:[2]

"One of the best things about growing up in a community is the amount of contact that a child gets with people from outside of the conventional family set-up. There is continuous contact and interaction with people of all ages and nationalities. This can lead to hugely enriching experiences, and many unusual friendships, not to mention the number of spontaneous multi-national football matches. It can also lead to even the most timid of children growing up to have an inner confidence, and an ability to communicate with a wide variety of people in all kinds of different surroundings."

"At the age of fourteen . . . I was living the life of an adult as we are all so eager to do at that age and with that I took on almost full responsibility for myself and my life. Often I would spend time in my space, usually with my best "friends who were all around me. This in itself was fantastic as there was no need for a phone call or any sort of journey. To get hold of my mates it was simply a case of going downstairs."

"There's a big garden and you just go to someone's unit to see if they're in, instead of planning to see each other in advance."

The book about Old Hall illustrates repeatedly how children who grow up in communities benefit from freedom and spontaneity. Compare this with the experience of children growing up in nuclear families in rural areas of Britain, who are dependent on their parents for lifts for many years, unless they are fortunate enough to have a good bus service. If parents are preoccupied with earning a living from the land, they are less likely to have time to drive their children around socially on a daily basis. There is evidence to show that children's emotional development is affected positively by growing up in an extended family or community.[3] The social engagement resulting from being surrounded by other women, men and children, as well as the parents, siblings and grandparents, enables children to develop their full human potential and become better able to empathise. Hildur Jackson, a pioneer of the co-housing movement in Denmark, notes the play opportunities, role models and freedoms available to co-housed children and compares them with the TV and electronic games-focused experiences of modern children, whose lives are circumscribed by traffic and other perceived and real dangers.[4] Growing up in a community thus brings significant social benefits, as well as reducing the carbon emissions brought about by endless ferrying of children around the countryside to see their friends. That is not to say that community children are cut off from the opportunities offered by the wider community, and many of those I encountered took part in local clubs, such as life-saving and football.

Communal living brings valued practical and emotional support. This ranges from a general appreciation of having like-minded people to talk to nearby, to an awareness of specific situations which are made easier by living communally. Some of the advantages cited were:

"They (the community) can be a safety net – if you're really stuck there is someone to help. (There are) more people to talk to – I think that's more natural, tribe-like – women talk to women and men talk to men."

"If you get back after a long day, there is someone to cook dinner. Someone nearby to pop round and chat to when you're having a bad day. Not even to chat to – just to be involved in their life for a bit."

"Shared strength in facing challenges – planning, grief from neighbours etc."

"When anyone has anything wrong with them, for example a hysterectomy, everyone rallies, takes meals to them, does their washing etc."

"Being in a community you have an intentional relationship with your neighbours – you have a commitment."

It seems a sad reflection on modern society that many of the functions mentioned above, in the past would have been carried out as a matter of course within the wider, local community – in rural areas, the village or hamlet. In some instances this still happens, perhaps more so among traditional rural people than people who have moved into the area more recently. Necessity causes people to reach out to their neighbours for help, and such incidents will occur more frequently for families and individuals who don't have the support of an intentional community.

I was made acutely aware of this recently when I heard that the Shire horse at my old community had fallen down and become stuck. It took six people and a lot of determination to get him onto his feet again. I found myself wondering how I would have coped with this situation were I on a smallholding on my own. I'd have had to depend on the good will of my neighbours to help me, which brought me to a greater understanding of the term 'social capital', a term which emerged in the early 1990s. It refers to the 'stock' of social relationships, built up over time, that enable productive interaction. In my case, the deeds I might have done to build goodwill amongst my neighbours would increase their willingness to help me in turn. Prior to this episode I had been aware of the concept in a theoretical way from the writings of Jules Pretty. In *The Living Land*, he identifies four aspects of social capital – trust, rules and sanctions, reciprocity and connectedness. "Diffuse reciprocity refers to a continuous relationship of exchange that at any given time is unrequited, but over time is repaid and balanced." [5]

The building and maintenance of social capital is vital for the success of an intentional community, but is of no less importance to families or individuals farming in the wider community. Intentional communities will also benefit from the conscious building of relationships with neighbouring farmers, both to gain acceptance in the wider community and as insurance for those times when help is needed. Residents at Laurieston Hall spoke of the help they received in the early days, when bemused neighbouring farmers lent machinery and gave advice to the novice farmers of the community. Thirty years later, the local farmers respect the community's determination to continue traditional methods of land management.

It was the residents of Laurieston Hall who readily pointed out the drawbacks of too much communality. From 1972 until the mid-1980s residents pooled their incomes and always ate together in one large, shared kitchen. With the advent of the housing co-op in 1987, people started to live in smaller units – singly, as families or in small communal households. This means that longstanding Lauriestonians have a good perspective for comparing different types of community life:

"Laurieston is less intense than a commune. When forced to live together and eat together it is much more difficult. Burn-out is more common. Being with people is tiring. I still find that in the summer [when they host courses]. [Now] it's like living in a village."

"There are a lot of pressures in a commune. It's stressful for everyone when sexual relationships change."

"Being in an income-sharing community is really hard. Being in a group is tiring. We're more like a village. This is a good compromise."

Many of these comments rang true with my experience of living in a community. I love the social aspect, the sense of belonging and the emotional support you gain from people who you see daily over breakfast and around the land. However, that close involvement can also limit the amount of time and energy you have for other activities, such as earning a livelihood and keeping in touch with friends and family outside the community. Any worthwhile relationship needs time and care invested in it and in a community it is possible to feel pulled in multiple directions by the demands of different people. My feelings were accurately reflected by the remarks of other community-dwelling women:

"You need to be self-disciplined. You can spend a day and feel you don't have much to show for it because you have spent so much time being considerate to others. It's just the 'peopleness' and the time it takes. I regret that I've not done more and get frustrated. You can't predict if you will walk into things that will delay you. I think people are a drain. They definitely are. They're both a drain and a support."

"A disadvantage of communal living is being answerable to others and time shortage. Dealing with other people's stuff. It's hard enough being a family, but when you've got four children and six adults it gets very complicated."

"One of the pleasures I gain from living in a community is knowing there are people around, though not actually interacting directly with them." This same woman cited, as a problem experienced in day-to-day life, "avoiding pointless conversations with people, ones that just waste time."

"I struggle with the number of things I want to do and the number of things I end up doing. To do the things that are good for me – maybe to achieve a certain amount of work. I like talking, but it doesn't get the work done. Clearing two days for a job can be difficult because of other jobs and social things. We have a lot of meetings. The lifestyle is very involving – time-wise, headspace-wise. It's not as easy as living in a flat and having a job."

These quotes illustrate that there is a tension between the valued emotional and practical support members gain from the community and the demands that these same interactions place on an individual's time and energy. Different personalities handle this tension in a variety of ways. Some people are able to balance the input necessary to maintain good relationships within the community with reserving enough of their time and energy to achieve in other areas of their lives. Others tend to get drawn into communal affairs at the expense of their own projects or personal emotional needs. And some people invest the minimum effort into communal activities and then wonder why they gain so little satisfaction from community life.

The deep-seated desire to feel 'part of something' was evident in several interviews:

"I've got a home with my tribal friends."

"We're social creatures, so that's what we yearn for. But because of individualistic society we're shackled and stopped from following what our souls yearn for."

"Being just a family can be lonely. We'd feel more comfortable as an ecovillage with people dotted around the land."

That sense of belonging can be a powerful source of energy. However, it can also be gained from belonging to the wider community. Many of the families and individuals I spoke to gained a similar sense of belonging from their village, local network of friends or extended family. It seems that the main social advantage of a community over a family or single person living alone is the geographic proximity to the people who can give emotional support, reducing the need to travel in rural areas.

The pros and cons of sharing

Four of those I interviewed had chosen to live in communities due to a philosophical belief in the idea of collective rather than private ownership. Another cited, "the joy of being able to share with people" as an advantage of living communally, and bemoaned the trend towards privatisation where he lived. Other people viewed sharing one or more of the items listed in box 10.1 (see right) as a benefit of communal life.

However, whilst mainly seen as positive, sharing can also be a source of frustration

Box 10.1 – Aspects shared within community life

- Cars
- Child-care
- Domestic duties
- Ethos
- Infrastructure
- Living costs
- Meals
- Responsibility
- Skills
- Tools and equipment
- Workload

and inefficiency. This theme of the ideals of sharing going hand-in-hand with an attitude of disillusionment echoes the experiences of the communards studied by Pepper in his book *Communes and the Green Vision*. Whilst sharing resources for greater efficiency was the most frequently cited eco-centric practice, at several communities collective resources such as cars, bicycles and tools were victims of the 'no-one owns, no-one cares' syndrome and suffered from a lack of maintenance.[6]

Pooling resources

The sharing of material resources, such as infrastructure, tools and equipment, is commonly viewed as being environmentally beneficial, since it results in more efficient use of primary resources. The materials and embodied energy used in making equipment such as washing-machines or cars mean that the more people who benefit from using them (up to an optimum level) the greater the benefit per unit cost to the Earth of using those resources. However, with the in-built obsolescence of many modern appliances, this theory only holds up to a certain point. If too many people use it, or the appliance is used too frequently, it might wear out more quickly and therefore need replacing more often. Sharing resources also has the potential to significantly reduce costs. Sharing cars, washing-machines, renewable-energy equipment and tools were all mentioned as being preferable to the duplication of resources that occurs in mainstream society.

It is not just the cost of buying and running equipment and tools that is reduced by sharing. Overheads, such as food bills, insurance and telephone line rental, spread between a greater number of people make for cheaper living. Three people mentioned that bulk buying of food made it easier to afford better quality, healthier food than if they were living alone. The largest shared resource of all is of course the land or property where the community lives. A number of people acknowledged that living communally gave them access to land, housing or a way of life that they would otherwise be unable to afford.

However, sharing things, especially tools, has a downside when they are not maintained properly or put back in their right place. One community member saw such problems as symptoms of a malfunctioning community and said, "When a community is functioning well no one with a lack of respect for communal stuff would be allowed to stay." Among the problems experienced in day-to-day life, issues that came up included:

"Tools not being in the right place, and deteriorating because they are not properly stored."

"Looking for things!"

"Someone else having the tool I want and not having replaced it."

As well as sometimes not receiving the maintenance they need, sharing cars also has the disadvantage of a reduction in flexibility, since the car has to be booked ahead and it is difficult to go away for more than a day at a time.

Shared responsibility

Many people recognised that sharing responsibilities such as land management, child-care and domestic chores enhance their quality of life. In some instances it gives people opportunities to live in a way they wouldn't have the skills or confidence to do alone. From the physical workload of managing land to the stress of trying to gain planning permission, sharing the burden on collective shoulders is seen as a definite advantage.

Whilst farming is not known for its compatibility with going away on holiday, being able to get away from time to time is vital for the long-term sustainability of human energy. Knowing there are people who have the knowledge and reliability to stand in for you if you need to go away, for example to care for an elderly parent or simply for an occasional relaxing break, can relieve stress. As such, sharing responsibility for tasks such as animal care, even if it is just intermittent feeding or relief milking, is a major advantage of community life. This is illustrated by a family farmer, who said:

> "In a community there is more flexibility about being able to get away and travel. On a bad day we can feel a bit trapped."

When asked to compare their social set-up with a more communal set-up, some single people and family farmers expressed regrets that they didn't have a wider range of skilled people to call on for help On a day-to-day basis, having other people around who can be called on to help is very useful, as is the pool of skills usually present amongst those living in a community:

> "There's a depth of experience and knowledge that is invaluable. Equally the wide range of skills and tools, the collective imagination vastly exceeds that of a family. That doesn't mean, of course, that it's the best ideas that get done." (community member)

> "Skills-sharing, blame-sharing, responsibility-sharing. They [the community] can be a safety net – if you're really stuck there is someone there to help." (community member)

> "Other people's energies – Stan's organisational and administrative skills, Rob's get up and go – different qualities that people bring. James is very good at putting emotions/thoughts into words." (community member)

> "Sometimes it is difficult finding people to help with heavy, physical things (lifting chicken-house, stacking logs, cutting grass). I have to wait for someone to come. I've developed patience because ultimately help will come. If I do the big

jobs, I'll use my energy up and won't have enough energy to pick the salad order. My fantasy is to sit down with others and allocate priorities." (single woman)

On the other hand, shared responsibility creates the risk of what one community resident described as 'social loafing', the idea that if you don't do a particular job someone else will, resulting in nobody doing it. This phenomenon will be familiar not only in intentional communities, but to people who work with others in any situation and can lead to endless frustration.

Community dwellers also appreciated the sharing of domestic duties such as cooking, cleaning, firewood and child-care. One man, who was in general very disillusioned with community life, still said, "There are utilitarian advantages to communal life – you can have a central fire that often stays going." Another person stated that she liked the fact that they used wood to heat space and water and that she would find this harder to do if she lived in a nuclear family situation.

Sharing child-care was seen as a big advantage. While at most communities shared child-care was an informal ad hoc arrangement, at a couple of communities sharing child-care is communal duty at which both parents and non-parents take turns on certain days (see Chapter Eleven, p.233).

On balance, it seems that the advantages of sharing resources outweigh the disadvantages, so long as it is recognised that a certain level of privacy is required by individuals and families. The close physical proximity of an intentional community makes such sharing easier, although the clustering of smallholdings or an eco-village set-up would also make the sharing of renewable energy infrastructure, expensive equipment or large animals (a draught-horse or a dairy cow) a possibility. Only one of the family farms mentioned experience of machinery-sharing with another local family:

> "We did try to link with another couple to share machinery, but it didn't work out. Each of us had their own agenda and there were flashpoints, such as haymaking. In UK society, each has their own little units and own things. It takes a lot to break down barriers. It's a bit daft not to share equipment that doesn't get used a lot, but it takes a lot of organisation."

Independence versus interdependence

"No man is an island, entire of itself." – John Donne, 1624.

As John Donne expresses eloquently, however individual we may feel we are, we are also highly interdependent, not only with those closest to us but with members of the human race as a whole. Joanna Macy, in her book *World as Lover, World as Self*, goes a step further, demonstrating the deep interconnectedness of each being with the rest of the world:

"The way we define and delimit the self is arbitrary. We can place it between our ears and have it looking out from our eyes, or we can widen it to include the air that we breathe, or, at other moments, we can cast its boundaries farther to include the oxygen-giving trees and plankton, our external lungs, and beyond them the web of life in which they are sustained."[7]

Whilst on a spiritual level, developing consciousness of our unity with the world is profoundly helpful as a motivation to live in greater ecological harmony, on a practical level there are barriers to be overcome on a daily basis. The society that most people in the Western environmental movement have grown up in is one that promotes individualism and for many it is a struggle to accept and embrace our interdependence with others. We therefore arrive at another apparent conflict of needs – the needs for independence and interdependence – expressed passionately by many of the people I encountered during my travels.

The related themes of control and freedom cropped up frequently during interviews. Control over time-use and standards of workmanship, and the freedom to choose how the land is managed were both valued highly. Self-employment was prized for the independence it gave from the constraints of employment. There was also, however, widespread acknowledgement of the benefits of interdependence with other people for practical, social and emotional purposes. It would seem at first as though independence and interdependence are opposing values, but it became apparent as I delved deeper into the subject that both are important and need to be balanced in order to achieve contentment.

A further, complicating factor is the issue of hierarchy. Compared with a conventional workplace, the communities I visited had no formal hierarchies, but it is natural that hierarchies arise, based on age, experience, skill and motivation. The presence of such hierarchies sometimes comes as a shock to new community members, who are attracted to alternative organisations by the ideal of equality amongst members. Yet it can be frustrating for senior or more-skilled members of a community to watch old mistakes being repeated by those who lack experience. Within groups that are trying to operate as a single unit, a balance must be found between willingness to accept advice from those with more experience and openness to fresh ideas from newer members. Where a group has the maturity to achieve such a balance, an informal and naturally developed hierarchy can provide a positive framework of social order. It is when hierarchy becomes a vehicle for power struggles that it can undermine and demotivate people.

Interdependence is a feature which characterises community life, whilst those who live and work alone or on family farms have relatively greater independence. Each brings its own advantages and disadvantages, and the bulk of this section will be based on a discussion of Table 10.1 below, which compares the experiences of people living in interdependent and independent situations. I should add here, that I do not mean to imply that communal life and individual life are completely analogous with interdependence and independence. People living and working alone or in couples are highly likely to have interdependent relationships with their wider community, friends or family, whilst individuals in communities are free to act independently to a greater or lesser degree.

	Interdependence	Independence
Pros	More people to do things Shared skills Shared responsibility Emotional support Sense of belonging Mutual aid	Control over time and land management Quick decision-making/less meetings Flexibility Personal/private space Diversity of work
Cons	Loss of independence and autonomy Long-winded decision-making Different ways of doing things/different standards Conflict 'Shoulds', guilt and resentment Letting people down Inequality of people pulling their weight	Necessary to 'buy in' skills and labour Very long working hours Stress/pressure shouldered alone Loneliness/isolation Risk of becoming a control freak

Table 10.1 – Comparison of the experience of community and more independent set-ups from the perspective of independence versus interdependence.

The interdependence of community life brings both practical and emotional advantages. On a practical level, there are more people to do the work and a greater variety of skills from which to draw. The converse of this is that for people managing the land independently there are fewer hands available, meaning that longer hours have to be worked to achieve the same amount, or labour and skills must be brought in. Several people working independently alluded to a desire to have others to help them, when asked about the disadvantages of their situation:

> "We haven't got enough arms! Manpower and skills-sharing. Someone who could help with the kids. I would ultimately like to be part of a community, but I don't think I'm cut out for it."

"The main disadvantage of our situation was the amount of work, work, work. If other people were around we could have delegated."

In reality, the relationship between the number of people available to do the work and the amount of work done is never as simple as a direct correlation between the two. Whilst one communard stated that, "I think you get more done in groups", this depends upon whether the group is in agreement about what needs to be done. My observations from visiting both community and individual/family land-based projects are that more work gets done per person in the latter. One reason for this is that it is easier to make decisions alone or in a couple, and therefore get on and do the work, whereas in a group decision-making can be a lengthy and sometimes interminable process. This was a point picked up by both community and non-community members:

"Less meetings. Ease of making decisions, getting things moving." (Couple)

"We don't have to talk about things all the time, we just get on with it." (Two couples)

"You lack the restraint of stasis from not being able to agree on something, although sometimes that happens between us as just a couple." (Family)

"You can get on with it. To be able to make decisions and act on them without co-ordinating, co-operating. You save time not having to discuss. There aren't many other advantages, but that's a big one." (Single person)

"Decisions take a long time to be made – because of consensus. Things can take longer to do in a group because of discussions." (Community member).

Decision-making takes longer in community because more opinions have to be taken into account. This reflects another challenging, but ultimately enriching feature of interdependent living – difference. All individuals are different, but those differences are brought into sharp focus when your lives are intimately entwined. Issues ranging from the mundane to the ideological were cited as areas of difference which caused tension amongst groups of interdependent people, and included:

"Other people's messiness, because I'm a very tidy person. Everyone has a different definition of tidiness."

"It's difficult living with people who are not on the same wavelength, e.g. watching TV, buying new clothes. We have different values. I worry about bringing up children here because there are only two other kids and one goes to school. I'd like to be a home-educating parent. Rick watches TV and I don't want my children to. There are two cultures at Brockhurst – I want my kids to be outdoor children, but fear they'd be indoor children if they wanted to be with the other kids in the community."

"I'd love it if we could provide all our own firewood from the woodland. We have a resource need and manpower, but I would like us to fulfil that need directly, rather than earning money and buying wood. It's very easy to find a way of earning lots of cash (as a therapist) and cheap to buy firewood, whereas its much harder to do it all yourself and its hard to resist these pressures inside a community."

"Control and accountability over what you produce. There's enormous variation in people's standards of what's OK and what is not. I would always be worried that by doing it in a community that one person's pulling harder than the others, that someone's understanding of the situation isn't clear and tensions arise. Even within our marriage we have different ways of doing things that we can't agree on. So we have our own roles. Tim does the cultivation and choosing varieties, I do the harvesting, quality control and marketing."

Trying to forge the opinions of a diverse group into a functional agreement is one of the greatest challenges to communal life, likened by some to 'herding cats'! How the disadvantage of difference is turned into a positive catalyst for personal growth is the subject of the next section.

Several people valued the general emotional support they gained from living communally, while people living alone stated that they missed the support network provided by a community. Those who had had opposition to their project, both from locals and planning officials, were particularly appreciative of the emotional benefits of being part of a group.

The emotional and practical support gained from interdependence has a cost, in that it requires you to be available to give help and support. Whilst this is entirely fair and reasonable, and in line with the concept of social capital outlined earlier, the intensity of demands on your time in an intentional community can make it difficult at times to pursue your own objectives. Above and beyond the formal work requirements of any community there is a grey area of willingness to help or 'be a good community member'. For a conscientious community member, this can be a cause of stress and ultimately exhaustion if you are continuously wondering "am I doing enough?" or regularly work overtime to ensure that your 'goodwill' balance sheet stays positive. Conversely, communities are renowned for including people less willing to carry their weight, causing resentment and ill-feeling, a feature mentioned repeatedly. The destructive emotion of resentment must be constantly guarded against when living communally, for as one interviewee stated, "If you feel resentment towards other people, all they do is take your dreams away."

Most people fall somewhere in between, teetering along the 'guilt-resentment' tightrope, as one member of Old Hall community in Suffolk describes:

"When I'm doing less than my whack (e.g. in deep winter), I find it hard to avoid feelings of guilt (brought up to do my duty, you see) and when I'm work-ing hard, especially on something necessary but unpleasant or boring, I find it hard not to be resentful of those who aren't and don't. And yet I must – because guilt and resentment are both corrosive. To live happily here you have to jump off this particular tightrope into the safety net of your own internal settlement. For me this goes something like 'I want the community to work well so I'll do what I hope everyone will do.'"[8]

Turning to the benefits of independence, control over land- and time-man-agement head the list. Living and working on the land alone or with a part-ner in a self-employed situation was seen as bringing greater freedom and flexibility. Reasons given for choosing their particular lifestyle included:

"I like being in charge of my own schedule and having flexibility and diversity in what I do." (ex-community member)

"Having worked for other people, which I found frustrating at times, I wanted to work for myself. We're in control of how we run our day." (ex-community member)

"Being in control of our lives more – control of physical environment. For a long time into the future we'll be managing these fields." (ex-community member)

"I'm experiencing a degree of freedom I've never known before."

This feeling of empowerment was not exclusive to people living singly or in families. When compared with mainstream life, involving being employed by someone else and being tied to paying rent or a mortgage, several people considered community life to be liberating. Often it had given them a sense of independence and control over their lives that they had lacked in their previous situations.

However, others said they felt they had lost a degree of control over their lives by choosing to live more interdependently. Disadvantages of community life included:

"Loss of autonomy. Looking at a piece of land and deciding what to do with it. You can't do that at Brockhurst."

"Not being free to make your own choices all the time."

"I find the loss of independence and autonomy difficult."

Another feature of living and working independently that several people appreciated, was the personal and private space that it gave them. Many people need to have somewhere to which they can withdraw and be protected from the challenges of difference which enter into every aspect of community life, especially in domestic life. The following contrasting quotes illustrate the difference between the independent and the interdependent living environment:

> "I'm a bit of a matriarch. I like to have my own home, to welcome people into it and then be able to say goodbye."

> "Laurieston used to be an income-sharing community. All those who did that are the ones who live outside the main house. That says something. It's difficult having to negotiate every aspect of your life. Its good that this place now has all sorts of living arrangements. Now regular meal-swapping goes on between kitchens, which creates links between people without the pressure of living together."

The security and opportunities provided by the interdependent nature of community have the potential to enhance quality of life. People who would not feel able to embark on a land-based lifestyle alone become empowered in a group to gain access to land and contribute to its management. Many of the community members said that living in the community provided them with opportunities such as running a smallholding, building their own eco-house and combining child-care with some form of meaningful work. For people wanting to provide for their own subsistence needs from the land communities are ideal, since a larger number of people can undertake a wider variety of tasks, such as fruit- and vegetable-growing, milking, cheese-making, preserving. However, a high degree of interdependence is less attractive to those aiming at commercial production.

A handful of the projects had managed to achieve a healthy balance between independence and interdependence. These included a family farm, where the children of the original farmers had been motivated to move back to the village where they grew up because of the support of the extended family. The two daughters and their husbands were raising their own families whilst managing to run successful agricultural businesses, since they were able to help each other and rely on the grandparents to help with child-care on a regular basis due to living a few minutes walk from each other. However, one daughter and her husband owned land and managed their business completely separately from the parents and the other couple managed a well-defined part of the main farm and were able to make day-to-day decisions without referring to the parents. The other place which stands out is Vallée de Mérens in the Pyrenees, where three generations are managing their own smallholdings and co-operating with each other when it suits them. As one of the original settlers said:

> "The hippies who came to live here came from different cultures/schools of thought and had to learn to live on the land again, so it's better that they did

this in separate households to avoid arguments. Then the children, who have grown up this way and learnt the skills, can work more closely together. Already three couples work together once per week on a large project to help each other out."

Personal development

Living in a community is a fast track to personal development, but the experience can be very tiring. The theme of personal growth resulting from dealing daily with the differences between fellow community members came up repeatedly in the interviews. Whilst there is the ever-present danger of coming into conflict with fellow community members, most people saw the challenges this presented as an opportunity to improve themselves and their ways of relating to other people:

> "A community stretches you on a personal level to deal with getting on with everyone. You have to make a big effort – have to face up to it. This is true in theory, but things can rumble along for years because it's too dangerous to rock the boat – too close proximity."

> "Dealing with other people's stuff. It's hard enough being a family, but when you've got four other children and six adults it gets very complicated."

> "Living in a community has helped with the journey of 'growing up' and becoming an easier person to live with. It has been hard, but done in a very supportive and loving community has really helped."

> "I get a lot from our talking circles – learning about myself, communication skills, all the challenges."

> "It's [living in a community] like living in a house full of mirrors – sometimes they're like funny mirrors at the funfair."

The last quote raises another feature of community life, that of being brought face to face with the realities of one's own limitations when they are reflected back in the irritating aspects of another person with whom you are in daily contact. Certainly I have found that living in a community has stretched me to reflect on my own weaknesses and strengths and has helped me become more assertive, less afraid of conflict and better at communicating.

Diana Leafe Christian calls this the 'rock-polisher effect':

> "The close and frequent interactions with other community members about how we live and work together," she says, "tend to evoke some of our worst and most destructive behaviours. And potentially it can heal them. In forming community groups and communities our rough edges are often brought up and then worn smoother by frequent contact with everyone else's. But the rock-polisher effect

can be so painful that it ejects people right out of the group, or the group becomes so fraught with conflict that it breaks up. Through good community process we can make the rock-polisher effect more conscious."[9]

While conscious personal growth is by and large a positive by-product of living communally, there is a danger that the effort required to sustain this growth and maintain harmony can detract from the other objectives of the group. Whilst all of the communities I visited were producing some food and fuel from the land, the actual proportion of their basic needs and incomes derived from the land varied considerably. My impression was that there seemed to be a negative correlation between the level of importance placed on personal development work and the proportion of livelihood that was being generated on the land. In other words, it seemed that the energy cost of maintaining a harmonious community detracts from the objective of achieving a land-based livelihood. On the other hand, ongoing resentment, conflict and bad relationships significantly reduce quality of life in a community and drag everyone down, not just the people specifically involved. Neglecting the emotional well-being of the community can be just as detrimental to the overall aims of deriving a livelihood from the land, as becoming too introspective. The all-too-elusive aim must be to find a balance between personal growth and outward action.

In contrast to community dwellers, those who are working the land alone or in families are able to invest a great deal more of their energy into their land-based projects because they didn't have to spend so much time servicing their relationships with other people. Of course, even in a couple or a family it is important for energy to be invested in sustaining relationships. However, living in a community can be like being married to several people at once.

Some communities have specific mechanisms for aiding clear communication and harmonious relationships. Feelings meetings or talking circles were a technique used by several groups as a way of intentionally creating a space to focus on emotional issues. At Steward Wood, a Talking Circle takes place at least every month and I got the impression that there was a deep sense of communication and harmony as a result. A Talking Circle involves members of the community passing a talking-stick around the circle, with whoever is holding the stick being able to talk about how they are feeling without being interrupted. Early rounds may provoke a fairly superficial level of communication, but as the stick continues to circulate and members respond to others a deep level of communication about emotional issues is achieved. One of the benefits of the Talking Circle is that it makes people listen more carefully because you are only able to speak when it is your turn to hold the stick. On the whole, I was told, people always finish the talking circle feeling better than they did when they started. One person described it as an "upwards spiral of emotion".

At Brockhurst, personal growth and clear communication have been a high priority since the beginning, with the four founders all being therapists and therefore deeply interested in emotional development. Over the ten years the group has developed a system of communication based on openness, honesty and careful use of language. The aim is for people to share how they are feeling, so that others can be understanding and supportive, rather than making assumptions because someone is behaving in a particular way. Often it is enough for the group simply to hear a person say "This is how I'm feeling", without needing to respond by doing anything.

A formal forum for communication has been built into the community's weekly general meetings, which begin with a 'go-round' in which each person can say how they are feeling. Community members feel that this 'checking in' process helps to deal with any emotional issues before starting on business matters, resulting in deeper communication for the rest of the meeting due to the improved understanding of each other's needs. I wondered whether such an approach led to extremely long meetings, due to the length of time it takes to address emotional issues, and was told that it is only once every couple of months that an issue arises that significantly lengthens the meeting. It appears that by regularly attending to the emotional health of the group a backlog of issues, which would take months if not years to deal with, is avoided, making for efficient and effective communication about issues when they do arise.

Two skills that are considered important in achieving communal harmony at Brockhurst are reflection and listening. Reflection, or thinking about what has been said, is a vital part of the communication process in that it helps people to consider issues from other people's points of view and thereby come to a better understanding. However, beneficial reflection relies on having accurately heard what other people are saying, which involves a process of active listening.

Listening is a skill taken for granted by most people, yet it was not until I took part in an exercise on 'Active Listening' on a permaculture design course that I understood the degree of effort required to really listen to another person. Arranged in pairs, one person had to speak for five minutes while the other person listened, and then that person had to reflect back what they had heard. All too often in group situations, while one person is speaking, others are thinking about what they are going to say next, rather than listening, leading to repetition of points and misunderstandings which may result in conflict. As one interviewee stated, "People are always making uncommunicated assumptions, which mean they don't understand each other."

The communication culture at Brockhurst bears many similarities to the system of Non-Violent Communication (NVC) devised by Marshal B.

Rosenburg, and outlined in his book *Non-Violent Communication: A Language of Life.*[10] In this book he teaches practical skills for enabling people to communicate about difficult subjects in a non-threatening and compassionate way. The technique is based on the idea that we naturally enjoy giving and receiving compassionately, but culturally learned, 'life-alienating forms of communication', such as making moralistic judgements or demands, block our ability to communicate from the heart. If instead we consciously observe and listen to the feelings, needs and requests in what the other person is saying, and demonstrate that we have heard and empathised, we are more likely to open up and enhance communication channels, leading to heartfelt understanding and better relationships.

"The overall purpose of communication is – or should be – reconciliation. It should ultimately serve to lower or remove the walls and barriers of misunderstanding that unduly separate us as human beings from one another." [11] It is the transcending of these barriers of difference that makes community life such hard work, but ultimately a process of personal growth and spiritual deepening. The theme of difference persistently reappears in any study of social dynamics, and is important in understanding how to live in harmony with other people. Difference, otherwise seen as diversity, is in fact key to the concept of sustainability. For, in the same way that biodiversity in ecosystems leads to stability by creating a wider range of evolutionary opportunities so diversity of skills, personalities and experience enables social groups (be they small communities or nation states) to respond more flexibly to change.

In his book *A Different Drum*, Scott Peck identifies a four-stage process of community building, through which any group must pass in order to become a true community.[12] The communities he speaks of are not restricted to the live-in or local communities that are the subject of this book, but extend from interest groups meeting weekly for some common purpose other than community building, to people attending a single intensive weekend course for the sole purpose of creating a community.

The four stages which Scott Peck describes are: Pseudo community, Chaos, Emptiness and Community. Pseudo community is the first response of a group trying to create community, in which they are extremely pleasant with one another and avoid all disagreement. A group moves into the chaos stage when differences start to emerge and members misguidedly attempt to heal and convert, in order to gloss over uncomfortable diversity. Underlying these attempts is not so much the motive of love, but the desire to make everyone 'normal', and the chaos stage is characterised by conflict as members fight over whose norm might prevail. It is only by emptying themselves of barriers to communication that a group can move from chaos to community. These barriers may include expectations, prejudices, differences in ideology and the need to heal, convert or control, most of which boil down to a self-centred desire to obliterate the differences between members of the group.

Emptiness is the most painful of the four stages, since it involves the 'letting-go' of beliefs, which in some cases define the individual. Emptiness can seem like a kind of death, and group members often seem paralysed between fear and hope because they incorrectly equate emptiness with 'nothingness' or annihilation. However, emptiness is necessary for rebirth into true community. The final stage, and in some cases end goal, is community. True community as described by Scott Peck is an experience of great joy, beauty and healing in which members of the group become able to communicate with each other on a deeper level.[13] He likens it to falling in love and notes that at the highest moments of community formation a supernatural feeling of ecstatic energy can be released. Forged into such a community, a group is better able to go on and achieve its collective goals.

The letting-go of the barriers to communication necessary to evolve into a community does not mean that the differences between members of communities are obliterated, resulting in a group members becoming the same bland average. In community diverse human beings are integrated into a functioning body, which benefits from the differences between its members. Appropriately to the vegetable cultivation theme of this book, Scott Peck says: "Community can be compared to the creation of a salad, in which the identity of the individual ingredients is preserved yet simultaneously transcended."[14]

Whilst useful in helping people to understand the dynamics of group development, workshops based on Scott Peck's theory are of limited value as a tool for solving problems in established residential communities. In an essay about the application of Scott Peck's 'Community-Building Process' to three British communities, Andy Wood concludes that for groups to benefit it needs to be introduced at the very start.[15] Even then, he adds, individuals must be willing to 'take part' in a process which challenges their core values, and in his experience most people were not.

Nevertheless, an appreciation of the role of difference causing conflict can go a long way towards a more mature approach to living in close proximity with other people. One woman who runs a farm together with her husband and parents – thus bridging a potentially difficult working relationship between in-laws – wisely remarked when talking about how they make joint decisions: "There's a lot of acceptance of differences between how people do things. We haven't really had times of great conflict because we accept and respect each other. The fact that we're happy and get on is more important than any of the decisions." She goes on to observe, however, that because they own the farm decisions are not as critical as if they were having to pay rent or a mortgage, which would push them towards having to get the best out of the farm all the time. Under greater pressure their differences in farm-management style might become cause for conflict.

According to Diana Leaf Christian only one in ten communities sustain themselves beyond the early years.[16] In her study of what enables communities in the United States to succeed, she notes that, "sustainable communities must be based on sustainable relationships – relationships that give more than they take – that nourish, enliven and inspire us. Such relationships are a continual source of energy." She goes on to outline some of the practices upon which sustainable communities depend:

- Sharing from the heart

- Listening to each other deeply

- Telling difficult truths without making each other wrong

- Speaking to and perceiving others in ways that allow us to stay in beneficial relationships with them while discussing even the most sensitive subjects.

- Using language precisely and replacing loaded words with neutral ones.

- Creating clear communication agreements to harmonise differing styles of communication. Some groups write down explicit communication and behavioural agreements, outlining for example whether swearing is tolerable or clarifying whether interrupting is unacceptable or just normal conversation.

- Check-ins – Creating a space at the beginning of meetings where group members can say what is going on in their lives at the moment and their feelings about it. Such a practice enables members of the group to be more sensitive to each other's personal needs.

It seems, therefore, that there are significant dividends to be gained from community life in terms of personal growth, energy and healing. However, as in so much of life, you reap what you sow. The fruits of communal harmony are hard-won and are dependent on all those involved being willing to give of themselves. One or two individuals cannot make up for the reluctance of others in the group to empty themselves of the barriers to communication, and sadly this all too often blocks the development of true community.

A paradox of needs

In the preceding discussions a theme that arises repeatedly is the juxtaposition of opposing needs. The need to have company and to be alone; the need to share resources in order to use them efficiently and the loss of control over belongings brought about by sharing; the need for practical and emotional interdependence and the need for freedom in one's life; and finally the need for energy to be invested in personal growth to create harmonious community, yet the energy cost of embarking on such personal growth. All of these apparently contradictory needs in fact form the basis of the dynamic, creative process that learning to live together with our fellow human beings represents, and have the potential to enrich rather than diminish quality of life if handled wisely.

It can be profoundly uncomfortable to be caught between two seemingly mutually exclusive concepts, yet, when unclear about which to choose, the very act of agonising between the extremes can lead to creative and enlightened solutions. I first became aware of the importance of paradox through reading Scott Peck's *A Different Drum*. In describing the psychological process by which true and lasting community is formed, he highlights that emptying of oneself of artificial boundaries between 'black and white' can allow a consciousness of the multiple dimensions to things, often with contradictory meanings.[17] He points out how mystics of all cultures and religions speak in terms of paradox, "not in terms of 'either/or' but in terms of 'both/and'." The capacity to accept ambiguity and to think paradoxically appears to be an essential pre-requisite of community.

With such fundamental challenges of living communally requiring a spiritual or philosophical approach, it is not surprising that it is spiritual and religious communities that seem to survive longest. From the ancient monasteries and convents of the middle ages to Gandhi-inspired communities of L'Arche and Steiner-inspired Camphill Communities, the evidence certainly seems to bear out an opinion I encountered frequently in my research, that 'only spiritual communities really work'. Other explanations for the greater success of spiritual communities over secular ones could include the fact that they are following a philosophy or belief system that has been passed onto them by a religious tradition or by a central founder (e.g. Lanza del Vasto or Rudolf Steiner), rather than having to make it up as they go along. As such, religious communities tend to be more hierarchical that secular ones. Hence there is less room for discussion and disagreement, or rather debate is held within communally agreed boundaries of dogma. A more positive explanation for the longevity of spiritual communities could be the emphasis on selfless love for one's fellow community members which, though in practice might sometimes be more theoretical than practical, is nevertheless more likely to hold sway when it is a central tenet of the community's belief.

The personal growth aspect of living communally has been compared above with a marriage. I don't think it is an exaggeration to extend this parallel to the extent of suggesting that this is why family farms work so well and have been the dominant model of land management for so long. I believe that the love within a couple or a family makes it possible to transcend the individual differences of opinion on how a place should be run. Although this is possible in a community, the energy that goes into decision-making and servicing relationships with so many different people is deflected away from physical activities. It is also more likely that a couple will be travelling in the same direction with regards to what they are wanting to do with their lives, and with their land. When the opinions of grown children come into the equation, matters can become more complicated. Still the bonds of familial love may well transcend differences of opinion and perhaps harmonious decision-making requires less energy than within a group of unrelated individuals, however similar their objectives may be from the outside. It is therefore easier for a family to run a commercial business than a community.

The longer a group of unrelated people live together, the stronger their bonds grow and the more like a family they become. Patterns of behaviour and agreement on overall objectives are less readily up for discussion and there are fewer decisions to make. This makes it easier for mature communities to sustain activities beyond maintaining themselves as a group. They are thus more likely to run successful commercial enterprises as a group. For example, at Laurieston Hall the early, energy-intensive experience of living as a commune has forged relationships of depth and familiarity which enable the looser-knit present-day community to carry out functions beyond community maintenance, such as running the People Centre (see Chapter Nine, p.185).

For those who decide to establish a project alone, there are a number of other alternatives for gaining some of the benefits of community without relinquishing control of your project. The most natural and traditional is the informal social network of rural areas, which may be based geographically around a village or town, or through common interest networks. Building up a strong customer base by inviting customers to help on the farm in return for produce or organising special events in which work (e.g. tree planting, barn-raising) is done in exchange for a meal or a party, as I have experienced at Fivepenny Farm and Vallée de Mérens. Such help, when given to other members of the wider community builds up social capital and increases the likelihood that when you need help it will be forthcoming.

Chapter Eleven

The Seven Ages of Men and Women

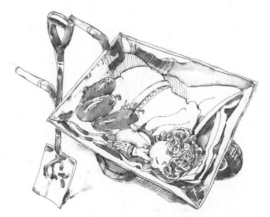

"All the world's a stage, and all the men and women merely players,
They have their exits and their entrances, and one man in his time
plays many parts,
His acts being seven ages . . . "
                                    – *As You Like It* by William Shakespeare

Human energy is a dynamic entity, changing on both a daily level and throughout a person's life. Whilst someone's energy levels, strength and health will vary according to their age, the amount of time they have to work on the land also depends on their role in life. A young, childless adult has greater capacity to throw him- or herself into a land project heart and soul, than a parent of young children, or someone who has responsibility for caring for an elderly parent. Yet the period during which many people choose to establish land-based enterprises often coincides with the time when they are starting a family, resulting in a potentially awkward energy bottleneck. In this chapter I will examine how people I visited managed their land-based activities at different ages and stages in life. Each life stage brings with it specific demands, and the responses of those I interviewed were strongly influenced by their current age and situation.

Although growing up on a smallholding has a significant impact on dependants, I am chiefly interested in the energy dynamics of the people who are responsible for running the holding. Thus, with apologies to Shakespeare, several of the 'ages of men and women' I refer to in this chapter relate to being parents of children of that age, rather than the child's perspective. Parenthood is a particularly significant role in the context of rural livelihoods, since the time of child-rearing tends to coincide with the most active working years. The joys and challenges of caring for children at different stages of development are ever-changing, and I discuss the 'ages' of pregnancy and being parents of babies, children and teenagers. I start the cycle at the stage before parenthood, that of being a young, childless adult, setting out to farm independently for the first time, and complete it with a discussion of the issues facing people who are growing older. The chapter ends by looking at the support extended families can offer to the smallholder, and the impact of gender on the division of labour.

Fledglings and young adults

Advice passed on to me by a person who had started market gardening as a second career, but had had to give up due to health problems, was:

> "I would recommend it [market gardening], but for young people. It's a young person's vocation. They've got the energy. The problem is there are so many people and not much space, so land prices have gone through the roof."

Likewise, a couple who bought a smallholding when they were in their late forties said:

> "Had we started ten years earlier, we would have had much more energy and wouldn't have got stressed. Had we been ten years younger it would have been easier."

In the past it was assumed that at least one of a farmer's children would take on the family farm. The decline in farming fortunes over the past two decades, combined with broadening career opportunities for educated young people, mean that the same is not true today. Many people who have grown up watching the relentless hard work and financial worry of their farming parents are keen to find other, more secure ways of earning a living. Hence, the level of entry into farming is very low, with ADAS finding in 2004 that between 1.4% and 2% of the farming population (including successors) were new entrants in the last five years. The lack of young people becoming farmers is reflected in the age profile of the UK farming community. Almost a quarter (23%) of farm businesses have a decision-maker involved who is over 65 years old, compared with only 3% of the general workforce.[1]

In contrast, organic farming is encouraging farmers' children to remain in the business, as well as attracting more new entrants. The average age of organic farmers and growers is 49, compared with 56 for commercial non-organic farmers, with only 6% being over 65 years of age.[2] Nevertheless, few of the teenage children of organic farmers I encountered during my research intended to follow in their parents' footsteps. They had witnessed first-hand the day-to-day realities of organic farming, which involves working long hours with the risk of losing your crops, and subsequent income, due to pests or frosts, drought or flood. Young people often want to strike out on their own path when they have the chance of independence, yet the lifestyle in which they have grown up will have had an influence. Later the desire to return to a more land-based way of life, especially when they in turn are raising a family, may lead them to at least growing a patch of vegetables and keeping a few chickens. Of the people I interviewed, six stated that a land-based upbringing was a factor in causing them to choose to live and work on the land as they were currently doing.

I came across few examples of children following their parents directly into a rural, self-sufficient lifestyle. One was in the Vallée de Mérens where, out of a family of eight children, three had chosen to remain in the valley where they had grown up and were in the process of establishing their own smallholdings. Although none was fully financially dependent on their own agricultural activities, undertaking seasonal shepherding, apple-picking and timber-framing work, they had built eco-houses, were growing their own vegetables and in one case keeping goats, rabbits and chickens. Their homes were either renovated stone shepherd's huts or self-built wooden cabins, and were barely visible amidst the dense beech woods covering the valley. It was an idyllic situation, but sadly unrepeatable in the UK due to the dense population and much stricter planning laws. At Tamarisk Farm, two of the daughters have chosen to follow their parents into farming. Ellen is now managing the main farm with her husband, Adam. The other daughter, Joy, and her husband bought Sea Spring Farm, a 15-acre smallholding in the same village, following careers in agricultural research.

In Britain, affordable opportunities to enter the farming business are scarce unless you are from farming stock. With declining numbers of children taking on the family farm, one might guess that there would be countless vacant farms ready to be taken on by eager young farmers. However, farms are often broken up when they are sold, to maximise the price of the farmhouse, meaning that there are fewer intact farms, with a house, buildings and land. Those farms that remain are getting bigger and bigger as they buy up spare land. The prices commanded by any land which has a house on it are way out of reach for prospective young farmers and growers, unless they have significant capital reserves.

Hence, many young people are looking for other options. Renting a farm or land is one possibility, and traditionally county farms were designed for just this purpose – to give young people a foothold in farming. These, by modern standards small (10-150 acre) farms, equipped with housing and farm buildings, are owned by county councils and let on five- to ten-year farm business tenancies to people with farming experience or agricultural training. The idea was that these tenancies would enable young families to establish a farm business before progressing onto larger, privately rented or owned farms. However, the increasing price of property and lack of capital to fund a move to a larger farm meant that tenants were 'trapped' on their county farms, and since the 1970s many county councils have sold much or all of their estate. Whilst some counties have retained estates comprising over 100 holdings, others continue to sell their farms to liquidate the assets, justified by the argument that the farms are too small to provide a living these days. Hence, the opportunity of renting a county farm is rapidly being eroded.

Another option is buying agricultural or forestry land with no house – a bare-land holding – and either farming it from a distance or building a house and other necessary buildings on it. The problem is that the former is extremely draining of human energy, whilst the latter raises a number of thorny planning issues, since residential building in the open countryside is strongly discouraged. There is a national planning policy (Planning Policy Statement 7, Annex A) which allows dwellings for those running economically viable agricultural or forestry businesses, but such development is so strictly controlled that it is extremely hard to convince planning authorities that the needs of the business justify a new dwelling.[3]

Another category of land dwellers is those for whom community and a sustainable lifestyle are as important as generating a land-based livelihood. As Chapters Nine and Ten demonstrate, there are clearly practical and environmental advantages to living communally or at least in close proximity to other smallholders. There is not yet national planning policy to allow for these developments, although a handful of projects have gained temporary permission after lengthy appeals. In these cases the mutual support within the communities, combined with technical planning advice from 'Chapter 7' (see Appendix 2, Resources) and moral support from a wider network of environmental projects, bolstered the individuals through the uncertainty and strain of the appeals process.

Land-based communities, such as Tinker's Bubble and Keveral Farm, provide valuable opportunities for young people to explore the possibilities for earning their living from the land without taking the financial risk of buying land alone. They are able to learn about the practicalities of living and working on the land by working alongside more experienced people.

The low living costs, enabled by the subsistence lifestyle and shared resources, create a sheltered, low-risk environment in which to establish micro-enterprises, such as salad-growing or green woodwork. At least four of the thriving holdings discussed in this book were helped by the fact that entrepreneurs had previously experienced similar work in a more sheltered setting, such as Tinker's Bubble, or as an apprentice on an established family farm. There is a desperate need for a planning policy that enables groups of low-impact developers to cluster together, to give each other the practical and moral support that enhances their chances of survival and success.

For those who are not yet ready to settle at a particular project, the organisation WWOOF (World Wide Opportunities on Organic Farms) gives people the chance to work on organic farms in return for board and lodging. Many aspiring smallholders now spend a year or two WWOOFing on a variety of different farms as a way of gathering experience and skills before they find paid work, buy land or join a community.

Parenthood

Pregnancy and babies

Women's experience of pregnancy varies enormously, and consequently so does their ability to work on the land before and after the birth of their babies. I asked eight women about how much they had managed to work on the land during pregnancy and during the early days of parenthood. Those who were fortunate enough not to have suffered severe morning sickness tended to carry on fairly normally until the later months of pregnancy. Gradually they noticed a decline in energy levels, and the need to rest more often and take naps. Energetic tasks like sawing firewood and carrying things uphill became difficult first, causing jarring and breathlessness. At Mulberry Tree Farm, both women were pregnant at the same time, which they found helpful as they had more sympathy for each other's condition. They said they felt more able to go and rest when they needed to, rather than soldiering on. One of them advised women to, "Enjoy the pregnancy. Don't try to be superhuman. Listen to your body and the baby." She used the winter when she was pregnant to create clear sets of instructions about how to run their box scheme, so that it would be easy for her to hand over the reins to her partner, when she wasn't able to work so much. Lambing was another job that women had to leave to their partners during pregnancy, due to the danger to unborn babies caused by diseases such as enzootic abortion and toxocariasis, which can be contracted from sheep.

A couple of women mentioned that their ability to work was only significantly affected when their bumps got to a size that made it hard to bend over. "At eight months, I got enormous," says one, "so I slowed down and stopped milking the goats because I was worried about getting kicked over and starting labour." Another woman went on riding horses and milking cows right up until the birth. One mother believed that it was really important for a healthy pregnancy and easy birth to carry on working. She particularly advised doing lots of squatting jobs just prior to the birth to build up muscles and open the birth canal. When her second daughter was imminent, she was squatting a lot, to plant garlic, and believes this really helped her have a smooth and easy birth. This woman also strongly recommended trying to have a home birth, having had three out of her four daughters out of a hospital, saying "It's really rewarding to have your child on your land, really special."

Another woman, Kerry, wasn't so lucky and suffered such extreme morning sickness that her partner had to take time out from his market garden to look after her. The situation was particularly acute during the first trimester of her second pregnancy because their older child needed looking after while Kerry was ill. "When Kerry was pregnant with Grace I didn't do any work apart from feeding the animals," her partner said. "Luckily it was the autumn. Had it been the summer, I would have had to employ someone." He advises parents to save some money ahead of time, not for buying baby things, but to be able to hire in help if necessary during pregnancy and the first few months of the baby's life. "When you've got little babies, remember they're little for such a short time and to be with them. I've employed people to work, just to have more time with the family."

Once the baby had arrived, several women started work again fairly soon, carrying their babies with them in slings or 'front-packs'. However one mother urged people to monitor how their body is coping following birth, after she worked too hard too soon. She succumbed to an acute and extremely painful bout of mastitis, which was possibly caused by leaving too long a gap between feeds. Another found that her ability to think efficiently and practically was significantly reduced when her daughter was really small. "My businesslike, rushing-around attitude was reduced. It was as if my Yang energy had gone down, and my Yin energy had increased and I just wanted to sit quietly and hold her." If it is your first child, adapting to parenthood will undoubtedly be a priority and a gradual easing back into work may be more appropriate than trying to pick up where you left off. As one woman said, "Be kind to yourself always. The land will endure. Enjoy your baby. Watch and learn." She told me of the pleasure she had gained once she let her garden go wild, since all sorts of unexpected wildlife arrived as a result.

All mothers sang the praises of slings, which enabled them to get on with many jobs while their babies slept or watched the world from their backs. "You put them on your back and pretend they're not there", advised one woman, "and keep them there until they're three and good at walking. Children know how to stay still. I milked the whole time with children on my back." Apparently, it is even possible to breast-feed whilst doing other jobs such as serving at a market stall or making apple juice, by carrying the baby in a snug front pack at breast level! As one mother pointed out, children are fairly weatherproof. She drags them out in all weathers, wrapped up well in waterproof coats, to get them used to being versatile. Carrying small children makes it possible to move faster than when they have just started walking, when progress can be painfully slow and they are more vulnerable to being knocked down by animals.

The amount you are able to do when you have a toddler at heel is greatly less than usual, and a couple of mothers stated that they were able to do only a quarter of the land work they had been able to previously. Others said:

> "Sometimes you just have to let go of things if you're struggling and ultimately prioritise the family if things are falling apart. Focus attention on the most valuable crops and let the others go. It ends up looking messy, but I think I'd rather stay sane!"

> "If you can't do something, then graciously let it go."

> "Keep things going, but be realistic about what you can do and downsize."

Some jobs would be downright dangerous to undertake with small children, and a previously very active woman at Tinker's Bubble listed carting (with a horse), tree-felling and working in the sawmill as jobs she was unable to do with her two-year-old daughter. However, she has gradually been able to do more gardening and make herbal remedies. She emphasised the importance of having your home central to your smallholding, so that your garden or animals are only a short distance away from the house. Having to walk up and down hill every time she wanted to work in her garden, milk or go out somewhere in the car was particularly exhausting, and during her late pregnancy she had to limit journeys up and down the hill to one per day, which seriously circumscribed her life. Had her garden been next to her house she believes life would have been much easier both before and after her daughter's birth. This point is reiterated by another woman, who observed that she was achieving more in the garden just outside her house after becoming a parent, since she could pop out and work for an hour while the baby was asleep, while she had to reduce her input into the communal garden.

As a new mother, however healthy and able to work you are, it is extremely hard, if not impossible, to do everything alone when you live and work on the land. This probably explains why the only single mothers I came across were living in communities. In all but one of the pregnancy examples above, the women were receiving huge practical support from their partners. For single mothers, and even where a partner was present, getting help from either the community, neighbours or extended family was considered invaluable.

The main roles of partners included keeping the agricultural/horticultural business going, chopping firewood and looking after the babies to enable the mothers to get onto the land. At Mulberry Tree Farm, the two fathers stepped into the breach to continue growing vegetables when their partners had babies within a month of each other. Previously one had been doing green woodwork and charcoal burning and the other undertaking community development contracts, both jobs that it was possible to put on hold in favour of the vegetables. Like many of the parents I interviewed, they were also benefiting from 'Working Family's Tax Credit' which, along with maternity allowance, replaced the lost income from the other work. Meanwhile they were able to maintain continuity for customers of the vegetable box scheme which their partners usually ran. Another grower adjusted his working patterns to do more during the early mornings and late evenings, and thus be available from time to time during the day to help his partner with the children.

Several people felt that the proximity of extended family or a supportive community was a lifeline in the early days. One mother regularly used to leave her children with their grandparents down the road if it was not appropriate to take them with her. When they got bigger, she devised a route through fields and back gardens so that they could walk to their grandparents without going on the road. Hence, she was able to leave the two older children alone in the house, if they didn't want to go out, knowing they were within safe reach of an adult.

A community can make a good substitute for extended family, and one mother appreciated the benefits of the community all the more since the birth of her baby. Two babies were born at the community of Brockhurst whilst I was writing this book. Whilst already a community that is especially supportive of parents, a significant change that came about after the births was that the number of shared meals increased from two to six per week, to save duplication of cooking. Knowing that the capacity of community members to do physical work was going to decrease as a result of the babies, the community had advertised for people to come and help with jobs such as milking the goats, chopping wood and weeding, and as a result gained four extra members.

Finally, a survival strategy recommended by at least four of the mothers was sleeping with your baby in bed with you. Being able to breastfeed without getting up alleviates the months of exhaustion from sleepless nights that are common to so many parents. There is no denying that the first two years of parenthood bring with them great challenges, as well as huge joy. Anything that can make those first two years easier is worth considering, and it is the time when all sorts of compromises are most likely to be made. There is no shame in this, if in the long term it means you are able to stay on the land, growing your own food and minimising your ecological footprint through low-impact living.

Caring for children

Many people choose to live out their land-based dreams at the same time as raising a family. Smallholdings, farms and rural communities can be ideal places for children to grow up in. They offer space in which to play, plentiful fresh and wholesome food and a practical introduction to many of life's most important lessons – birth, death, sex and care for the environment. Yet, establishing and sustaining a rural business, whilst learning the ropes of parenthood, presents significant challenges of time and energy management. Most of the couples I visited were either in the process of raising children, or had done so in the past, and issues relating to children were the third most commonly cited reason for choosing to live and work on the land.

People appreciated that being self-employed and working from home enabled them to spend more time with their children. Compared with a desk job or many technical activities, the nature of gardening and animal-care is such that it is safer and more fun for children to help their parents, or at least play around the edges while they work. The flexibility of self-employment makes it possible to spontaneously take the children for a bicycle ride or go blackberry-picking when the weather is good, rather than being restricted to weekends. For the parents who are the primary child-carers, it is more pleasant to have your 'other half' working nearby and the chance to integrate some land-work with domestic activities, than to be stuck at home all day every day with just small children for company.

The space and resources available to those who grow up on a farm enables them to experience freedom, play opportunities and responsibilities that are rare for children in today's cautious culture. Both parents and children appreciated the quality of life and outdoor fun that their chosen lifestyles offered:

> "We loved it. Playing in the river, having rope swings, building dens. As a kid the quality of life was brilliant. Until we got to secondary school age, and then we stopped wanting to be in a field."

"I value being able to give [my son] this lifestyle – running through meadows, playing in the woods, putting up swings."

"I grew up on a smallholding. I wanted to bring my children up like that so they could grow up outside, lots of space and natural surroundings. I wanted to work where I live so I could see my family more."

"[The community] is a safe, enriching, creative place for my son to develop."

Communities offer further advantages, in that both children and parents have friends and practical help there on the spot. The fact that children can go off and play with other community children, or hang out with other adults takes pressure off their parents. Both formal and informal shared child-care arrangements mean that children have a range of adult influences. Occasionally the distractions of informal child-care can be a cause of tension for community members who don't have children, but on the whole these times are balanced out by the enjoyment and spontaneous energy that children bring to a community.

At several communities, children were being home-educated and the varying skills of other community members were drawn upon. For example, at Steward Wood adults other than the parents are playing an increasing role in teaching subjects such as maths, computer technology and woodland survival skills, and I witnessed a couple of close friendships which had developed between particular children and adults. This feature of community life could be seen by psychologists as particularly beneficial, since there is evidence that it is healthier for children's emotional development for them to be brought up in an environment where there are other women, men, children and grandparents, than in a nuclear family.[4]

"We're in a very isolated rural area. If I didn't have Kathy and Tristan I'd go nutty. I see Tristan and another neighbour each day to have a chat, and ring up to borrow things. The kids get to see each other."

However, the alternative lifestyle that the children of organic farmers, or those who grow up in communities, experience can be potentially isolating if they become too cut off, physically or culturally, from their peers, as several people were at pains to point out. Worries expressed by interviewees included:

"The stress of getting the children what they need. We don't want to impose our lifestyle on them. Sometimes we stretch our financial resources to give them what they need. The children's needs have defined our approach to life. We try to live a middle-class lifestyle."

"What impact our lives are having on [our son] and how he'll be able to integrate with wider society and culture, especially if he's not at school."

"Be aware of what you're putting the children through. Young people take more risks with children. How do you envisage children fitting into your project?"

One of the biggest challenges for farming parents is dividing their time between work and caring for children. Paradoxically, whilst working from home enables them to spend more time with their children, at busy times of year the demands of a garden or livestock can be highly disruptive of family life. Trying to work and look after children simultaneously is a skill that some people find easier than others. I observed various approaches to childcare, ranging from involving the children in farm tasks, to sending them to a nursery or child-minder for several mornings a week so the parents could work without interruptions. Parents at both communities and family farms mentioned the difficulties of juggling work and care of young children.

A classic example of the establishment of a new smallholding coinciding with bringing up a young family is the case of Pentiddy Woodland Project. The 27-acre holding was bought in 2001, and in 2004 Ele and Anthony Waters gained five years' temporary permission to live there in a mobile home, while they established their woodland permaculture project. When I visited in 2005 the family had been living on the land for three months and were finding the combination of establishing a smallholding, earning a living from rustic furniture-making and caring for their two children (four and two years old) very demanding. Two sets of adult hands just never seemed to be enough, when the list of things that needed to be done kept growing and growing. As Anthony said, "The kids dictate the way the day goes. I have a problem focusing, even with a list, because there are so many small, diverse things to do." Chronic sleep-deprivation from interrupted nights and having to work one-handed with constant interruptions meant Ele found that, "Trying to achieve anything that is useful is hard." She told me that she sometimes envied communal set-ups, where there was more manpower, a pool of skills and the responsibility could be shared with others. As primary child-carer, she was becoming frustrated that she was unable to develop their vision for the land. She had the skills and the planning permission but no spare time, leading to a sense of disempowerment. At the time of my interview they had recently agreed that Anthony would look after the children to free up some time for Ele to work on the land. As they acknowledged, "We're still in the early days of living here, as well as being new to the parent thing, so are trying to find a balance." Two years later the acute stress of that time had subsided.

In communities there is a wider pool of adults to look after children. While most of the communities I visited had informal arrangements for sharing child-care, two operated systems which provided all parents with some child-free time in which to do land-based work. At Mulberry Tree Farm, the introduction of the workers' co-op (see Chapter Nine, p.186) included an agreement that each of the four community members (two sets of parents) would look after all the children for one day each week. This freed up three days per week for each adult to work and had, in the eyes of one member, "completely opened up our lives. I don't know why others don't do it. We can both be mother and father and our individual selves. We don't have to give one thing up for another." At Brockhurst, where only some residents are parents, one task on communal work-days was looking after the children. Hence, all community members – parents or not – were encouraged to think of creative things to do with the children, since it counted as part of their work contribution, and parents had their hands free to do other work fairly regularly. Such a system bypassed the stress expressed by a resident at a community where parents were in the minority, for whom a daily struggle was, "getting everything done. It's a fine balance between bringing up kids, earning enough money and trying to do your work-share. There's a lot of negotiation. You've always got to account for yourself. There's very little room for spontaneity. I would drop the 2.5 days of work-share to make it more family/relationship friendly and put more emphasis on what people can do."

Another solution, where parents are in a minority and other community members haven't the time or inclination to help with child-care, is to use commercial child-care services such as nurseries and child-minders. This is only viable where the parents are earning sufficient income to pay for child-care. However, it was opening up work-time for two couples who were running successful businesses from within communities.

Other parents were managing to combine child-care with their work. Until children are about three they can be carried in a backpack or sling, but later they need to be entertained or become involved in the work. The strategy of one smallholder was to fill a wheelbarrow with toys, books and sleeping equipment to use as a mobile base for her young children. "I did a lot of work when they were asleep," she said, "Being self-employed as, what we'd call in the States, a 'Ma and Pa' operation is hard. In many ways it's brilliant because you're always at home. It requires an enormous amount of time-management. We learnt about videos, for keeping the children entertained, early on."

The alternative strategy to distraction is involvement, and this is carried out very successfully by one smallholder. Jyoti has given her children tasks to help with from a very early age, reasoning that they are happiest when they are copying adults and made to feel useful for the part they are playing. "The whole first stage of a child's life is imitative and that's incredibly important", she stated. For example, if she is cooking she will give her children a vegetable to chop, or when sowing they would be encouraged to use their nimble little fingers to place seeds in the module trays. When, as frequently happens, they initially moan about having to go out with her and do something, she is firm and explains that "this is how we get our money to buy other food." Usually she finds that they quickly get involved in the task and seem to enjoy it. Giving her three-year-old daughter small responsibilities, like going to fetch elastic bands for bunching carrots, makes her feel important. This approach is a practical manifestation of her belief that an adult-centred universe, rather than a child-centred universe, is good for a child's well-being. That way children learn and benefit from what their parents are doing, rather than developing the belief that the world revolves around them.

As her children have grown older they have started their own mini-enterprises, such as growing flowers to sell on the market stall or keeping bantams to produce eggs. Hence, they have learnt the connection between work, money and the independence to buy things that they want from an early age, whilst developing practical skills that will last them a lifetime.

Despite the advantages of involving them, Jyoti acknowledges that small children do slow you down considerably. "You've got to be really, really patient. Pick up just a few tasks and keep plodding on until they're done." Children remain children for such a short time it is important to design your life around having enough time to spend with them, and not wish away their childhood in frustration at all the things you can't do. If that means delaying the commencement of enterprises that demand the sacrifice of family time, then so be it. As one parent advised, "Unless you want to put your child in care you have to live within limits. A more stress-free option is not to try and squeeze in more than you can manage." Another couple, who are still running their market garden after 50 years and raising a family of six, recommended gradualism. "We started with nothing and built it up. Don't set up a scheme for making a living wage and depend on it straight away. Try this and try that and see what works. We grew organically. I came into it gradually because of the children." Such an approach meshes well with the time that becomes available as children go to school and spend increasingly longer parts of the day away from home. In no time they become teenagers and their needs will change accordingly.

Teenagers

Despite their increased independence, teenagers still require significant amounts of parental time. Their needs are different, but no less important, and it can be hard to predict when they are going to want attention. The conflict between work demands and time devoted to parenting was a concern raised by several people in my survey, notably those living and working on family farms, rather than in communities:

"My main worry is the children – that I'm not spending enough time with them."

"I worry about how [our lifestyle] has affected {our daughter], but she's at a funny age now. We thought she'd just love it. We didn't realise what a time-consuming thing it is growing vegetables. We now realise how committed we've been to it and how she got sidelined a bit, which I regret."

"Our daughter has chronic fatigue syndrome. We were down at the field so much and she felt so alone and neglected. It wouldn't have happened if we'd lived on site because we could just pop in and out of the house if it was nearer, but it gave her the message that the field was more important than her. You get caught on the conveyor belt, feeling you have to do it [i.e. work in the garden]. Since she got ill I've had to divide my loyalties between her and my husband and the field. I spend my life having to justify loyalties to the other side."

One parent consciously creates time to be with her teenage and adult children through selecting particular activities to do with them when they are at home, such as riding out to check the cattle and sheep. However, some teenagers are loath to participate in farm work, and other ways of spending time together must be sought. Simply being together at meals is important for building family solidarity, and taking care to plan morning and evening farm work around meal times is a non-verbal indication of where parents' priorities lie.

Other issues for teenagers living in rural areas can be mobility and isolation. The absence of rural bus services in many areas means that, until they learn to drive, teenagers are reliant on either cycling or being driven by another adult. Whilst driving children around to enable them to have a social life is another good way for parents to spend time with their increasingly independent offspring, it can create ecological dilemmas and sometimes necessitates the keeping of two cars on the road. Transport was considered a primary day-to-day problem for one mother, who pointed out:

"We've got two cars. [My husband] needs one for work and I need it for markets and for our daughter. There are no buses, so we have to take her to places. Some neighbours of ours moved out of the area because they had three adolescents who needed ferrying around everywhere, and they wanted to be somewhere less isolated. Transport is especially an issue with adolescents."

"I don't meet up with friends very much because its secluded here. I bumped into some friends in [the local town] the other day and had a really good afternoon with them, but they don't tend to come out here much. They're not in the psychological pattern of leaving town." (teenager)

Equally, the difference in lifestyle between rural and urban children, especially those whose parents have chosen a very low-impact existence, becomes significantly more pronounced upon reaching adolescence. As mentioned in a previous quote, whilst an outdoor lifestyle seems fun as a child, dens, swings and mud lose their attraction for most teenagers. The desire to live like one's peers can temporarily over-ride deeper-held environmental values in the drive to fit in and not become culturally isolated. As one mother, whose teenage daughter was longing to leave home, said:

> "It's hard to live lightly with a teenager. Yet, when our son was a teenager we were uncompromising – not driving him around."

> "We strive to be mainstream for our children's sake. Our daughter has only just stopped worrying about the untidiness of our house when her friends come round. Before we always had to tidy it up before they arrived."

Despite these frustrations, I got the impression from most of the teenagers I spoke to that they valued their upbringing and the opportunities it offered, compared with a more conventional, town-centred life. They seemed particularly mature in outlook and engaged in the realities of modern farming, whilst appreciating their sense of belonging to a place, the quality of their home-grown food and their detailed understanding of the countryside, compared with their peers.

Single parents

During the course of my research, I met five women who were bringing up children without partners, and all were living in communities. This reflects the ultimately supportive environment and opportunities provided by communities, as expressed by all among their reasons for choosing to live communally:

> "It was very appealing as a single parent. I didn't want to go out to work and leave [my son]. Here I could live and work and be with the family. Living and working in the same place. It's fantastically secure. Very safe. Mutual support was very appealing with a kid."

> "I wanted to have other adults and kids around."

> "My daughter was three when I arrived. There was another kid of the same age with a single mum. I came here out of a housing need – not out of high ideals. I was unable to afford a house, so it was amazing to become my own landlord."

> "Being a single parent is easier in a community, financially. Otherwise, I'd have to work and have less time with [my son]. Here we have so many resources. He'd be a TV kid if we didn't live in a community."

> "If anything, the practical and emotional problems of being a single parent are less from living here because there are other people around and other children for my son to play with. We do co-operate – sharing cars and lifts to school, cooking meals together, sharing the burden."

Various themes are evident in these quotes, the most striking being the better quality of life that communities offered to single parents, compared with living alone. Communities enable parents to integrate meaningful work and child-care in a way that is harder in mainstream society, enabling children to spend more time with their parents. They offer an affordable and secure place to live, with the benefit of a close support network of other adults and children. Hence, in the absence of a second parent, children have a host of adults to befriend, teach and look after them. Without community support, living the dream of rural self-sufficiency would be significantly harder, if not impossible.

Adulthood without children

Not all adults have children living with them. This may be because they have chosen not to have children, their children have left home, or they are waiting until their business is established before they start a family. From a practical perspective, life is probably easier for couples without children, since they have more time and energy to focus on farming. They may also be under less financial pressure, if they have no dependants to support. However, whilst the early stages of parenthood may be demanding in terms of time and energy, there comes a time when children can help out on the holding, offering a valuable source of support. When grown children leave home, the sense of emotional loss for the parents may be compounded by the loss of labour and their contribution of ideas. For single people without children, isolation is a potential problem, due to the time-consuming nature of land-based work.

Growing older

Old age comes to us all in the end, and even those who have lived the healthy outdoor lives of smallholders and farmers eventually have to scale down their operations or hand them over to a younger generation. Several interviewees had passed their youthful years and were considering how long they would be able to continue farming, as their energy declined and they became more prone to physical ailments. It seemed that after the age of about 50 people were becoming aware of the fact that the physical demands of their chosen lifestyle were such that some sort of change would be necessary, yet for many this was a problem to which they were still searching for a solution.

When asked, "What are the main worries you have about your life here?", issues relating to getting old were mentioned by 16 different people, the third most common response after community conflicts and financial issues. Typical answers included:

"Creeping old age."

"Getting old, staying strong. Maybe we wouldn't want to carry on. If I look after myself I won't need new hips in ten years time, but if I don't, I will. I have to look after my back. I have to have the presence of mind to realise I'm 55 and look after it."

"Being able to physically maintain this lifestyle. [My wife] had a slipped disc six years ago and I increasingly suffer from asthma."

"I'm unsure about my physical capability to live like this in the future. Old age – people are skipping round the issue and not addressing it." (community dweller)

"As we age, I question how sustainable some of our practices are (e.g. carrying and chopping wood)." (community dweller)

Yet people were also aware that their active lifestyles were keeping them healthier and fitter than they would be if they were more sedentary:

"Living here is tiring, but that physicality can be good for keeping old people going." (woman, late 60s)

"If I hadn't been living here I'd be a lot sicker than I am because of the exhausting physical work. The work here keeps me fitter. I make it a mission every day to be exhausted at some stage – by carrying something up the hill, chopping firewood." (man, mid-60s)

"My health has been affected positively without any doubt. My knees are wearing out with osteoarthritis from working on them. But then we are older and this is the first time, in the last two or three years, that we've acknowledged that. I never sit and do nothing. It's a feature of this life." (woman, mid-70s)

"Health is positively affected by working on the land. The physical work one does and diet one has as a result of the produce is a good thing." (man, 80)

An allied concern was that the low financial returns possible from farming had made it impossible for many people to make financial provision for when they grew too old to work. Whilst some people had planned for their old age, or had other occupations to fall back on if their health failed them, others were entirely dependent on the income generated from their physical labour, and were asking:

"How long can we earn a living doing this and if we don't, how can we afford to stay here? I'm 60 years old and have no pension plan. We're looking at creative ways to make [our holding] work for us."

"We're worried about our pension plan. We cashed ours in to buy this place. I'm seriously worried about when we're too old to work."

"My main worry is the future. We don't earn much money, no pension. I don't think I'd want to be living this way here, maybe in Spain. [My husband] doesn't trust the economic system not to collapse, but what happens when we're 60?"

For those who owned their holdings, one option was to sell up and live on the proceeds in a smaller property, but such a decision is heart-wrenching due to the attachment that develops when one has loved and tended a piece of land for years. Responses from some of the older interviewees to the question, "How long do you think you will live like this?", included:

"I'll stay here as long as I can see a logic to how the land will be utilised in the future. I couldn't go on under-utilising the land ad infinitum because it's against my principles. I gave so much of myself for so many years, but my love affair with the land has waned."

"This property is valuable. I don't want to be attached to the property. I don't want to be market gardening in ten years, or even five years. We'll live here as long as we can financially. When you own property there are options."

"In five years time we hope to downsize, so we're just a little smallholding selling some vegetables – special vegetables like salad, but not potatoes and carrots. I don't know how sentimental I feel about it. I'm working on myself to keep an open mind. I love it. The hardest thing would be to leave the trees we've planted."

To which her husband replied:

"I can't see us spending the rest of our lives here because it takes time to maintain and look after the place itself, quite apart from the vegetables."

For those who were living in communities, the issues are somewhat more complicated. When land or homes are owned communally, the option of selling up and living off the proceeds in old age is not available. This situation provoked some strong feelings, even amongst some of the younger people I spoke to, who saw themselves becoming trapped because they wouldn't be able to afford to leave the community:

"I worry about the economic trap, because you put in a relatively small amount, which gets less and less. As time goes by it gets harder to access land anywhere else. The more trapped people feel, the more that can antagonise frictions between them."

"I worry about having to stay here when I don't want to stay here, about not being able to afford to leave."

In theory the community could be seen as an insurance policy/pension in itself. A number of years of active service could earn you the right to work less hard as you grow older, whilst enjoying the benefits of mutual support and the fruits of the labour of younger community members. In practice, the financial situation of most people living in communities left them little spare time or money to significantly support older members. As one woman living at a community said:

> "For someone with a long-term health problem, it's their friends who'd help them out, not the co-op. It's more like a village here than a big, happy family. You need to make a strong connection with people to get reliable help."

The issue of old age was most prevalent in the established communities, where the advent of a generation of dependent community members was provoking debate about the amount of work people were expected to do as they became less able. People within the same community reported mixed experiences, including:

> "I haven't any other options [of where to live]. I feel like people are very tolerant of my being unable to do things."

> "The physicality has such a value. When you're seen to be working hard you're liked."

> "Older people tend to feel guilty for not doing enough work because they're incapacitated in some way (e.g. bad back, bad foot, etc.), even though other people say its fine for them to stay, even if they're not able to do the range of work. One couple, a 75-year-old woman and a man, left to live in the local village last year. Work is the main thing people do together, so if they can't do it, they may not feel valued in the community. It's important to accept that although people may not be such hard workers they can offer things such as a caring, humorous or celebratory role."

However, an equal barrier to the traditional community-care model for older people was the reticence of older people themselves to be dependent on their fellow community members.

> "I wouldn't want to be dependent on others – I'm too independent."

> "I worry about the burden of concern you leave on your community as you get less physically capable."

> "Hurting my foot and not being able to work freaked me out because of dependency."

Although some older people may be unable to engage in heavy manual work, there are usually lighter tasks that they can usefully perform around a farm. In traditional rural societies, old people would be the ones who stayed home to look after children and domestic fowl, prepare food and mend clothes. Today, all farmers are required to spend a considerable amount of time working on accounts, keeping records for DEFRA and their organic certification body, and dealing with a constant stream of new regulations. Administration is a valuable service that people can offer when they become too old for heavy labour, freeing up time for the younger members of the family or community to devote to physical work.

What seems to emerge is that while there are some conventional strategies people adopt as they become less physically able (pensions; moving to a smaller place, being cared for by family, carers or in a home), we still have much to learn about how to grow old whilst living sustainably on the land. The subject of how to cope with old age is beginning to be discussed in some communities, but on the whole there is still a gulf between reality and the ideal, traditional vision of old people remaining with their extended families or communities, where they are valued for the wisdom and light services they can offer.

Extended families

With the mention of older people helping to care for young children, we have come full circle to the neat and natural way for all ages to have a place and a role in farming communities. In the past, when most farms were handed on from one generation to the next, there would be a mixture of ages involved in day-to-day life, and it made sense for grandparents to do the lighter work of child-care, to free up fit young adults for the fields. Everyone would turn their hand to whatever they were capable of, and skills and knowledge were passed on like a relay baton between generations.

Today, many people live at a distance from their extended family, making it difficult to enjoy the benefits of that support. Several generations of mobility, caused by moving for work, travel opportunities and cross-cultural marriages, have scattered some families across the globe. Yet, in traditional rural communities of the UK today, inheritance is still an important aspect of farming, keeping families tied to a particular place for generations. Such families are usually deeply embedded in the local area, and hence the extended family is more likely to be close at hand than for the average young couple. In a survey comparing organic and non-organic farms it was found that 16.7% of non-organic and 11.5% of organic farmers had family living at the same location. Non-organic respondents had family living within 25 miles in 66.7% of cases, compared with organic farmers for whom the same was true in 51.6% of cases.[5] These figures reflect the fact that organic farmers tend, more often than non-organic ones, to be new entrants to farming, and have frequently moved into the area when they bought the farm, rather than being indigenous.

The holdings within this study are virtually all being managed by first generation or second generation farmers or growers, and hence few people were from the local area and surrounded by extended family. In one case, two siblings had deliberately chosen to move back to the family farm with their young families to be able to benefit from the mutual support of extended family. Whilst one family went into partnership on the family farm, the other bought land in the village and established their own horticultural business. Both valued having grandparents close at hand. In turn, the grandparents enjoyed regular contact with the grandchildren, as well as practical support from their children as their health and energy levels declined. In at least two cases, parents of community residents had moved on retirement to be closer to their children and grandchildren, and were offering regular child-care support.

Another benefit of living close to extended family is that it is easier to care for elderly parents, which is a real consideration for people working the land. Compared with other jobs, it is much harder to drop everything and take a few days off if a parent has a stroke or a fall. There are animals to feed, crops to water and customers to satisfy, and going away takes considerable forward planning to find and teach someone else how to manage in your absence. Living in a community increases the chance of finding someone to cover for you in an emergency, but it can be disruptive to have to repeatedly call on others if ongoing problems mean you need to be away frequently. When parents live nearby it is possible to integrate helping them into the regular routine, and they may well enjoy spending time on the holding participating in daily life. How many of our parents would be willing to live with us and adapt to a low-impact lifestyle in their old age remains to be seen!

In the absence of extended family, it seems that a community can offer an admirable substitute. Two mothers of small children mentioned how the support of their communities made up for their mothers living far away. Certainly a functional community, in offering mutual practical and emotional support, sharing child-care and cooking, plays a similar role to that of an extended family. Whilst several people were quick to state that nuclear families need space within intentional communities, to develop their relationships and avoid friction, the value of community in helping the very young, the old and those who are caring for them is a theme that has arisen repeatedly. It seems that mutual support, be it from blood relations or a close-knit community, smoothes the passage through life and makes it easier and more enjoyable than struggling on alone or as an isolated nuclear family.

Gender roles

The division of labour in farming communities has always been dependent on gender, and in some ways the same is still true today. This is perhaps because, of all modern professions, farming is one of those that still require significant physical strength alongside the ability to spend long hours outside the domestic realm. The first time I became acutely aware of the difference in strength between myself and men was when I was working on a mixed farm, some ten years ago. We spent a great deal of time moving bales, both small rectangular ones and large round ones. At the time it seemed that the dimensions of awkward and heavy things such as bales and filled sacks coincided with what it is easy for a man, rather than a woman of average strength to lift. I have since learnt that technique rather than brute strength is the secret in lifting heavy weights. Health and safety regulations have led to a reduction in the weights that both sexes are expected to lift. Today there is no reason why a fit woman shouldn't, with practice, participate in all the same aspects of farm work as men.

Women's emancipation has led us a long way from the past, when women were seen as little more than servants of their farmer husbands. As Jefferies stated in *Toilers of the Field*, his description of the lives of farm workers in the late nineteenth century:

> "Farmers are decidedly a marrying class of men. The farm is a business in which a wife is of material service and can really be a help mate. The lower class of farmers usually marry quite as much or more for that reason as any others."[6]

In those days women's and men's work was strictly demarcated, with women working in the domestic realm as well as doing some poultry-keeping, milking, calf-rearing, haymaking and tending the kitchen garden. Only men undertook work such as ploughing and mowing. Whilst women participate in a much wider range of tasks today, modern farming is still male-dominated, with a recent study showing that 85% of decision-making farmers are male.[7] Another significant change in working patterns on today's conventional farms is that farmers' wives often go out to work or establish their own rural enterprises at home, to supplement the farm income. This can sometimes lead to stress as they try to reconcile their roles as bread-winners for the family and 'appendant' to maintain the status of their husband or partner in what remains a fairly 'patriarchal' way of life.[8] Research suggests that organic farmers are more likely to be women than non-organic farmers.[9, 10]

It was noticeable that at many of the family farms I visited, and even at some of the communities, traditional gender roles were in place. At places where young children or babies were present, this is understandable, since breast-feeding means it is necessary for the woman to look after very small children. However, after they have been weaned children can equally easily be looked after by the men in the household, giving the mother a chance to work on the land. Whilst this occurred in some instances, for example at Mulberry Tree Farm where each of the two sets of parents look after the children for one day per week, at several other farms the women remained the prime child-carers. This is perhaps a sign of inertia, whereby the man who has been doing the farm-work/growing while the children were small, knows the system best and it is more efficient for him to remain in charge.

The replacement of machinery with manual labour seems to accentuate gender roles, perhaps due to differences in average strength between men and women. I was particularly struck by the fact that at two of the four places that were more or less fossil-fuel-free, very traditional gender roles seemed to be in place. The women were in charge of cooking, cheese-making and poultry, while the men cared for larger animals, cultivated arable crops and carried large loads. In most cases this reflected the fact that women were integrating child-care with farm-work. However, at the smallholding where I stayed in Vallée de Mérens, where no children were present, the man was the one who had lived there longest, and whose principles had shaped their farming system. He was the one who milked the 32 goats, carried vast bundles of dry bracken across the mountain to use as bedding, and spent two months each summer making hay with hand tools due to their policy of not using machinery. His partner spent a large proportion of her time processing milk into various cheeses, as well as preparing meals, caring for the poultry, dogs and parts of the vegetable garden. I got the impression that there was a delicate power balance within their relationship, which relied on each sticking to his or her role. In other instances, traditional divisions of labour are perpetuated by women not having learnt the skills that would enable them to do the same jobs as men, rather than due to any physical inability.

In most developing countries women tend to be the main farmers in the household, whilst men migrate outside the family to supplement the household income – a direct contrast to the more conventional farming families in the UK, where it is the wives who go out to work. In rural communities in Africa, Asia and Latin America, the extended family plays a crucial role in the household's livelihood strategy, with older girls, grandparents and great-grandparents supporting the mother by taking care of domestic duties and helping with farm-work. There is much we could learn about how to sustain our human energy whilst using simpler farming methods, from these traditional cultures in developing countries. I have not spent enough time in developing countries to be able to write authoritatively about how people's differing working patterns affect their energy use. However, I believe there would be great merit in further exploration of human energy use in developing countries.

A *dynamic pattern*

For families, communities and society to function optimally, there needs to be a dynamic pattern of changing roles and responsibilities as people grow older. One young father in a community was troubled by the lack of allowance for the needs of different generations, saying,

> "What I'd like to change is that standards have become high, but because of ageing people there's less energy and its hard to say we'll do less of this. Having created a very efficient system, we're now finding it very hard to maintain it. There's not a lot of leeway for doing things badly. The original people made mistakes, but there's not much tolerance of younger generation's mistakes. There's not much willingness to be radical, try new things, be creative, because to run the system is about all we can manage. This is a common frustration amongst the young folk."

Each age group has its contribution to make, and nowhere is this more true than on the land. However, the last 50 years of agricultural modernisation have changed the order of power and responsibility, as one of my older respondents observed:

> "Traditionally there must have been a dictatorship with a dictator family member in charge. It's all a bit different with the rapidity of change – it's less appropriate for the old to be in charge because technology changes and everyone is doing it differently now."

Technological change, alongside the succession of farms from one generation to the next being less certain than ever, and the decline of the extended family, means that the rhythm of changing roles that carried our predecessors through from one generation to another has been lost. Now we will have to adapt to further changes in technology if we are to stabilise the climate by cutting emissions of greenhouse gases. In some cases this may mean a return to more traditional practices, while other solutions will combine new knowledge and materials with old ideas. Whatever the technology, we are going to have to learn to function without depending so heavily on fossil fuels and, like our ancestors, will have to invest more of our own physical and mental effort than hitherto into the task of cultivating the land. We have strayed so far from the traditional model of close-knit communities and extended families helping each other, that it is impossible to simply revert to traditional farming methods. The social fabric that allowed agricultural techniques to function has been allowed to fall into disrepair. Yet there is much that we can learn from our ancestors and other cultures about how a sustainable rural society can function, so that we can choose social structures that will support the farming methods of the future.

Chapter Twelve

Siestas and Fiestas: Balancing work, rest and celebration

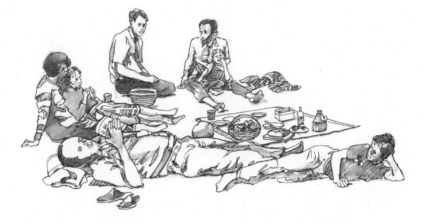

Central to the long-term stability of any smallholding, farm or community is finding an appropriate balance between work, rest and play. Herein lie the secrets of success and the stumbling-blocks that can cause an otherwise well-designed project to falter and fall. Achieving such a balance is just as important, though more challenging, where fossil fuels are being replaced by manual labour. The severity of the climate-change situation and the imminent fuel price rises resulting from declining oil reserves seem powerful reasons to work even harder to produce food sustainably, distribute it locally and attract more people to land-based occupations. Yet if small-scale, local and organic food producers are going to become numerous enough to make a significant impact on cutting carbon emissions and finding alternatives to our oil-addicted economy, it is vital that the task of running such outfits is seen as enjoyable and fun. Only by people seeing what fine quality of life those who've chosen the low-impact, land-based path are enjoying, will enough people be tempted away from the ease and convenience of 'high carbon' consumer lifestyles.

So, how is it possible to create enough space for fun and relaxation, when you're struggling to earn a living, do the best for your land, your animals and the wider environment, and offer those around you (your partner, children, community, friends and neighbours) the care and attention they need? This is the question with which I started researching for this book and in this chapter I will share with you the harvest of advice, observations and discoveries that I made during my journey.

Work

The value of work

A wise book by John O'Donohue, which draws from the Celtic tradition, describes work as "a poetics of growth".[1] By this he means that work is a way in which we grow, develop and give expression to our souls. For this to be possible, it is necessary that the work is meaningful and provides opportunities for imaginative creativity. Sadly, many people in the modern world simply work in order to earn the money they need to survive. Work is seen as a necessary evil to be endured and forgotten about at the end of the day, a place of repetition, anonymity and powerlessness, or perhaps even an activity to feel ashamed of. Even some people who work on farms feel disenchanted by their work, when they are required to spend long hours doing highly repetitive activities, are exposed to dangerous chemicals or are producing commodity foodstuffs for a faceless customer. It is hard to view your work as an expression of creativity when your back is aching from picking fungicide-drenched strawberries for hours on end!

Working on the land has different connotations when it is your own or collectively shared, when you believe in the system of production or when your harvest will be enjoyed by people you know. Although organic and small-scale hand-based farming systems require enormous amounts of repetition, the fact that you are working with living materials (soil, plants and animals) in a natural environment and that your activities are meaningful (producing healthy food in a way that is kind to the environment) places tedious activities in a wider picture of personal growth.

Gandhi also made the connection between work and spiritual growth. Here, Lanza del Vasto describes the distinction between the work of slaves and free men:

> "A man makes himself by making something. Work creates a direct contact with matter and ensures him precise knowledge of it as well as direct contact and daily collaboration with other men; it imprints the form of man on matter and offers itself to him as a means of expression; it concentrates his attention and abilities on one point or at least on a continuous line; it bridles the passions by strengthening the will. But in order that work itself, and not just payment for it, shall profit a man it must be human work, work in which the whole man is engaged: his body, his heart, his brain, his taste. The craftsman who fashions an object, polishes it, decorates it, sells it and fits it for the

requirements of the person he intends it for is carrying out human work. The countryman who gives his life to his fields and makes his flocks prosper by work attuned to the seasons is successfully accomplishing the task of a free man. But the worker enslaved in serial production, who from one second to another repeats the same movement at the speed dictated by the machine, fritters himself away in work which has no purpose for him, no end, no taste, no sense. The time he spends there is time lost: he is not selling his creation, but his very lifetime. He is selling what a free man does not sell: his life. He is a slave."[2]

Such observations are as pertinent today, in this world of mass consumerism, as they were over 60 years ago, when Lanza del Vasto lived and worked with Gandhi. Tragically, a large proportion of the human race has been drawn into 'slavery' as defined by Gandhi, cutting them off from the potential source of personal fulfilment provided by work. As I consider the people I encountered, one unifying feature between them is that all were seeking work which, 'engaged their bodies, hearts, brains and taste'. Whilst their motivations for choosing a land-based livelihood and lifestyle were stated in various ways (to take environmental action, to have "greater autonomy over how I use my time and resources" and to do something that is "real and tangible"), they boil down to the same need to be working at something worthwhile and creative.

In contrast to the virtual world in which many people now work, manual work puts people directly in contact with real materials, which can be profoundly healing and mentally restful. The monastic tradition of manual labour recognises the concept of "laborious leisure, in which the hands and muscles are at work, but the spirit is at rest."[3] The Cistercian abbot André Louf once wrote, "We must work with some material that resists us, and against which we have to pit ourselves to reshape it. We will thus be kept in contact with reality."[4] As he travelled between contemporary communities, in search of idealism as an antidote to cynical and speedy modern culture, Tobias Jones observed the importance of physical work in sustaining individuals, healing the troubled and building community. "Physical work used to be a sacred activity because it turned the body into an instrument, something which could subtly be worked upon as we were moulding our material. That is why various writers have insisted that physical labour should be the spiritual core of a community."[5]

Manual and mental work

In my experience manual work is invaluable as an antidote to mental work. Having grown up in a generation where studying to degree level is almost a right of passage for young people from middle-class families, I believe we're developing an imbalanced society which is top-heavy in people who can write essays and short of those who can cultivate a field or install plumbing in a house. Moreover, I think that focusing too much on mental work at the expense of manual work is unhealthy for the individual, resulting in information overload without sufficient time to contemplate and rest the mind, whilst working the body. I have found that whilst studying or undertaking any sort of writing work, I perform best when I integrate regular bouts of hand-work in amongst the head-work. Whilst writing this book I have enjoyed the near perfect balance of working in a market garden in the mornings and writing in the afternoons, giving me ample time to mull over ideas whilst picking salad leaves or hoeing weeds. It seems that inspiration strikes more often when away from the computer than when sitting struggling with the next sentence.

That is not to say that manual work does not employ the brain. Indeed it does, and as such seems a more balanced and healthy activity than pure head-work. To perform physical work efficiently requires thoughtfulness, observation and forward-planning, and running an environmentally sustainable, economically viable farm is not something that can be undertaken successfully by a fool. The skill in running a diverse land-based business of the sort described in this book requires the ability to juggle a range of enterprises, to prioritise jobs and to imagine innovative ways of presenting and selling your produce.

Motivation

I have observed over ten years of working at a variety of different farms, market gardens and communities how my motivation varies according to my relationship with the work and the person I am working for. I have worked in employee situations, where my role has ranged from straightforward worker to supervisor and planner of future crops, and as a WWOOF volunteer, as well as managing my own small market garden whilst living at Tinker's Bubble. I find my energy and desire to really apply myself to the work increases in proportion to the degree of control and responsibility I have over the garden. I contrast how I felt whilst hoeing weeds as an employee, when it seemed to go on forever, and in my garden at Tinker's Bubble, where there never seemed to be enough time to get down to some straightforward hoeing, and am reminded forcefully of the benefits of private enterprise.

The motivation arising from self-employment could be explained on a superficial level by there being a more direct correlation between how hard you work and the income you will be rewarded with, compared with when you're working as an employee. However, there are so many variables involved with earning a living from the land (weather, pests, price of crops etc.) that many of the farmers and market gardeners I know earn much less per hour than they are paying their employees. I believe that true motivation wells up from the fulfilment of living out dreams or life aspirations. Where people are fortunate enough to be realising those dreams, they are willing to work hard for very little financial return, at least in the early stages. As one smallholder I interviewed said about her work:

> "It's totally absorbing of time and thought, but it's a challenge I enjoy. On a soul level I needed to do it for me. I've spent most of my life outside and increasingly couldn't resist the pull to buy my own land. I wanted an adventure. This seemed like a great adventure."

Conversely, when people are obstructed from following their dreams it can have a profoundly negative impact on motivation. I encountered two community dwellers who felt disempowered because either the reasons they had joined the community had failed to materialise, or the nature of the community had changed. One man had hoped his community would offer him the opportunity to combine self-sufficiency with being an artist, in a way he had witnessed in some 'primitive' cultures he had visited. However, the community's main emphasis was on earning a land-based livelihood and he found that the low returns on his gardening efforts and "being niggled at by other people when you're working hard" made him feel apathetic and unhappy. The other man was worried that many of the values for which he had chosen his community (home education, vegetarianism and spirituality) were being eroded by new members who were trying to make the community more mainstream and businesslike. As a result he felt ill, emotionally exhausted, and disempowered.

Another cause of motivation loss can be boredom. A man who had spent the best part of his life at one community weighed up the pros and cons of remaining in the community or leaving:

> "I feel very safe and secure here, but also very stuck and caged. They're both valid feelings. What if I live 20 or 30 more years here? Will I just keep doing the same things as I decline? It's very difficult to be passionate about things after being here for so long, and I don't think lack of passion is good. But leaving would involve taking risks."

Maintaining motivation amongst members of a community is a fragile balance. Although in theory, working co-operatively and having a stake in the decision-making process is a motivating force, in practice creating a totally equal and harmonious system is difficult due to the differences in people's personalities and levels of experience. It seems that in some communities, hard work is a commodity that can earn you status. However, it can equally be divisive if it is used to belittle others, especially those who are unable to work due to ill health or child-care responsibilities. As one community member remarked,

"You need to value people for their different strengths. You can have hard workers who demotivate people and vice versa. Over time you can see how getting on with people, rather than being demanding, motivates people more. It pays dividends. If everyone's miserable, what's the point of achievement? Keep asking the big question (what's it all for?) in front of each thing you do and it'll sort out the important things from those that aren't."

In contrast, another man found the lack of a formal power structure in his community frustrating compared with a conventional employment set-up, where there is a boss in charge of a group of people. He noted that in the latter case, the situation is only as good as the boss. However, he couldn't think of any advantages of an egalitarian community over an employment situation with a good boss, saying that:

"[My community] is better than working for a bad boss, but worse than working for a good boss. A good boss will take suggestions from the workforce. A communal system could work well if responsibilities were delegated to different people, and the whole thing was run on a co-operative basis where people could take charge of their own areas. I feel happier about the work performed in commercial employee situations than the work that's been done at [my community]."

Traditionally the position of employers over employees is one of power, since they are the paymasters, are able to hire and fire, and have the final say in deciding what should be done. Such power, if misused, can become control, placing the worker in an infantile role of dependence and reduction of autonomy. Thankfully, the relationship between employer and employees is often more sophisticated, involving a two-way flow of communication and respect between the two. As the community member quoted above points out, a good boss will be open to ideas from the workforce. Ideally, an employer is caring and thoughtful of the workers' needs and will manage in a style that seeks out the workers' strengths and interests. However, ultimately in an employee situation, the employer still has the power to choose what is to be done and to what standard, since by paying his employees he is effectively buying their time.

The situation is different with volunteers and fellow co-operative or community members, and successfully motivating either is a skilful art. By definition, a volunteer is working out of choice rather than for reward. Hence, the supervisor has a different relationship with workers compared with an employer with their paid employees. It is even more crucial to discover what the volunteer hopes to gain from their work, since rewards other than money are usually the motivation for offering their services. It may be that they are wanting to gather experience or learn new skills, or meet new people. Alternatively, volunteer work might be viewed as an act of service, of giving to the local or global community.

Cultivating volunteer enthusiasm

An interesting blend of motivations is found in the WWOOFer, a common variety of volunteer found on organic farms. The organisation WWOOF (World Wide Opportunities on Organic Farms) creates opportunities for people to experience life on organic farms and smallholdings by bartering their work for accommodation and meals. Likewise, the services of WWOOF volunteers can be invaluable to host farms, as well as providing new and usually interesting company. However, the relationship between WWOOFer and WWOOF host is fragile, and positive WWOOFing experiences rely on a conscious effort of give and take on both sides. Although many WWOOFers are motivated by a desire to learn about organic farming, a large number of people also see WWOOFing as an affordable and more enriching way to travel. Staying on a farm and working for your keep is an ideal way to gain insights into rural culture or to practise a foreign language, when travelling abroad. By finding out when they arrive why a WWOOFer has chosen to come and help, WWOOF hosts are more likely to understand how best to motivate their volunteers. Equally, WWOOFers need to remember that even if they are on holiday, they are entering the life of farmers or a family who are busy trying to earn a living, and sensitivity to that fact will be appreciated.

I have experienced both sides of the WWOOF coin (as host and WWOOFer), as well as talking to numerous WWOOFers as we have worked together. In doing so, I have gleaned a few insights that might be helpful in making the best of interactions between WWOOFers and their hosts:

- *Working Hours* – The WWOOF guidelines suggest that working 6 hours per day for six days per week is a fair exchange for bed and board and a friendly welcome at the farm, and recommend negotiating before arrival how many hours are expected and what sort of work will be entailed. Usually the host is working far longer hours than that, but it is unreasonable to require WWOOFers to work the same hours as their hosts when the stakes are so different. A more common situation, and one I realise I have been guilty of, is to say to WWOOFers that they are welcome to stop after six hours, but can continue if they wish. Unless they are confident and assertive, this can result in the WWOOFer feeling pressurised to continue working beyond their allotted time in order to please the host.

- *Instruction and Motivation* – Most WWOOFers will be relatively inexperienced at farming or growing and will be hoping to learn from their hosts. Ensuring that they are given a wide range of activities during their stay, rather than continuing all day every day in the same occupation, can make the difference between enjoyment and feeling exploited. Clear communication about how a task should be done avoids expensive mistakes, such as a valuable crop being mistaken for a weed. Ideally the host will work alongside the WWOOFer for at least a short time, as a demonstration and to provide a sense of solidarity. In the absence of financial reward, praise for work well done can go a long way towards motivating WWOOFers, who may be feeling insecure in a new working environment.

- *Accommodation and Meals* – Accommodation will vary from farm to farm, as will eating arrangements. One comment I have heard from both WWOOFers and WWOOF hosts, relates to the need for longer-term WWOOFers to have some personal space. This can be difficult when you are sharing a small house and three meals a day together. If at all possible, arranging for some meals to be self-catered in a caravan or cabin can be a relief to both parties, allowing the host/couple/family to have some private time together and to relax from hosting, while the WWOOFer can have a little more independence. Whatever the living arrangement, making a WWOOFer feel relaxed and trusted by the household is key to a long-lasting, harmonious working relationship. From the hosts' perspective it is important to feel that the home and its culture is respected by the WWOOFer, if not agreed with, and occasional offers of help with domestic duties will be warmly welcomed. It can be quite tiring having to entertain a visitor at the end of a long working day.

- *Reliance on WWOOF help* – It is important to remember that WWOOFers are essentially volunteers, and may come and go at will. Designing a business to be reliant on WWOOF help is unwise and can lead to frustrations when they don't appear when you need them, or leave in the middle of a busy period. Treat them as a bonus that relieves you of pressure or enables a little more than you expected to be done.

The list of Do's and Don'ts (opposite) were compiled by an interviewee, Patsy Chapman of Longmeadow Farm, when she and her husband went travelling and became WWOOFers for a few months. Having run a market garden themselves, the experience of being a WWOOFer reminded them of what it is like to be dependent on your hosts, not only during work-time, but for food, accommodation and local knowledge. She kindly agreed to share this list of her observations of what makes for a good WWOOFing experience.

Do	Don't
When they arrive, spend 15-20 minutes just talking about the place, plans for the week etc. Hopefully have time to walk around and ask the WWOOFer about him- or herself.	Set people to work the minute they arrive.
Have available old work clothes for WWOOFers to borrow. Also work gloves, kneeling mats and a bucket for each person to carry around tools, water etc.	
Explain as clearly as possible the boundaries between WWOOFers' space and family space.	Have too many 'grey' areas, such as: use of the phone, internet, washing-machine etc.
Make sure there is plenty of nice food. Simple, but a bit fun too and try to get them all to cook at least one meal during their stay.	Put out nearly empty jars, bowls etc. Makes people feel they are being given scraps, even when actually there is plenty of food.
Make time to keep the kitchen tidy by explaining its workings to everyone......recycling etc.	Have a shambolic kitchen so it's difficult to keep order and discouraging for people who WANT to be helpful.
Be decisive about jobs. Organise the day in advance.	Argue with spouse about priorities in front of helpers
Have definite breaks for water or tea so people know where they are and feel secure. Have elevenses out in the field where the work is happening whenever weather permits (it's nice to enjoy the place during relaxed moments too).	Be a clock-watcher.
Have contingency plans for surprise weather.	
TRY TO ALLOW PEOPLE THE SATISFACTION OF FINISHING A TASK. Respect people's schedules for travelling and be helpful about transport to buses, trains etc.	Chop and change tasks from hour to hour or day-to-day before they are completed.

Table 12.1 – How to keep your WWOOFers happy.
(courtesy of Patsy Chapman of Longmeadow Farm)

Discipline and Order

One feature which I noticed was common to many of the more successful case studies was the degree of tidiness and organisation. The businesses that were really thriving were those where the land was impeccably weed-free, and tools were well cared for and tidily stored. This outward evidence of order seemed to reflect an inner discipline, which characterised the work attitude of people who were able to juggle multiple projects and sustain their energy. A couple who have grown and sold vegetables for over 20 years said that one of the things they would find hardest about living in a community would be the mess. They had observed that the communities that have prospered are the ones that are very disciplined, a view which is supported by the evidence in my study, in which the two longest-running communities – La Borie Noble and Laurieston Hall – were both very well organised.

Untidiness and disorganisation result in wasted time and frustration, as things get lost or broken, or jobs take longer because they weren't done at the right time. This is particularly true with weed control, as summed up by the old saying, 'one year's seed, seven years' weed'. An impressive example of efficient weed control is Charles Dowding's 1¼-acre salad garden at Lower Farm in Somerset, where there is barely a weed to be seen. Having focused on removing all seeding weeds during the first two years after establishing raised beds, Charles now only needs to hoe over the entire garden once every ten days, for two to three hours, to keep it weed-free. He emphasises the importance of actively searching for weeds to remove, for example by crawling through the asparagus bed in its off-season 'jungle period', rather than simply casting an eye over the garden. In doing so, he points out that one often sees other things needing attention, supporting the old expression, "There is no manure as good as the farmer's boot/shadow." Compare this with the time spent hoeing or hand-weeding when weed seedlings have been left to grow for a couple of weeks too long, and the wisdom of making the effort to weed in good time is clear.

On the other hand, a valuable skill to cultivate is the judgement of how thoroughly a job needs to be done. I have noticed that people who are new to gardening are often very meticulous and slow when they are weeding. It is counterproductive to spend too much time weeding one part of a garden, whilst the rest becomes overgrown and runs to seed, and over thoroughness can lead to small jobs becoming overwhelming. It is worth considering what you are trying to achieve, when starting a particular task, and choosing the most appropriate level of thoroughness. For example, if you are trying to stop tall weeds overwhelming a crop, it is more important to roughly weed the whole crop than to get out every last little weed, whereas in a seed-bed or salad garden a more thorough approach pays off. With practice it is possible to become faster at weeding and other activities, and to evaluate the level of thoroughness called for.

Time management, list-making and prioritisation

One thing is for certain – the work of a smallholder is never done. The sooner that lesson is learned and the goal of getting to the end of the 'to do' list is relinquished, the greater the chances of success and sustainability.

There is nothing wrong with making lists. They are a very useful tool for organising your thoughts, reminding you of what needs to be done and helping you to prioritise tasks. One smallholder stated that she often loses the lists she has written, but finds that it is the mental process of prioritising that's important, not the actual list. Several people, especially those with young children, mentioned their reliance on making lists for the next day as a way of keeping focused amidst the chaos and clamour of interruption. The mistake is when you expect to get to the end of the list.

"Expectations – don't have them," was the advice I was offered by one friend, who is involved in building a very stable and productive land-based community. He stated that:

> "The only deadlines we have are natural. There's an issue of expectations and use of words like 'should', which makes people guilty if they don't do things. I do things because I need to do them or want to do them, and when both together that's when I have my real motivation. I manage my time very thoroughly. Everything I do is because I intended to do it that day, but I never expect to do all of the jobs written down in the diary for that day."

Another friend, who worked as a computer programmer before he took to the land, spoke to me of a similar strategy for avoiding burn-out, whilst we weeded broccoli together. He sets his goals for each day at zero, meaning that if the sum total of what he achieves in the day leaves him in a better position at the end of the day than he was at the start, then the day was successful. He acknowledges that it sounds terrible to have such low expectations, but pointed out that when people are rushing to get a large number of things done fast they are more likely to set themselves back by making mistakes. At least by achieving nothing in a day you haven't undone previous achievements. He found that in the computer industry, which is renowned for its high-pressure contracts, his attitude of setting low expectations made it easier to do each job really well.

Applied to working on the land, the kind of day you want is having not broken any tools or caused physical injury to yourself, but having still accomplished something. For example, that extra hour's weeding that you shouldn't have done at the end of the day because you were tired could cost you six weeks of recovery from a back injury. By allowing natural priorities to show themselves, or simply by choosing the job on the list that you feel like doing that day, the chances of accomplishing something worthwhile are greater than if you undertake a task reluctantly because you feel under obligation.

Of course there are always jobs which are less pleasurable, but those that absolutely must be done will push themselves up the order of priority, whilst some eventually drop off the list because they aren't really that important. Others will appear more appealing at some times than others. For example, doing paperwork on a rainy day is preferable to doing it when the sun is shining!

The other nugget of wisdom my ex-computer programmer friend shared with me related to scheduling. He bemoaned the planning sheets that project managers made. When things went wrong, as they inevitably do, and deadlines were passed, the whole schedule would have to be rewritten, wasting time that could have been spent working on the project itself. He spoke of one brilliant manager who would always double the amount of time his programmers estimated that they needed to do a job. The beauty of this system was that it was almost always possible to finish ahead of schedule, if all went according to plan, and if it didn't go well, the chances were you'd still be on target. Such a strategy builds morale, since success was the outcome more frequently than if deadlines were consistently missed. Constantly feeling that you're running to catch up, and never quite getting there, is exhausting and demoralising. Sadly it is a common situation, on the land as much as in the office, since the seasons never stand still. One of my interviewees, when asked how often she felt too tired and overworked to enjoy her life on the land, replied:

> "Often. It's mental tiredness, because you're just struggling so much and there's always something else that needs to be done and that weighs on you – for example, I'm really behind with my paperwork at the moment."

For certain personalities, mine included, the temptation to plan your day, week or season, is very great. The problem is, life invariably gets in the way, sending broken-down cars, spontaneous visits from friends, escaped animals and patches of weeds that take longer to subdue than you ever thought possible. Then there is the familiar situation, described by one market gardener:

> "Your whole life is slightly out of control. You have a task in mind to do, but on the way to do it you see another, more urgent job."

Her solution was similar to that of my two friends, in that she would plan to do only one task each day, so if she got another done it was a bonus, rather than trying to do too many things in a day and being disappointed.

So, continue to write lists, but don't expect to finish them. With lists it is a case of having a 'the glass is half full' attitude of appreciating what you have achieved in a day, rather than having a 'the glass is half empty' attitude of looking at all the things on the list you still haven't done.

Mental attitude

As I've pored over the transcripts of the interviews and pondered about what makes some people more able to sustain their energy than others, I have noticed certain personality traits that seem to tally with success and longevity on the land. The first thing to strike me was the response of certain people to the question, "What are the main worries you have about your life here?" A handful of people answered with words to the effect of, "I don't really have worries," and these tended to be the people who were thriving, rather than merely surviving. Whilst some of them expressed frustrations or annoyance about some aspect of their life, they genuinely seemed to be free of worries. Now, their lack of worries could be interpreted as being a result of the fact that their projects were going well in the broader context of a straightforward, problem-free life. However, there were also indications that their personality and attitude to life played a part in creating the circumstances which enabled them to be laid back. For example, three of those who stated that they had no worries were living in situations with fairly precarious planning status and were experiencing significant hostility from local people. A couple of people told me that they consciously don't allow themselves to worry, saying for instance that, "I don't focus on problems, I look for solutions," or "I'm not a person that worries."

On the other hand, a few people appeared to be weighed down by worries. Whilst the issues they were concerned about were perfectly valid, their lives, on the whole, didn't seem to be particularly more problematic than those who don't worry. As a person who tends to worry myself, I feel there is a lesson to be learnt here about the energy draining nature of worry, and the choice we have about how we approach problems. A common phrase amongst permaculture designers is, "There are no problems, only solutions." It seems that whilst problems do inevitably arise, we have power to control how we address them. Rather than seeing them as negative obstacles between us and progress, they can be viewed as opportunities for imagination and creativity.

In his book *Anam Cara: Spiritual wisdom from the Celtic world*, John O'Donohue introduces the French proverb, *"Une difficulté est une lumière/Une difficulté insurmontable est un soleil"* (i.e. a difficulty is a light, an insurmountable difficulty is a sun).[6] He explains how blockages often arise not because an actual piece of work is impossible, but because we have constructed an image of the task being difficult, saying "the image is not merely a surface; it also becomes a lens through which we behold a thing. We are partly responsible for the construction of our own images and completely responsible for how to use them. To recognise that the image is not the person or the thing is liberating." He goes on to describe how awkward and difficult situations can turn out to be great gifts, because they encourage us to think laterally. Using a beautiful metaphor of the soul being like a tower with many windows, he explains how lateral thinking occurs when we draw back from the window we usually look out of and choose from all the other windows, which offer alternative views of possibility and creativity.

Another familiar attitude I encountered during the interviews was that of the driven personality or workaholic. Environmental and social activists have a tendency towards this condition, due to the enormity of the tasks they are addressing, which seemingly have no end. Whether you are focused on global problems, such as climate change and poverty, or the local solution of producing affordable, organic food for local people or creating a harmonious community, it is possible to get so caught up in chasing goals that you forget to stop and rest. However, being an "achievement junkie" can be internally as well as externally caused if you habitually value yourself according to what you have achieved. The psychological complexities of low self-esteem and the causes of workaholism are too huge a subject to delve into here. However, just questioning why you are so driven to achieve can be helpful in breaking unhealthy work patterns.

Allied to the driven attitude is the issue of resentment, which frequently arises in those who are working hard alongside others who are not pulling their weight. It is an especially common sentiment in communities, where people with a variety of attitudes to work are put in close proximity whilst working towards a common aim. Several community dwellers mentioned negativity originating from themselves or other people being a significant drain of energy. Another community member observed that in the past she based her expectations of achievement on other people's rates of work, and found that she often became tired and stressed. Now that she recognises her own capabilities, she is more realistic and gentle on herself, and manages to avoid becoming overtired.

Those who were thriving appeared to have a fairly relaxed outlook on life, even though to me they seemed to be achieving more than I could achieve in my wildest dreams within a single day, year or lifetime! For instance, when I visited Dun Beag in 2005 David Blair was juggling forestry, building a guest cabin, maintaining his renewable-energy systems, organising an ecovillage project and a community composting scheme, teaching permaculture, keeping poultry and maintaining a small forest garden. When I commented about how much he was achieving, his response was, "I just try to keep the mindset of thinking I'm just pottering about in the woods." When I probed him further about his relaxed attitude, he told me that it is the very diversity of his occupations that keeps him going. Another woman, whom I also admire for her seemingly endless energy and ability to run a mixed farm, raise a large family and continue land-rights campaigning, stated that she enjoys the diversity, flexibility and challenge in her life. This brings to mind another old truism, "A change is as good as a break." Being able to choose between a range of possible activities, or even moving from one pressing kind of work to another, can be as refreshing as taking some time off. For example, a market-gardening friend saw returning to work on his land as being like a holiday after spending six weeks behind a computer putting together his case for a planning appeal!

Rest

Whilst discipline and motivation go a long way towards managing a productive garden or running a viable land-based business, there comes a time when it is necessary to stop and rest, in order to sustain your energy over the long term. Breaks vary in scale and frequency from daily tea, coffee or lunch breaks through days-off to full-blown annual holidays. All are equally important in their turn for resting the body and refreshing enthusiasm for the project concerned.

Break-times

Over the years I have observed with interest different workplace cultures, and have come to the conclusion that people are most productive when their days are punctuated with regular breaks for tea, coffee and lunch. To be more precise, a routine of working in two-hour bouts and then taking a 15-30-minute break before resuming work again, seems to be a successful formula at several places where I have worked both on farms and in offices. Such a regular routine, when known about and accepted by all the workers, gives a framework for the day and can help with motivation, especially when the work is monotonous or physically demanding. At Tamarisk Farm, we always know there will be a tea break at 10.30am and that we will stop for lunch at 1.00pm, and hence can plan our work around those times. A recent introduction when I visited Brithdir Mawr was the 11.00am coffee break, to which community members were called from wherever they were working by a conch shell. This new institution seemed to be a significant ingredient in creating a strong community identity, since it gave people a point in each day when they knew they would see each other.

Another work culture, which I find less satisfactory but seems to suit some people, is to work at each job until it is finished or you feel tired and then stop for a break. This is all very well when you are working alone, but when groups are working together it can be disruptive to have people stopping at different times. It is also demoralising, when working for someone else, not to know when your next break is going to be. I remember one farm job, where my employer would often think of another job which needed doing just when you thought you were about to go and have lunch. Of course farm work is frequently unpredictable, especially where animals are concerned, and sometimes it is necessary to delay break-times to deal with an emergency. However, where employees or volunteers are involved, trying where possible to keep to a regular schedule of coffee, lunch and tea breaks is a valuable way of making their work-life more pleasant.

Break-times can be enjoyable social occasions, especially where workers are spread out doing different jobs across the land and they come together for refreshment. They are a time for exchange of information, light banter or deep philosophical discussions, as well as replenishing energy levels with food and drink. I can remember countless occasions when I have felt as revitalised by the humour, camaraderie and stimulating break-time conversations with my fellow workers, as by the refreshment. However, being offered good quality food prepared by the employer, whether it be freshly baked bread with cheese, fruit or cake, will also make workers feel valued and motivated. Many years later I still recall with a watering mouth the rich yellow-yolked, garlic fried eggs that one grower used to prepare for the workers at Friday lunchtimes!

The supreme example of a place where a timetable determined the daily and weekly pattern is the community of La Borie Noble, in south-west France. Here the day is divided into two four-hour periods of work, whilst each morning and evening includes times for meditation and prayer, and a hot meal is served at lunchtime to all residents and guests. The times when each activity begins are marked by a bell, which rings out across the valley from its tower. The bell is also rung once per hour during working hours as a signal for a moment of silence and recollection – a 'rappel' – to call people to 'be present at the present'. I particularly liked this institution, since it is all too easy to get wrapped up in whatever you are doing and forget to be present. To be reminded to just stand and take in your environment, notice how you are feeling and who you are working with, seemed to enrich each day. I can still recollect my time at La Borie Noble with great clarity, partly as a result of the 'rappel'. Whilst to some the idea of such a timetabled existence may appear oppressive and impractical, I was impressed by how much seemed to get done at La Borie Noble in a relaxed and unhurried way.

The tea and coffee culture, however, does not suit everyone and some of my interviewees had other ways of taking time out during their workday. For example one woman said that when she feels really tired during the day she walks to the river at the end of her field to paddle, takes a nap or chooses a gardening job, such as sowing seeds, which she knows will revitalise her. Despite working a gruelling schedule with daily 4.30am starts in the summer, she stated that between March and November she is tired, but to a level she can handle because she's become good at taking time out when she needs it .

Power-napping is an art well worth cultivating, since it can refresh you quickly and without the awful groggy period that follows a full daytime sleep. A large proportion of the brain's activity is caused by visual stimulation, so by just lying down and closing your eyes for ten minutes it is possible to gain some of the benefits of sleep. I have found doing a ten-minute deep relaxation a very effective way to refresh myself before an afternoon's work. I lie on my back with my arms laid out from my sides, allowing the bed or ground to fully support my weight. I then mentally think through every part of my body, relaxing first each finger, the back of the left hand and palm of that hand, wrist, forearm and so on all the way to the toes, before repeating the routine down the other side. Once your entire body is fully relaxed you can just lie there and enjoy it, before slowly bringing yourself back to the present and opening your eyes.

A step further is to make the time to meditate each day, which is a profoundly effective way to rest the mind, and find clarity and an alert attitude. A market-gardening friend told me that the secret of his sustained energy is a daily meditation practice. From time to time he treats himself to a full retreat at a Buddhist meditation centre, which helps him release mental clutter and thereby boost his energy level. Similarly, the space timetabled for meditating at La Borie Noble seemed to contribute to the calm, orderly and centred attitude of many of the community members.

Days off

Self-employment enables you to step outside the framework of weekdays and weekends. This may be welcome, but the down-side is that, especially in busy seasons such as the spring and summer, it is possible to lose yourself in an endless sea of workdays. If you continue working for too long without a break, productivity tends to go down whilst the risk of injury, breakages and costly mistakes increases as a result of tiredness and loss of focus. Whilst there are certain tasks which it is necessary to do each day without fail, such as milking, feeding animals and watering seedlings, I believe it is important to plan a regular day off work into the weekly routine in order to sustain your energy and enthusiasm. This can, however, be difficult when there are urgent jobs crying out to be done and there never seems to be enough time within the week to do them.

A solution to this conundrum is the idea which Patrick Rivers described in his very helpful book *Living on a Little Land*. He and his wife Shirley bought a cottage and seven acres of marginal land, which they turned into a self-sufficient smallholding that enabled them to significantly cut their need for an outside income. Patrick noted that in their first year there they happily worked twelve hours per day, seven days per week, but then started to slow down and achieve less and less because they were becoming 'stale'. They then tried taking Sundays off, but found themselves getting bored and frustrated when "the carrots were crying out to be thinned and the hay whispered 'Turn me'". The compromise they hit upon was the creation of 'Special Days':

> "Once a week – on Sundays when possible – we have our 'Special Day'. We get up a little later. We put a cloth on the breakfast table; have coffee and maybe hot, buttered, honey buns for a treat. We make no plans, but linger afterwards. We do just what we want to do. It might be nothing or we might thin those carrots, or do something frivolous like making a flower bed. One of us might be working while the other loafs. It matters not. Special Day has only three rules: firstly, short of essential, routine jobs, like milking the goats and collecting the eggs, and short of some exceptional event such as getting in the hay before a storm, we do just what we like; secondly, if we do work we must not feel virtuous; and thirdly, if we do not work we must not feel guilty. Shirley and I have found that in the end we usually work pretty much the same as most days, but what we do hardly feels like work. We look forwards to Special Day; it renews us."[7]

The subject of days off arose several times along my journey, with people mentioning that if they ignored their body's signs of tiredness and didn't take a day off, they risked injury or illness. One man mentioned how he felt overtired more often since his son had been born, because he no longer "had space to enjoy his tiredness". He used to have a rest day, when he claimed he did nothing all day. He said he was learning the detriment of not having that any more and noted the importance of recognising his natural body rhythms as he gets older. Even partial days off can be helpful. As one farmer noted, "Having something regular you do each week, preferably off-site, punctuates the week and forces you to take a break. It is important to make a conscious effort not to miss such breaks, however busy you are, since they can force a sense of perspective on your busy-ness."

Holidays

Everyone needs a holiday from time to time, but agriculture is a profession that makes going away difficult, and many farmers go for years without taking a proper break. This was certainly true of several of the smallholders I visited, who mentioned that they rarely or never go away on holiday. The effort of finding a capable person to look after the holding, teaching them all the intricate details of daily management or rearranging marketing systems to work without you, can be so stressful that some feel it's not worth the bother. Yet getting away and having a change and a rest is a crucial ingredient in the human energy equation. The sense of revitalisation that a good holiday creates makes people more alert, productive and open to new and beneficial ideas. It is all too easy to get stuck in a rut, working hard because it is what needs to be done, and forget the potential energy and insights that a thorough rest can release.

One of the advantages of working outside on the land, compared with a man-made environment, is that the variety and amount of work changes with the seasons. Day length, light intensity and the cycles of nature profoundly affect both human energy and the rate of growth in the plant world. Hence, different kinds of land-based work have their slack seasons to compensate for the times when life is almost unbearably busy. For example, for a vegetable grower the busiest season is between April and July, while the winter provides opportunities for times of rest. Conversely, a coppice worker would find October through until March the busiest season, since this is when the sap is down and wood can be cut without harming the tree. The quiet times of year are invaluable for recharging the batteries, and if more than one enterprise is planned, it is well worth thinking about when will be the best time of year to take a holiday, to ensure you benefit from a slow season.

As one smallholder said, "In a community there's more flexibility about being able to get away and travel. Part of it is sharing. On a bad day we can feel a bit trapped." Communities and ecovillages offer the benefit of having a reservoir of capable people nearby who can cover for you when you go away. Whilst it may still be difficult to negotiate help from other busy smallholders, the potential of reciprocal cover arrangements between neighbouring landowners provides a powerful incentive to carve out some time to look after your friend's goats or seedlings. One community member pointed out that holidays can offer a valuable opportunity for those in a very small, close-knit community to have some more personal space when the other family goes away.

Finding the balance

In considering how work and rest can be wisely balanced, the phrase 'less is more' comes to mind. Several people stated that they rarely became overtired because they had learned to pace themselves and take regular time off. However, what can you do when you're in the position of this community dweller?

> "I've got myself into the habit of not getting really tired, but that means I'm not getting things done that I want to and that's making me unhappy"

Sometimes it feels as if you can't win whichever way you try to balance work and rest – there just never seems to be enough time. In this situation, it may be that it is necessary to re-evaluate what you're trying to achieve. By prioritising the activities you are involved in, it may be possible to select certain ones that you can drop or delegate to someone else, and thus prune down your commitments to a more manageable scale. However, this is sometimes easier said than done, when working with other busy people.

The ideal balance between work and rest varies greatly between individuals, and whilst some seem to thrive on very little sleep, whilst packing their time to the full, for others it is vital to create enough space for rest and relaxation. It can be particularly hard to achieve your own personal balance when working closely with others, particularly in a community or co-operative situation, where the pressure to 'keep up' and 'pull your weight' can be immense. In this situation, it is important to be firm about where your own personal boundaries of capacity lie, or you can find yourself being drawn into unhealthy work patterns, as these community dwellers have discovered:

> "If I base my expectations on other people's rate of expectation I'm bound to get tired and stressed. Whereas, if I base them on what I know my capabilities are, then I'm more realistic and gentle on myself."

> "I seldom feel too tired and overworked to enjoy life. I feel it's up to individuals to learn their boundaries and then communicate them to others. It's part of being an adult. Sometimes it's harder to say 'no' than 'yes' ."

> "I've decided that my health is better preserved by pacing my life, which means learning to say 'no'. The change came about with someone who wasn't pulling their weight. I realised I wasn't going to die making life easier while he sat there doing nothing, and thought, 'Why doesn't he carry some wood? He's 25 years younger!' Afterwards, I realised it wasn't just him, it was the structure of the place without equitable distribution of responsibilities."

Indeed, using your energy prudently when working in any group situation relies on developing a sense of what is a fair proportion of the work to undertake personally, together with the confidence to assert your need to stop and rest when you need to. Again, as on the personal level, if the group is struggling to achieve its aims – for example, running a viable business or managing the land in a sustainable way – it may be necessary to re-evaluate whether those aims are realistic. Sometimes the whole group may be relieved if one person says, "Enough is enough, we can't carry on like this" and that can be a prompt towards positive change. However, so much hope and effort may be invested in a group enterprise or project that it can be daunting to be the person to challenge whether it is feasible. In such a situation, good communication skills, such as those taught by Marshal B. Rosenburg in his book *Non-violent Communication: A language of life*, are valuable for getting the message across in a way that is non-threatening.[8]

Play

Having fun

Alongside work and rest, play is a vital ingredient for a happy and sustainable life. By play, I mean any activity that involves the pleasure of having fun. Many of those I interviewed mentioned their particular ways of unwinding and having fun, which included cycling, dancing, playing tennis or going to parties. However, they acknowledged that exhaustion resulting from their work or general business often got in the way of these activities. All too often the urgency of land, livelihood, family or community-based tasks mean that fun slides quite a long way down the priority list. As one community dweller said:

> "It's hard graft running the People Centre – it can't stop when it's started. I'd like to have more fun. I worry about how serious and critical we are, how grumpy and cynical we all get. We chose this life so we could have a balance between work and play, but sometimes it's hard to do that. Some of us – including me – are workaholics."

When working or living as a group, creating the space to have fun together can be particularly valuable, since it is these times that bond people and provide an incentive to keep working at relationships during the tough times. These can be spontaneous, such as moments of hysterical laughter during a shared meal, or they can be planned. For example, a couple of communities had taken to going to the beach *en masse* from time to time. A traditional opportunity for employers to treat their workers is by throwing a Christmas party or arranging an evening out at the pub. Whatever the vehicle, being together in a different, more relaxed context can change the energy dynamics of a group, usually in a positive way, as these people recognised:

> "I think we should dance more at [our community]. We used to dance in the big room and people would join in. We were together, not in a work way or a food way, but just having fun."

> "Mental and emotional energy could be increased by more stimulation in some areas – I do feel a bit stagnated sometimes. I think a start would be a regular games evening, so we have more fun. Storytelling sessions, reading aloud."

Celebration

Another aspect of play is celebration, whether it is the celebration of a particular achievement or just a way of creating solidarity within a group. Celebration is a particular feature of community-supported agriculture (CSA) schemes. CSA involves customers becoming 'members' of the scheme and thereby sharing in the financial or work responsibility involved in running a farm in return for a share of the produce, or simply the sense of greater association with the farm. Whilst the organisation of CSA schemes varies from place to place, part of the idea behind them is to build a network of supportive individuals who can help sustain the farmer through being more understanding of the seasonal variations and risks inherent in farming. Organised celebrations are a wonderful way for farmers not only to say thank you for the support from which they have benefited, but also to reinforce the social connections between members of the CSA, thus building community.

EarthShare CSA in north-east Scotland organise the Tattie Festival to celebrate the end of the potato harvest in October and in the summer, subscribers get together to enjoy strawberries, cream and cucumber sandwiches at the annual garden party. At Stroud Community Agriculture, a monthly social event is organised to bring members together. This has resulted in new friendships forming over activities such as barbecues, harvest supper, bonfire night and snail races! Even CSA schemes which are less hands on than EarthShare or Stroud CSA have events which bring together subscribers. Plaw Hatch and Tablehurst Biodynamic farms in East Sussex organise an annual barn dance for the 400 shareholders who helped them to raise capital to buy their land. Since there is no arrangement at this CSA scheme for shareholders to receive the farms' produce free of charge or at a discount, events such as the barn dance, open days and farm walks are an important part of building the sense of being part of a valued community enterprise.

Celebration is a way of expressing gratitude, not only to people but to the Universe, or God if you're a believer, for the abundance of produce that springs forth from the Earth. It is a way of acknowledging the things that have gone well, as an antidote to the awareness of things that have gone wrong. It is easy not to notice the success of systems (whether they are a marketing scheme or a yoghurt-making operation) when they are working well, because they are simply doing what they are designed to do. Problems, when they occur, are more noteworthy since they demand attention, yet usually only happen occasionally compared with the majority of the time when the system is running smoothly. Hence, making a conscious decision to celebrate the satisfactory day-to-day running of a project can raise morale amongst those involved, as well as acknowledge the fortune that has prevented potential problems from arising. People love traditions, so creating a particular annual celebration which is unique to your project is likely to attract a loyal following amongst fellow workers, community members or customers. A regular fixture on the calendar of all those associated with the community of Steward Wood is their annual party, which celebrates the anniversary of the group purchase of the land. It involves a camp fire, food, singing and an opportunity for visitors to see whatever new developments the last year has brought forth.

Celebrations can also be a way of building links with the wider community and letting them know what goes on at your farm. In recent years, the celebration of Apple Day on the 21st October has raised awareness of the diversity of apples that are available from UK orchards. Members of the public are invited to apple tastings and identification sessions at fruit farms or gardens, where they are able to walk around the orchards or watch a cider press in action. Whilst living in Somerset and Kent, I attended several Wassailing Ceremonies in January, where apple trees are doused in cider to encourage them to fruit well and evil spirits are driven out by making a racket with whatever instruments or voices are available! Wassailing is an ancient tradition with a host of songs and apple-related drinks to go with it, and shows the deeply engrained human need to link social festivities to the agricultural year.

Lanza del Vasto, who founded the L'Arche communities, considered celebration to be central as an ingredient for keeping communities together and established a culture of celebration which lasts to this day. Those who take part in haymaking at La Borie Noble mark the end of each day's work bringing in the hay by sitting in a circle and sharing wine, nuts and other treats. Throughout the year traditional festivals such as Easter, Christmas and Summer Solstice are celebrated, alongside customs concocted within the communities, such as Women's Day and Men's Day, which involve a special day of events being organised by the opposite sex to provide fun and relaxation.

Festivals, whether they are public ones such as Christmas, New Year or Bank Holidays, or annual celebrations which are unique to a particular project, have an important role as markers, punctuating the year. By forcing people to step out of their usual routine and take a day off, they create a space to reflect on the time that has passed since last year's festival and the progress, losses, joys and grief which have been experienced within that window of time. The increased intensity of activity around a festival such as Christmas, both in trading produce and socialising with family and friends, may make it hard to find time to reflect. However, there are numerous other opportunities to create a quieter space for reflective celebration. A beautiful little book by Glennie Kindred, called *The Earth's Cycle of*

Celebration, offers a host of ideas for seasonal celebrations based on the Celtic Calendar.[9] Whatever your spiritual beliefs, the annual cycle of growth and decay which takes place on the land, provides a wonderful framework for creating private or group celebrations which can help reconnect us with the passing of time.

Blurring the boundaries

Over the years I have had various discussions with friends about the importance of leisure time and days off. Several people have held the view that the division between work and leisure is an artificial construct, and that within their chosen lifestyle work is leisure since it is enjoyable and fulfilling. As a fruit-grower once told me, "I have a true peasant attitude. I work all day in the orchard and then I return to work there in the evening because I enjoy it." I have discovered that they are not alone in this view as I have delved more deeply into the characteristics of people who are successful at sustaining their physical, mental and emotional energy.

Although Patrick Rivers and his wife Shirley devised the concept of 'Special Days', described earlier in this chapter, they found that their self-sufficient lifestyle led to the division between work and leisure becoming so blurred that it almost disappeared. As Patrick says,

> "I used to think that work was essentially an activity you were paid for and reluctantly performed usually between set hours – say nine to five – between Monday and Friday; that it was useful; and that you went away from home to do it. Now I'm not so sure. Most of my work earns us no money; I do it at any hour of the day, and day of the week; much of it I enjoy more than my previous 'leisure'; all of it I do within the farm boundary, and often alongside Shirley and other people of my own choice. Moreover, its end product is unquestionably useful. There is no set time for 'leisure'. Certainly there is time for doing what we want to do, but if what we want to do is as likely to be planting some crop as reading the paper or planting some flowers, how can we split our lives on two? And even though it has become an imposed convention to do so, just how natural, we ask, is such a split life for any species? We have found that the way we live uses all of ourselves: our heads, hearts and bodies and this is surely a very healthy way."[10]

The psychologist Marshall B. Rosenburg advises readers in his book, *Nonviolent Communication: A language of life*, "Don't do anything that isn't play."[11] Whilst this may seem a radical, if not irresponsible, statement to make, when its meaning is explored further it can be seen as a recipe for leading a happy and fulfilled life. For what Rosenburg means is that actions motivated purely by our desire to contribute to life, rather than out of fear, guilt, shame, duty or obligation, will lead to enrichment. In his words, "When the soul energy that motivates us is simply to make life wonderful for others and ourselves, then even hard work has an element of play in it. Correspondingly, an otherwise joyful activity performed out of obligation, duty, fear, guilt or shame will lose its joy and engender resistance." Such an idea echoes the observation made by Patrick Rivers that, "We have found, paradoxically, that the more seriously we take any activity, the more fun there is to be had from it." [12]

A delightful passage from a book about peasant smallholders in the Dordogne region of France in the 1930s, illustrates how this blurring of the boundaries between work and leisure is a characteristic of traditional rural life. It describes how a spontaneous social gathering occurred at the house and inn of a particular woman, Clelie, at corn-husking time: "Such a gathering of folk is normal here. That is the way in which work (many kinds of it) gets done by co-operative amusement, for such it is. No one was asked to come and work at a price per hour. No one was asked to help at all. One by one, Clelie's clients, as they came in for refreshment or a chat, proceeded to join in, contributing a joke or a story or a little piece of news as well as a pair of hands." [13]

Perhaps this attitude of turning work into an agreeable social occasion helps explain why, even though manual labour made tasks more onerous and time-consuming prior to the availability of oil, traditional rural cultures were able to sustain themselves for many hundreds and thousands of years. Certainly the adage 'Many hands make light work' rings as true today as it did in the 1930s and I'm sure I'm not the only one to have experienced the joy of accomplishing a large task in the company of friends or community members. A memorable example is when a group of the younger people in the Vallée de Mérens, in the French Pyrenees, gathered together to dig the garden of the family I was staying with at the time. Despite not being able to understand much of the relaxed banter between the French diggers, time seemed fly by in the merry and energised atmosphere. At lunchtime and in the evening we were rewarded with a feast, washed down by home-made cider.

Which brings us back to the Findhorn motto, 'If it is not fun, it is not sustainable.' As Dr. Chris Johnstone notes in his book, *Find your Power*, "Personal power is sometimes associated with images of strict discipline, grim determination and self-denial. If the process of improving our lives, work or world gets too grim, we won't last the course. To stick with a journey of change, it needs to be attractive to us. Making what we do enjoyable is therefore deeply pragmatic." [14] He outlines a number of principles which can help bring joy into an activity, including breaking tasks into smaller chunks so you can experience 'mini-victories' every day, watching for when your enthusiasm for a task starts to wane as a signal that you need a break, and finding the right level of company to turn a drudge into an enjoyable social occasion.

Engaging the spirit

In exploring the subject of the relationship between work, rest and play, the spiritual source of energy is a theme that arises repeatedly. It seems that the energy which gives us the power and enthusiasm to live life to the full, to be able to offer help and achieve our aspirations, is a life force that needs to be nurtured and fed. It is almost as if such energy is a divine gift, which if treasured will multiply, but will wither and disappear if neglected and abused. The secret to sustaining your energy, therefore, lies in being in touch with its spiritual source, whether you believe it to be the internal essence of who you are or an external God or interconnective force that flows throughout all living ecosystems.[15] By taking time to understand and become engaged with that which motivates you at a deeper level, you will gain the power to sustain yourself through the day-to-day demands and challenges that life throws up.

This is perhaps one reason why those communities which are centred on a shared spiritual belief system tend to be the ones that endure over time. Whether it is simply because of the spiritual practices, such as meditation, prayer and celebration, which keep people in touch with the source of their energy, or a supernatural power guiding and protecting them is not for me to judge. However, whether it is an overtly religious or very grounded love of humanity and nature, it seems that engaging with the spirit is an important component of land-based initiatives that hope to endure over time.

Chapter Thirteen

Surviving or Thriving?

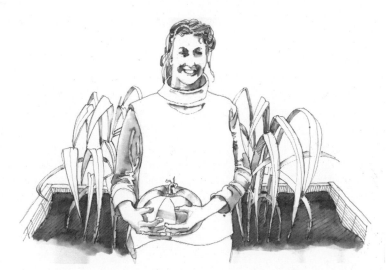

The ultimate aim of any long-term project is that it will not only survive, but thrive. In contrast to the concept of surviving, which means 'continuing to live or exist, to be still alive or existent', the word 'thriving' implies growth, prosperity and enjoyment.[1] It is vital that any scheme which has sustainability at its heart provides the people running it with a quality of life that enables them to grow and flourish in body, mind and spirit. Not only that, but it must provide a level of enjoyment that makes involvement a more attractive proposition than other, competing opportunities. As I have said before, 'If it is not fun, it is not sustainable.'

Although on the surface it may seem clear which case studies are doing well and which are struggling, to categorise them definitively is more difficult. The places I visited are so diverse that one is not comparing like with like. Their objectives range from providing food for the local community via an economically viable business, to minimising personal environmental impacts by living communally and being wholly or partially self-sufficient. People's priorities and measures of success therefore vary according to their aims.

In evaluating whether the smallholders I visited were surviving or thriving, I used the following as indicators of success:

- Level of sustainability – Use of resources (energy, soil, water), emissions of greenhouse gases, conservation of biodiversity.

- Quality of life – Time spent with family, health, independence, security, pleasant environment, enjoyment.

- Economic viability – Are businesses breaking even? Are subsistence needs met by land-based activities? Is project as a whole generating a surplus (of money, food, timber etc.) or is it running into debt?

- Longevity of Project – How many years has smallholder been operating? How long do they think they will continue to live like this?

- Successors – Do the children of the smallholder wish to live and work on the land?

For those living in a community, other measures of success will also apply. The levels of harmony, trust and communication between community members are good indicators of a functional community. The greater inter-dependence implied by sharing resources such as land, housing and equipment, means that stability is an important aim for those trying to live together.

Drawn together, these indicators add up to a general picture of whether the smallholding or community is doing really well, just getting by, or seriously in danger of having to be wound up.

Another consideration is the fact that projects and people's experiences change over time. From one month or year to the next a smallholding or community can move between a state of struggle and one of vitality and enjoyment. The passing seasons bring with them different pleasures and demands, whilst certain phases in life bring with them greater challenges than others. My visits to each smallholding enabled me to observe them at one point in time, but evaluation of their success at sustaining human energy relies on a longer-term perspective. It should also be noted, that my analysis in this chapter reflects my interpretation of how each project was faring. In retrospect, it would have been interesting to ask each interviewee whether they felt they were surviving or thriving, but in the absence of that question I have had to deduce an answer from observation and the interviews.

Thriving

Only a few projects stood out as thriving on all fronts at the time of my visit. They include Mulberry Tree Farm, Fivepenny Farm, Dun Beag, and the Trading Post. Some had clearly flourished over a long period, but were looking for new directions as old age approached, while others, although going through temporary difficult patches showed promise of becoming successful and happy places to live and work. Examples of the former are Longmeadow, Tamarisk Farm, Sea Spring Farm and Laurieston Hall, while the latter are represented by Pentiddy Woodland Project, Tinker's Bubble and Keveral Farm. Like people, every project has its ups and downs, and it would be unrealistic to expect them to operate at their optimal level all the time. A better measure of success is stability – whether those running the smallholding have the resilience to bounce back from temporary periods of stress, conflict, ill health or financial hardship. The fact that four of the projects listed above were still thriving after 20 years or more is a sign of stability.

Long-lasting success

The nine-acre holding at Longmeadow has provided a reliable full-time income for Hugh and Patsy Chapman since 1986. They have produced a significant volume of organic vegetables for local people and sold them through their box scheme (140 boxes per week), wholesale deliveries to shops and restaurants, and latterly their farm shop. Compared with other holdings in my study, the Chapmans use a relatively high degree of mechanisation to cultivate 6.5 acres of vegetables each season. Cultivation, some weed-control, transplanting, irrigation and mowing all involve diesel or electricity to provide power. During the early years, the Chapmans combined their work with raising two children, and latterly have inspired and trained up at least three of the next generation of organic growers. At times, the relentless hard work and stress have led to temporary illness and injury, but through measures such as stopping the box scheme for three months during the 'hungry gap' (March-May), they have been able to sustain their energy and enthusiasm. Other factors contributing to their success include their disciplined and orderly approach to work, the fact they live on site, having a supportive organic farmer next door, and their ability to make decisions without referring to a group.

Arthur and Josephine Pearse, who have been farming at Tamarisk Farm since 1960, have the distinction of having attracted two of their children back to the land, both of whom have now been farming in their own right for over 20 years. In the early years, while Arthur worked as a sociology lecturer and managed the market garden in his spare time, Josephine ran the farm and raised six children. Over the decades the mixture of enterprises at Tamarisk Farm has varied, and has included arable, pigs, milking goats, vegetables, sheep, cattle and holiday cottages. Having another source of income (Arthur's lecturing) allowed the Pearses to let the farm evolve according to the time and energy they had available. Significant thresholds, such as the children going to school, Arthur's retirement from lecturing, and the return of their daughter Ellen and her husband Adam to farm in partnership with her parents, coincided with developments in the business. For example, after Arthur's retirement a vegetable box scheme was started, intensifying production in the market garden for nine years, until age and ill health led them to a less demanding way of selling the vegetables. The close proximity of extended family has created an invaluable support network, enabling a diverse range of farming activities to be closely integrated with child-care.

Although from the same family, and operating in the same village, Joy Michaud (née Pearse) and her husband Michael have ploughed an independent furrow at Sea Spring Farm. Adaptability, specialisation and a blend of land- and non-land-based incomes, are the keys to their staying power over 22 years. When general market gardening proved insufficiently profitable, Michael worked as a Soil Association inspector and later Joy began editing for the organic press. In 1996 they started 'Peppers by Post', their mail order chilli pepper company, which has gone from strength to strength, and Michael has diversified into running courses and horticultural journalism. Meanwhile, in response to a need for a horticultural photo library, Joy has branched out again and combines this with her editing work and cultivating, picking and packing peppers.

The longevity of Laurieston Hall community, which was established in 1972, can also be ascribed in part to its combination of adaptability and a disciplined, orderly approach. When communal living became too intense during the mid-1980s, they reorganised to enable people to live in family households or smaller, communal units. Thus, the hub of communal activity shifted from living to working. Over the years, the emphasis of the residential camps and courses run by the People Centre has changed according to demand. In the 1970s they were mainly political (women's lib, gay weeks and anarchist camps), moving during the 1980s to become more therapy orientated, and in the 1990s towards dance camps and holidays mixed with occasional conferences. After 30 years of honing, the People Centre is run efficiently by a core group of six, and provides casual paid work for other community members. The management of the livestock, the vegetable garden, the firewood, the hydroelectricity and the maintenance of the buildings rely on the careful division of labour between members of the community during their weekly workdays (2.5 per week). The place appeared to work like clockwork, but during my visit I was aware of a level of concern about how this scale of work could be continued as they all grew older, and whether the current structure could attract younger people.

Another long-lasting community, in the wider sense of the word, is composed of the individual smallholders who lived in the Vallée de Mérens in the Pyrenees. Since 1978, individuals, couples and families have colonised old stone farm buildings and established a network of independent, yet co-operating, self-sufficient smallholdings. Although most people there are motivated by a desire to live a simple, ecologically sound life, they are not ruled by a collective dogma and are free to earn their living and manage their land however they choose. Hence, a subsistence lifestyle can be supplemented to a greater or lesser degree by other income-generating activities. Whilst enjoying a higher level of individual freedom than people in other communities, when support was needed in times of trouble, hard work or to celebrate a joyful event, such as a birth, I witnessed the community pulling together as one. The beautiful surroundings, combination of freedom and community, and subsistence opportunities, contribute to a high quality of life, which is attracting a second generation of younger people to remain in, or move to the valley. Sadly, in the stricter planning environment of the UK, it would be hard to replicate this model of land-based living.

A bright future awaits

The Trading Post (1999), Mulberry Tree Farm (2001) and Fivepenny Farm (2003) are more recently established, but all appear to have positive futures due to their dynamic approaches to meeting the need for local, organic food. Each combines successful commercial elements, of varying scales, working co-operatively with others and a degree of low-impact development. They are all driven by a strong vision, shared and deeply held by those responsible for both the decision-making and the bulk of the work. However, they are also flexible enough to adapt to new opportunities and challenges. Although many of the skills they have needed have been learnt 'on the job', each individual brought relevant experiences of low-impact living, marketing, gardening or eco-building. Also driven by vision is David Blair, who has developed his permaculture project, Dun Beag, with the intermittent help of others since 1995. Despite initial local opposition, planning obstacles and a fire which destroyed his home in 2006, he has maintained an optimistic, flexible and relaxed attitude to managing his 30 acres of Atlantic oak woodland, adding value to Sitka spruce and minimising his personal ecological impact.

Flourishing communities

Keveral Farm, Brithdir Mawr and Tinker's Bubble have all experienced periods of turmoil and instability, but I am left with a feeling of optimism that all three will endure. Forging independent, and often strong-willed, characters into a cohesive body to achieve lasting change is not easy. Despite the theoretical benefits of collective action – a greater pool of skills, more people to do the work, shared resources and responsibility, and sense of belonging – the reality all too often involves long meetings, heated discussions and disillusionment. Added to these challenges, each of these communities has faced local opposition and lengthy planning battles in their attempts to provide affordable opportunities for people to live and work on the land in a low-impact way. Each has overcome these challenges to become a vibrant community, where small-scale, land-based enterprises can thrive. At Keveral Farm, the change from the collectively run box scheme to a system of private rental of plots of land has given individuals more control over their livelihoods. Debate at Brithdir Mawr centred on differences in the ways people approached low-impact living. The division of the land into three separate holdings has allowed some to engage in a simpler, more spiritual existence and avoid electricity altogether, while others live more mainstream lifestyles, using electrical appliances powered with renewable energy and producing a proportion of their food and fuel from the land.

I was unable to visit the two community-supported agriculture schemes, Earthshares and Stroud Community Agriculture, but both appeared to be thriving. I would attribute this to the fact that the responsibility and work of running the schemes was shared between the producers and consumers in a way which enabled each to be very clear of their roles. In addition, the emphasis on social events and the sense of belonging to a supportive community which is working towards a common goal (growing and distributing fresh, locally grown, affordable organic food) seemed to contribute to generally high morale.

Successful in parts

An element of compromise was present in all of the projects I visited, but in some this was more marked than in others. It is easier to be successful in certain areas if you are willing to be more relaxed about other principles, and this pragmatic approach had been taken by several of the communities and smallholdings.

For example, Steward Wood and Brockhurst are highly successful as communities, but less emphasis is placed on earning a land-based livelihood. Both demonstrate many of the best features of living with others, including a friendly, harmonious and supportive social network, clear communication and the sharing of facilities and responsibility. However, although they are meeting some of their subsistence needs (some vegetables, eggs and firewood) from the land, most residents still derive a large proportion of their income from non-land-based sources. Both communities have several members whose primary responsibility is caring for small children, meaning that family time, a stable income and ease of cutting fire-wood to keep the home warm are high priorities. Living communally enables them to co-operate and thereby reduce their ecological impact, but compromises between principles and pragmatism are a daily reality.

Steward Wood focuses on low-impact living and generating electricity using simple and small-scale, renewable technologies. Over the eight years since the community was established in a Devon woodland, they have built their own simple homes using local and recycled materials, used only wood for heating and cooking, and curbed their electricity use to that which they can generate themselves. A significant development was the decision to compromise their policy of not using fossil fuels, to allow a chainsaw to be used for cross-cutting firewood. An independent study of Steward Wood's environmental impact, calculates that the average ecological footprint of a resident is 2.05 global hectares (gha), which is 39% of the typical footprint of a UK citizen (5.29 gha).[2]

The community estimates that about 65% of their basic needs are met by subsistence.[3] However, although increasing quantities of vegetables are grown each year and they now keep hens for egg production, a large pro-portion of their food is still bought in. Furthermore, at the time of my visit, few residents were earning their living on-site directly from land-based activ-ities. Instead, they are 'selling' their experience of low-impact, subsistence liv-ing, by running courses on renewable energy, low-impact building, bush craft and permaculture design. In the future they aim to generate livelihoods from a diverse range of direct and indirect land-based activities (courses, forestry products, vegetables and eggs), and employment within the local community, for example teaching computer courses and work at a recycling centre. It could be argued that by influencing other people, through the courses they run and their integration with the local community, the community are hav-ing a more widespread positive effect on the environment than if they were solely occupied with earning a land-based livelihood.

At Brockhurst, the community is also gradually increasing the amount of food and energy it derives from the land, and now produces vegetables, fruit, eggs, goats' milk and cheese, to meet the community's needs for much of the year. Like Steward Wood, they are placing more emphasis on sub-sistence and environmental education, than on selling produce from the land. A grant from Cyd Coed, a fund aimed at opening up woodlands to the public, has enabled them to improve footpaths and build a roundhouse and a 'welcome shelter' in which to host school groups. These facilities will make it possible to run green-woodworking courses and forest school ses-sions, with classes from local schools. I find it interesting that, in the absence of the financial and time pressures of running a farming business, both Steward Wood and Brockhurst were able to focus more effort on low-impact living and community cohesion.

On the other hand, some of the couples and families running agricultural enterprises are living more mainstream lifestyles and buy much of their food, apart from the produce they specialise in, from elsewhere. An extreme example of this situation, which I have come across elsewhere, but not amongst the smallholders in my study, is where organic producers have such a low income and feel so pushed for time that they live on non-organic convenience food from the supermarket. Most smallholders I visited tried to supplement their own produce with other local and/or organic food. However, it commonly seems to be the case that smallholders focus either on subsistence production, supplemented by another income, or on fairly specialised commercial production which brings in sufficient income to pay for other goods and services. There just do not seem to be enough hours in the day for a single person or couple to operate all the elements of mixed subsistence smallholding (cow, pigs, chickens, vegetables, grains) and to operate a commercially competitive business. For a community, where different people can take responsibility for individual elements of a mixed system, it is easier to combine partial self-sufficiency with commercial production. However, then it becomes necessary to devote a greater proportion of time and energy into communication, group decision making and maintaining harmony.

Surviving

A number of projects I visited could be described as surviving rather than thriving, since current circumstances meant day-to-day life was an endurance test rather than a pleasure. Such circumstances included not being able to live on the land due to planning restrictions; chronic injury or illness; the stress of raising small children whilst establishing an ambitious low-impact project and unstable community dynamics.

Planning

The struggle to gain planning permission to live on the land is a common cause of stress among smallholders who cannot afford to buy land with existing accommodation. Among the twenty-eight projects I studied, at least twenty were affected in some way by planning issues. Most had succeeded in gaining planning permission after a lengthy appeals process, some had temporary permission and were currently having to prove the viability of their business, and two were struggling to manage their land whilst living in a nearby village.

These two smallholdings were seriously in danger of folding due to stress. Firstly, trying to run a land-based business when you do not live on site is even harder work than when you do live there, due to the number of jobs that need to be done throughout a very long day. For example, watering polytunnels and harvesting salad leaves need to be done early in the morning when it is cool, whilst hens need to be shut in at dusk, which can be as late as 9.30pm in the summer. Long hours are manageable if they can be integrated with domestic activities, but become exhausting and unsustainable if home is a long walk or a short drive away. Not living at the holding is particularly disruptive to family life, since sharing meals together and keeping an eye on small children whilst working, becomes virtually impossible. Secondly, the costs of living in an ordinary house (i.e. rent/mortgage, utility bills etc.) are out of proportion with the average income of self-employed land workers. Hence, it is usually necessary to maintain another source of income by working part-time or full-time elsewhere, thus reducing the amount of time available to work on the holding.

At one holding, the couple lived only a ten-minute walk away from their land, but the cost of servicing the mortgage on their house meant they had to keep a full-time and a part-time job on top of their vegetable and sheep business. Being split between two centres of operation, even only a ten-minute walk apart, meant that extra organisation was needed to ensure they had the right tools with them, and that none was left on the land due to risk of theft. They had to give up keeping chickens, due to not living close enough to be able to protect them from foxes. Furthermore, the long hours they worked during the summer to fit in around their other jobs meant they were seldom home in time to eat supper with their teenage daughter. They were on the brink of having to give up commercial vegetable-growing due to the mental and physical strain of juggling jobs and not being on hand to sort out emergencies when they arose. Yet their produce was in great demand, and the service they provided by growing affordable vegetables for local people would be sorely missed were they to give up.

Injury and illness

At the time of my visit, Gitta Wulf, who runs Les Jardins de Mondoux, was recovering from a back problem which had incapacitated her for much of the previous summer. There was a question-mark over whether she would be able to continue with her mixed farm, where she produces vegetables, eggs and bread made from home-grown and milled wheat. I was thus heartened to find out that, three years later, she and her husband are persevering with their project, having adapted it to lessen the strain on her back. She has reduced the area of her garden and started using black plastic mulch to prevent fallow beds and pathways becoming over-run with weeds. By sharing a market stall with a neighbouring organic grower she is able to specialise in tomatoes, salads and other light crops, thus avoid-

Box 13.1 – The Problem with Planning Policy

National planning policy does, in fact, allow for new dwellings to be built for agricultural, forestry and other rural workers, provided the business is financially viable and it is absolutely necessary for the functioning of the business that a worker lives on site.[4] Personal preferences or the circumstances of individuals, such as parenthood or a desire to live sustainably, are not deemed to be sufficient justification for a rural dwelling. In their zealous protection of the open countryside, development control planners rarely award planning permission for rural dwellings, since they are suspicious of people trying to speculate on land. However, their rigorous application of the functional and financial tests often results in bone fide projects, which would have contributed greatly to the sustainable development aims of planning policy in general, being refused permission.

As a result, some people move onto their land first, establish their agricultural or forestry project and then apply retrospectively for planning permission. This approach is fraught with problems, since it is necessary to be discreet about where you live, there is often great local opposition to any new form of development, and there is the risk that refusal of planning permission and enforcement action could bring the whole project to a halt. The insecurity and stress of living in hiding can take quite a mental toll. The opposition to new rural developments, especially when they are surrounded by rumours and misunderstanding, can be vehement, personal and very unpleasant. It can take years to break down barriers, become accepted by neighbours as a valued part of the community and demonstrate that you are not a threat, but a potential asset to the area. Finally, the paperwork, expense and emotional demands involved in trying to gain planning permission create huge amounts of pressure and take up weeks of time that could be spent working on the land. For those projects that had had a struggle to gain planning permission, this was considered to have been the most stressful aspect of establishing the business.

ing too much digging, and focus more on egg and wheat production. Gitta's husband, David, works abroad as an engineer for two or three months per year, bringing in a supplementary income which pays for the development of the farm.

Even the most stable of farms can be caused to struggle by an injury that puts a key person temporarily out of action. As I was finishing this book, Ellen Simon, at Tamarisk Farm, broke her leg badly just as lambing was beginning. Hence, her husband Adam had to manage alone throughout much of the spring and summer. Fortunately a support network of family, friends and workers from the adjoining market garden were able to help when extra people were needed, but he missed Ellen's skills and judgement for many of the more specialised jobs. Furthermore, there is only so much you can encroach upon other people's time, and to make up for Ellen's absence he has had to work longer hours than usual during this particularly busy time of year. Although working longer hours is manageable for a limited time, sustained lack of sleep over a period of two to three months can wear down even the healthiest of people.

Two of the smallholders who were working alone also appeared to be working absurdly long hours, to ensure that their businesses proved their financial viability to the planning authorities. One was getting up to start work at 4am in the summer, and during the year of my interview became seriously ill for a time, while the other resented the fact that despite producing organic food he was eating unhealthily, because he rarely had time or energy to cook himself decent meals at the end of a day's work. Both seemed lonely, and at the time of their interviews were wondering how long they could continue. However, two years later they are both still in operation and one considers that she is now thriving. She told me,

> "There are good years and bad years. It's about holding on through the rough patches and believing that it will get better. Even at its grimmest, I remind myself, I'm not hungry, I still have fire, and I still have friends. I have total belief in the way I live, and it brings me pure joy."

Young families and young projects

The establishment of any smallholding, particularly from scratch (i.e. building the home as well as managing the land) is hard work. When this coincides with the early years of parenthood, the demands can seem gruelling. Two couples among the case studies were finding the simultaneous demands of small children, developing a holding and earning a living pretty tough at the time of my interview. In both cases, the mother, who was doing the majority of child-care, was feeling frustrated that she was able to achieve very little land-based work. The fathers were trying to offer support, but also needed to continue developing the infrastructure of the holdings and earning a living. Add to this the exhaustion caused by regularly disturbed nights and two-year-old tantrums, and the stress escalates pretty quickly.

At Fivepenny Farm, Olly tries to work in the garden early in the morning and late at night, while the children are asleep, so he can spend time with the family during the day. He also recommended that parents save money with which to pay extra workers when the children are small, to free up more time to spend with them. For women, to be financially dependent on a partner, and limited in the number of practical things you can do, is disempowering. One of the benefits of communities is that child-care can be shared more easily, but for couples it is equally important that from an early stage the mother is able to participate in work other than child-care. In these cases, both couples acknowledged that their troubles were temporary, and would ease as they learned better how to combine child-care with their land work. As I finish this book I am happy to report that life is easier for them.

Community dynamics

The most recently established of the communities, La Sorga (2002), in the Dordogne region of France, still appeared to be somewhat unstable when I contacted them three years after my visit. Previously they had a relaxed policy of welcoming everyone, and asking for voluntary donations of work and money. Two of its original members remained, but they had had troubles with people coming and going and not contributing enough to the project, which caused conflict and almost led to its collapse. To protect themselves from exploitation, the founders have introduced a trial period for people who want to join the community. They have also agreed that all members will work six to eight hours per day, and contribute 100 euros per month or at least one third of their income towards communal expenses. The introduction of these basic rules means the community has survived those difficult times and is now feeling positive about the future.

When enough is enough

Sadly, the stresses and strains of living and working on the land sometimes cause people to give up and seek an easier way of life. This can be intensely disappointing, because such a change of lifestyle usually involves relinquishing long-held dreams. There is rarely one single cause of people deciding to stop, but rather a collection of contributing factors, one of which may finally tip the balance.

Among the people I interviewed, only one smallholder had had to give up completely. Sue Williams, of Meadows Farm in Dorset, kindly agreed to talk to me about why she and her husband had decided to call it a day with their market-gardening business in 1994. For eight years they rented 18 acres about five miles from the town where they lived, and grew field-scale organic vegetables, as well as keeping a few pigs. The smallholding was their main livelihood, and they sold their produce at a twice-weekly market stall in the town. During the summer they would camp on the holding, but most of the year they had to live in town, since there was no residential planning permission, mains water supply or electricity at the land. This in itself put both a practical and a financial strain on the family, because it was necessary for the holding to generate enough to cover their mortgage and utility bills, as well as running two vehicles. From a practical perspective, living five miles from the holding meant the Williams either had to spend very long working days at the holding, or drive to and fro several times per day in order to balance work and family life.

During the early years, the couple's children were small and were happy to spend their spare time playing in the field while their parents worked, but on rainy, winter days, and as they became teenagers, they wanted to stay in town more. It was often not worth Sue returning to the holding after she had collected the children from school, and her husband, Richard, often found himself working alone. Although a tractor was used to cultivate up to eleven acres of vegetables, a high labour input was still necessary, and left to cope alone for long periods of time, Richard found it hard to keep on top of the weeds. Had they lived on site, it would have been possible to leave the children inside, but keep an eye on them whilst continuing to work. They would also have found it easier to host WWOOFers or, due to reduced overheads, have been able to employ people to help. Another problem, which arose from living at a distance from the holding, was not being present to deal with emergencies, such as escaped pigs, meaning that the animals had usually travelled a considerable distance by the time they were discovered. Security was another issue, and a number of petty thefts meant it was necessary for all valuable equipment to be transported home each night. As Sue said, "It was just very tiring, like fighting a losing battle."

Eventually it became necessary for both Sue and Richard to supplement their income with other jobs and although they kept going with the market stall, they stopped growing the vegetables and bought from a wholesaler instead. However, their customers started to dwindle, especially after a new supermarket opened on the outskirts of the town, and finally they stopped trading altogether. Sue identifies a number of factors having contributed to the demise of their business, but feels that not being able to live on site and the lack of finance were the two main problems. From a historical perspective, the early 1990s were a hard time for organic growers nationally, since an economic recession temporarily curtailed the growth of the organic market. However, being unable afford a smallholding with an existing house, and being prohibited, by local planning authorities, from living on site is a problem that continues to have a negative impact on many potentially successful rural businesses.

For Simon Sleigh and Jennie Gettens of Little Farm, a chronic back problem was a major factor that led to their having to dramatically scale back their vegetable enterprise. They were able to afford a house with eight acres of land, due to having had a well-paid career and some capital, but this meant that they were older when they started their growing enterprise. For eight years they ran a very successful, all-year-round box scheme (over 100 boxes per week), selling vegetables grown on up to four acres, with no other workers except their trusty David Brown tractor. Theirs was the first box scheme in their area and it proved very popular, as well as being financially sustainable. However, when Jennie developed a back problem, Simon

Box 13.2 – Tips for successful smallholder relationships

- Before you embark, make sure that you both want a similar outcome from your life on the holding, and speak regularly about progress towards, and threats to, this outcome.
- Don't get too wrapped up in the holding and its needs. Try to develop the ability to maintain perspective under pressure.
- Make sure that the decisions on the holding are joint decisions.
- Find time to talk and listen – even when the needs of children and the holding seem pressing. Not listening and talking could jeopardise everything that both of you are trying for. If you can remember this before a conflict arises, it can be enough to make you realise that the docks/greenhouse/fence really can wait, otherwise you might end up with none of the above!
- Take a break. Go away to somewhere special for both of you and get friends to come and keep an eye on the place. When you get back, your friends will tell you how wonderful your place is and you'll have had time to realise how wonderful you both are and what you have to lose.
- When personal trouble does loom, try to use the plus points of the holding to diffuse it rather than allow the negative points of the holding to escalate it. Use the holding as a source of strength, not weakness in your relationship (go sit in a favourite tree together, spend time feeding the chickens together, jump in the pond together, with children in tow too).
- Don't lose sight of the fact that you are doing this for emotional fulfilment!

was left alone to do all of the heavy work and found himself working longer and longer hours. After two years of working alone, Simon found that the continuous stress and exhaustion were affecting his health and taking the enjoyment out of the growing. Now, they no longer run the box scheme, but still grow some vegetables, which they sell at farmers' markets, and Simon has another job as a social worker assistant. Although it was difficult deciding to stop the box scheme, since they had to admit that their dream of earning a land-based livelihood wasn't working, now the pressure is off, Jennie's back is better and they are able to enjoy the holding in a more relaxed way. However, they feel uneasy about not using their land efficiently and are searching for ideas to develop its potential in a less physically demanding way.

Sometimes just one of a couple decides that enough is enough, while the other remains committed to the dream of living on the land. The precise circumstances that lead to smallholders' splitting up vary, but often frustrations relating to the land get confused with problems in the relationship. I have observed that the pressures of caring for children under the age of two, in combination with the day-to-day realities of living a low-impact rural lifestyle, especially in the winter, can lead to relationships crumbling. Babies and toddlers, especially when they cause sleepless nights and are prone to tantrums, seem to magnify the cracks in a relationship. When the mother is feeling disempowered, because she is unable to earn a living and is dependent on her partner, and the father is having to shoulder many of the, previously shared, practical tasks alone, tempers can quickly become frayed. Ideally, clear communication will lead to a solution, such as the father taking on more of the child-care so the mother can contribute work on the land. Sadly, clouded by exhaustion, conflicts sometimes escalate to a point when they become unbearable, and one person decides to leave.

In a functional community or extended family, that situation can be relieved by a support network of friends, who can help with child-care, cut firewood, cook meals and lend a sympathetic ear at times of acute stress. This need not be an intentional community, but such a support network does need to be easily accessible, rather than geographically distant, to be able to offer the necessary practical support. Conflicting objectives within a community who have decided to share land can cause serious stress themselves, and lead to disillusionment. I came across several people who had left communities because their needs were not being met or their aspirations were stifled by the group process. For most of these people, however, leaving the community and setting up alone was viewed as a positive natural progression, rather than a sign that the community had somehow failed.

There are usually several, interlinked causes for a smallholding failing to thrive, but it is possible to identify a number of individual factors which have contributed to the struggles of the projects discussed above. Likewise, by observing successful smallholders at work, and analysing their answers to my questions, I have identified certain ingredients for not only surviving, but thriving. These stumbling-blocks and keys to success are summarised below in table 13.1.

Significant stumbling-blocks	Keys to success
Loneliness and isolation	Positive and relaxed, 'can do' attitude
Low food prices not covering labour costs	Adaptability and flexibility
Long hours lead to exhaustion	Tidiness and efficiency
Injury and illness	Clear roles and delegation of responsibility
The demands of small children	Keeping the 'day job'
Conflict within communities or couples	Trust and communication
Stress caused by bureaucracy	Integration with the wider community
Logistics of having to live off-site	

Table 13.1 – Significant stumbling-blocks and keys to success.

Overcoming the obstacles

Despite the growing urgency to find ways for people to radically reduce their carbon emissions and fossil-fuel dependence, there are a number of significant barriers that are stopping people from returning to the land. They include:

- A scarcity of affordable small farms and housing with sufficient land for self-sufficiency.

- Strict application of planning policy

- Lack of skills to carry out efficient manual work

- A culture of individualism which makes it hard to co-operate effectively

- The times when stress, exhaustion and ill health outweigh the enjoyment of living and working on the land.

None of these barriers is insurmountable, but they require the combined efforts of individuals, local communities and national government to be overcome.

Affordability of land and accommodation

Unlike during the 1960s and 1970s, when the first wave of 'back to the landers' was in full flood, there are now few abandoned farm labourers' cottages, let alone small farms, available for less than £250,000, even in more remote parts of the UK. Buying a house with sufficient land to provide for subsistence needs, or to set up a land-based business, is now beyond the means of a large proportion of the population. However, people are finding other ways to access land and low-cost housing. Three possible options are, the collective purchase of farms or land, the establishment of community-led CSA schemes, and buying a bare land-holding on which to set up a smallholding from scratch.

Groups of people, who alone would be unable to afford a farm, are pooling their resources to buy land and smallholdings which they will manage collectively. Once a significant proportion of the finance has been raised, it is often possible to draw in further finance through loans from family, friends and ethical banks. Mechanisms such as loan stock, a form of fixed term loan devised by Catalyst Collective to help co-operatives raise finance, are a useful way of formalising loans from family and friends who wish to support an initiative.[5] People buying land together would also be wise to invest considerable time prior to buying land in discussing their aspirations, agreeing on a legal structure and finding a method of conflict resolution. The most stable communities and group land projects I encountered were those which shared a vision, had built a deep level of trust and communication and had invested time at the beginning in choosing an appropriate legal structure.

Until fairly recently, the price of an acre of agricultural land or woodland was within the means of many people. Even now (in 2008), when it has risen to over £5,000 per acre, land without buildings is a fraction of the price of land on which there is a house, or simply planning permission for a house. A number of the case studies featured here bought bare-land holdings, and built up the necessary infrastructure for a smallholding from scratch.

Towards a more balanced approach to planning

There is an inherent tension within land-use planning policy, which seeks to simultaneously protect the natural environment and encourage economic activity. The two need not be mutually exclusive, as most of the smallholdings in this book demonstrate. Indeed, the Government's current planning policy for rural areas (Planning Policy Statement 7) recommends that decisions on development proposals should ensure an integrated approach to social inclusion, protection and enhancement of the environment, prudent use of natural resources and maintaining high and stable levels of economic growth and employment.[6] However, planning policy, as currently applied at local level, emphasises protection of the countryside and reduction of road traffic, whilst viewing the efforts of smallholders as economically insignificant compared with large-scale farmers. People are viewed as predominantly consumers of resources, rather than being seen as potential producers of at least the resources they need for subsistence.

Small-scale, mixed enterprises that are producing food and other goods for local people in an environmentally sound way need to be recognised for the contribution they are making towards sustainable development, and allowed to live on their land, rather than being viewed as blots on the landscape. They can then not only minimise their car use and be present to attend to night-time emergencies, but meet their subsistence needs for food, fuel, rainwater harvest, renewable energy and timber from their land.

There is at least provision in planning policy for rural dwellings for people earning a full-time living from agriculture or forestry. For those wishing to retain an alternative part-time income, keep their hand in at some other occupation or supplement their subsistence production or land-based income, there is no such provision.

This dual-livelihood lifestyle was in evidence at the communities of Laurieston Hall, Keveral Farm, Brithdir Mawr and Mulberry Tree Farm. The quality of life experienced by residents at these places indicated that they were sustainable in terms of human energy, as well as being productive and environmentally sound. For example, half of the residents at Keveral Farm combine land-based occupations with other work. By living co-operatively and meeting many of their needs from the land individuals living there have succeeded in reducing their ecological footprints to 38% of the national average. One parent who lives at Keveral Farm said to me:

> "It's the ideal way to live in the countryside for people who want to grow their own food. You can share resources, help each other and share transport. Lots of farmers are isolated, bogged down by paperwork. I'm just surprised the Government doesn't do more to encourage it. It makes sense."

A more positive way to protect the countryside would be to recognise the contribution that smallholders can make towards achieving sustainable development. For over ten years, 'Chapter 7', the low-impact planning advisory organisation, has been lobbying central and local government for changes to planning policy which would encourage the practical manifestation of sustainable development. Their document, 'Fifteen Criteria for Sustainable Development' lists points which can be used by local planning authorities to distinguish between land speculators, and genuine smallholders and low-impact developers.[7] These points have been incorporated into policy by a handful of local authorities, but there is no national policy as yet which is equivalent to these local policies.

The art of manual labour

The age of abundant oil has done much to erode the ability of the average person living in Europe, the United States and Australia to carry out manual labour over a prolonged period. In fact, the majority of westerners are pretty feeble in comparison with our forebears, and lack the fitness, physical strength and technique to work manually at the speed necessary to be economically competitive. Through much of society, machines have replaced manual work, and even in poorer countries, those who can afford machines have been forced into using them in the name of global competitiveness. Many of the skills required to farm successfully without fossil fuels, which were honed by our forefathers over centuries, have been virtually wiped out since the 1940s. Although tractors were used on farms in the UK in the 1930s, the drive to increase food production after the second world war forced all farmers to become 'more efficient', with threats of land confiscation if they failed to modernise.

One decision facing smallholders today is what level of technology to use to manage their land. This will depend on their objectives, the scale of operation, the type of farming, whether subsistence or commercial production is planned, and the relative availability of labour and capital with which to buy machines. The replacement of agricultural machines with hand tools may be seen as foolish, commercially uncompetitive, and a romantic luxury to be enjoyed by the 'hobby farmer'. However, the small-holder, who combines thoughtful, energy-efficient design of their holding with lessons in how to use hand tools effectively, may find themselves in a secure position as the price of oil rises. For, whilst the terms 'unskilled labour' and 'manual labourer' are frequently used interchangeably, in the days when all labour was manual, farmers were capable of prodigious per-formance with the tools available to them. For example, the standard rate for mowing grass with a scythe was between one and two acres a day, while a good pair of foresters with an axe, bucksaw and team of horses could cut six cords (768 cu.ft) of timber in a day.[8]

Manual work relies as much on technique as on strength and fitness. After more than ten years of working on farms, I have developed a range of skills that my office-working peers lack. I have learnt not only some spe-cific manual skills, such as how to weed efficiently and to mow with a scythe, but also strategic skills. For example, significant time and energy can be saved when moving materials from one place to another by avoid-ing double handling. This may seem obvious, but the conscious application of such principles on the small scale – such as when building a compost heap – is often overlooked. The best way to learn how to use your body and mind to perform manual work is to get on and do it, whilst con-sciously studying how technique can be improved and jobs made easier.

Experience is a great teacher, but can be usefully supplemented with instruction from people with superior skills. People who worked the land with hand tools in the past are sometimes only too delighted to pass on their knowledge to the next generation. Meanwhile, growing interest in the use of traditional tools such as pole lathes, scythes and horse-drawn equipment is leading to courses of instruction becoming more widely available. There is little that can beat the satisfaction of completing a task by applying personal skill with a well-designed, properly adjusted hand tool and I would encourage anyone who has never had that experience to seek it out.

Working harmoniously with others

Working on the land requires co-operation with other people. Whether you opt to live in an intentional community, or to manage land individually, you will be connected into a web of interactions with your neighbours. In the past, when populations were more settled, villages had strong commu-nities of interdependent individuals. Even today, farmers are less mobile than the rest of the population, and traditional farming families tend to be deeply embedded in the local community as a result of decades or even generations of interactions with neighbours. The fact that the only places I visited where fossil fuels were not being used were self-sufficient communities indicates that co-operation is a prerequisite to reducing our dependence on oil. Living costs are less when you are collectively self-sufficient. Furthermore, subsistence production means it is less important to be commercially competitive, and therefore removes the necessity to use machines.

Within the wider community, farms and smallholdings may trade with each other, thereby building local economic resilience, help each other in emergencies and provide a supportive social network of like-minded people. A future involving more people working on the land, using less fossil fuels, to create local self-sufficiency is going to require a higher level of co-operation than exists at present.

However, the benefits of co-operation come at a price – loss of independence. This presents a significant challenge in a society where freedom and autonomy are highly valued by individuals. In this book, I have tried to present a menu of graded options for collective land-management, so that readers can choose the level of sharing and interdependence they feel comfortable with. At all levels of co-operation, good communication skills and trust are invaluable to overcome the hurdles of difference. Too often emotions, such as fear, greed and insecurity, threaten projects which are technically feasible.[9] If small-scale, organic food production on a network of farms and communities is to provide a significant solution to the problems of climate change and peak oil, smallholders need to make a conscious effort to learn the skills of co-operation and conflict resolution. Such skills are equally valuable to the farmer wanting to collaborate with others to sell produce to a larger market and the young family hoping to live in a self-sufficient community. The rewards, in terms of increased access to land or markets, affordable organic food, sense of belonging and joy through working together, are well worth the exertion.

Surviving the 'bottle-neck' periods

As I draw this book to a close, the busy season in my other job, market gardening, has come around again. I am reminded why I started research into how smallholders can sustain their human energy. Nature waits for nothing, except, perhaps, the weather. In the UK, April, May and June are the months when plants are growing at their fastest. For the market gardener this means seeds need to be sown, weeds are growing rapidly, threatening to swamp young vegetables, and dry, windy spells require more time to be spent watering. Every way you turn there are jobs requiring immediate attention. Other operations have their own 'bottleneck' periods. Lambing requires extra long hours, and sometimes night-time attendance.

Haymaking and grain harvest entail intense bouts of work, starting early and ending late, while the weather stays dry. For the coppice worker or hedge-layer, late winter becomes a race against time, as all work must be completed before the sap rises and the nesting season begins. Fortunately, the pleasures and excitement that attend these times compensate for the stress and lack of sleep, and the fact that they are finite means a less intense period is usually within view. The real challenge is to keep going when unforeseen circumstances compound a busy period, or when the busy period seems unending. For example, when an accident takes a key person out of action at a critical period or when multiple enterprises mean there is no let up between busy phases. It is at these times that the true sustainability of a project is really tested.

No matter how well-organised you seem to be during the slack periods of the year, there are always times when the number of things that need to be done seems greater than the time available to do them all. Like objects flowing through a narrow gap or bottleneck, fitting multiple tasks into a narrow time-frame requires the release of pressure, so they don't cause a blockage or a breakdown. One of the valuable lessons I have learnt is to take a step back when a situation gets stressful, and look at all the competing demands on my time from a wider perspective. The deliberate analysis of priorities usually shows the natural order in which jobs should be done, and eliminates those that are not necessary.

Another lesson has been the importance of acknowledging personal needs. The need to have a good night's sleep, regular breaks for refreshment and a dose of fun can easily be neglected during busy periods. Of course, it is sometimes necessary to compromise on these needs, but each person's level of tolerance to compromise will be different. People's personalities have a significant effect on their attitude to stress. Some thrive under pressure, and are not worried if jobs are not done perfectly, as long as they are done. Others like to get things right, and feel unhappy if they are forced to cut corners. Knowing your own limits, in terms of your desired levels of thoroughness, the amount of sleep you need, how you react when your blood-sugar levels are low and how often you need to take breaks from heavy labour, can help you to assert your needs. If you know that the consequence of overstepping your boundaries is a poor day's work the next day, illness, grouchiness or depression, then it will benefit not only you but those you work with, if you stay within your limits.

A more abstract mechanism for surviving the bottlenecks is to plan for unforeseen events or tasks that take longer than expected. If every hour is already accounted for, then there is little time margin for work to expand into, besides that which you need for resting, eating and spending time with friends and family. Frequent erosion of time set aside for meeting your own needs or those of your family can lead not only to exhaustion, illness and injury, but also resentment and conflict if those you love feel they are less important than your work. Realistic time-management, which acknowledges the likelihood of unforeseen events or problems, means that if everything does go according to plan you have the bonus of extra time left over either to do something else or to rest.

The ideal smallholding?

One lesson I have learnt whilst studying smallholdings is that there is no single recipe for sustaining human energy. Instead there are many ingredients that may be combined in a variety of ways to suit the needs of the individual – subsistence or commercial, machinery or hand tools, community or family farm? Then, there are trade-offs to be made between advantages and disadvantages of particular models. For example, communal living may create a wider pool of skills and readily available help, but it can make decision-making more complicated and lengthy. Earlier in this chapter I identified several of the features which distinguish projects which thrive from those that merely survive. To conclude my study of human energy I will describe the kind of smallholding I hope to establish as a result of my research. Of course, for other people with different aims, the details will vary.

As a single woman, wanting to grow organic vegetables and fruit to sell to local people, I would like to combine the benefits of managing my own land with the availability of a close support network of friends and neighbours. It is important to me, to be able to choose how to use my time efficiently and make decisions without referring to a meeting, yet to know that in an emergency or if I need to go away, there are people I could call on for help. I would also value the social aspect of being able to visit friends without having to drive, and perhaps being able to share meals on a weekly basis with a neighbour. This could be achieved by finding a smallholding that is close to people I already know, or in a locality with a culture of smallholders. Alternatively, such a situation could be created by buying a larger farm or plot of land with a group of people, and then dividing it into several smallholdings. I call this the 'cluster' model, since it combines the benefits of community with those of autonomous smallholdings, by creating geographically clustered holdings.

Ideally, my neighbours would be farming in a diversity of ways, and it would be possible to trade the goods in which we specialise, such as vegetables, dairy products, herbal remedies or woollen garments. It would also be possible to co-operate with them to market produce, for example by taking it in turns to tend a weekly market stall, or delegating crops to different growers to ensure that a delivery scheme has a wide range of vegetables, fruit and perhaps eggs or meat. Where I encountered box schemes on my journey, those who took a three-month break during the hungry gap (April to June) seemed to be better at sustaining their energy and enthusiasm than those who continued all through the year. Yet customers need to eat during the hungry gap, and may not want to revert to the supermarket to supply their vegetables. A coalition of neighbouring growers, such as that developing at Keveral Farm, would be able to maintain a continuous supply of produce, without putting the strain on a single person.

Other forms of co-operation could include monthly work parties to help each other with bigger, more daunting tasks, such as tree-planting, coppicing or hay-making. I would like to be able to steadily reduce my dependence on fossil fuels, by using horse-drawn tools for cultivating vegetables and using wood to cook with and heat my house. However, it would be hard to undertake haymaking or coppicing alone, without the use of machinery. It would be easier to rely solely on hand tools in a woodland collectively owned and managed by neighbouring smallholdings, where coppicing was undertaken as a group activity over three or four winter weekends. By combining work with a social gathering, fuelled with lots of good food and drink, and perhaps music around a fire in the evening, other non-land-dwelling friends could be encouraged to come and lend a hand. The annual coppicing weekend at Tinker's Bubble usually attracts 10 to 15 visitors, and results in enough wood being cut, using hand tools, to supply the community of twelve adults for a winter.

Untapped sources of experience

My investigation into human energy use has been limited to projects currently operating in the industrialised countries of the United Kingdom and France. I am well aware that whole continents of farmers could teach us about how to manage the land without fossil fuels. In Asia, Africa and South America there are countless examples of land being managed sustainably, using simple technologies, and the people living in those societies have a wealth of experience about how to use their own energy wisely. Closer to home, in Eastern Europe, one can encounter villages where horse-drawn tools are used instead of tractors, and hay is still cut with scythes and turned by hand. These are the people we really need to be studying to learn how to live in a post-peak-oil society.

Such rural societies are under threat from the pressures of modernisation, global agribusiness and bureaucratic legislation.[10] By taking an interest in the skills and experiences of farmers in Southern or East European countries, not only would smallholders in Western countries benefit, but they would provide encouragement to such farmers that there is value in maintaining their traditions. If, rather than being viewed as 'backward peasants', traditional smallholders start to see themselves as repositories of knowledge that holds a key to future survival, they are more likely to resist the powerful pressures to modernise. There is great potential for two-way flows of information through networking, communication and exchanges between smallholders in different countries. I hope that this book will provide a stimulus for further research into how people all over the world sustain their 'human' energy.

Another way we can learn about how people live without oil, is to look to the past. There are still people alive in the UK who can remember the days when labourers and horses worked the land, rather than machines. During the second world war, food security was maintained through the 'Dig for Victory' campaign and the mobilisation of the Women's Land Army. Some older people have fond memories of their days working on the land, whilst others remember endless toil, but many would be willing to share their memories if asked. Especially valuable are the memories held by individuals about particular pieces of land they have worked, and an informal chat with a long-standing local can yield a wealth of information about local climate anomalies, soil conditions and farming traditions.

One piece of advice I would offer to any aspiring smallholder, is to go out and explore the various options yourself. There is nothing like direct experience for showing which models work and appeal to your particular circumstances. Before taking on a piece of land, I would urge anyone to spend at least three years visiting and working on different smallholdings. The first year, I would recommend going on a tour of organic farms through WWOOF, to get an insight into the different ways people operate. I think it would then be worthwhile to spend a couple of years working at one particular holding or community, to get an idea of the full cycle of work through the seasons. There is nothing like seeing a crop through from sowing to harvesting, or getting to know farm animals through daily contact. Staying at one place for two or more years has value, in that it becomes possible to learn from your mistakes, and see improvements, year on year, as your skills develop. Working on a farm or smallholding for a longer period also enables you to become part of the wider community, and can sometimes yield useful contacts when it comes to searching for land. I would, however, encourage readers to look far beyond the case studies featured in this book, so as not to put those farms and communities under undue pressure from visitors. There are many other interesting smallholdings and communities who host visitors through WWOOF or the communities' directory, *Diggers and Dreamers*.[11] and they are usually happy to share their experiences with aspiring smallholders.

Towards high-quality, low-impact lifestyles

People have many reasons for choosing to live and work on the land. One powerful motivation for smallholders, as reflected in my survey (see Table 4.3 p.72), is the desire to address environmental issues through positive action. The environmentally sound provision of food, fuel, timber and other fibres for local people is a direct way of addressing problems such as long-distance transport of goods, biodiversity loss, soil erosion and water pollution. When a land-based livelihood, whether subsistence or commer-cial, is combined with living in a simple, well-insulated house, built from local or recycled materials that uses renewable energy, it is possible for an individual to dramatically reduce their environmental impact. However, for individual action to have significant impact on a national and global scale, to combat climate change and create resilience to 'Peak Oil', there needs to be a major increase in the number of people living in such a way.

There is a general perception that the reduction of our environmental impact requires a drop in our standard of living. In a society where many forms of enjoyment involve the consumption of goods and services, the curtailment of consumption is viewed as tantamount to the loss of quality of life. Yet, those who choose to simplify their lives and become net pro-ducers rather than consumers, experience many improvements to their quality of life. When asked about the main pleasures in their lives, the smallholders in my survey spoke of a sense of achievement, spending more time with their families, having more control over their time, regular access to fresh, home-grown food and a pleasant living/working environment. These, surely, are the features of life that most people ultimately aspire to.

It cannot be denied that such quality of life is hard-won, due to the work involved in earning a land-based livelihood, and the challenges faced in gaining access to land and an affordable home. Furthermore, techno-logical changes that could reduce dependence on fossil fuels, such as replacing machinery with efficient hand tools and animal traction, have to find ways to become commercially competitive in a fossil-fuel-based econ-omy. In this time of adjustment, as we prepare for an age when energy and food are no longer cheap and it is necessary to share limited environmen-tal resources with a growing global population, an element of compromise is necessary. The point at which compromises are made will vary between individuals, according to their values and circumstances, but there is no shame in accepting temporary compromises within a wider context of pos-itive action.

Even Mahatma Gandhi, who is well-known for his strict adherence to vows of simplicity and nonviolence, in his efforts to create a more just society, had a pragmatic approach to life. When his young disciple, Vinoba Bhave, was about to set out and establish a new ashram, Gandhi advised him,

"The beauty of compromise consists in a deed's being done. What are fine words if they are void of thoughts, and what are thoughts if they are void and correspond to no deed? The deed may be small, but it is full. It is far from perfect, but at least it is something done. In order that it may be done, it must limit itself to time, place and people, and compromise with what is there. If the thought inspiring it is perfect, the commonplace deed is a great step and a beautiful compromise. The beauty of it consists in today's compromise being less impure than yesterday's; it consists in our eyes being carried in a straight line towards something beautiful when we look, not at the deeds, but at the direction in which they are set. The work for which you are setting out should consist in living a sane and lasting, and, therefore, a model life, and not in killing yourselves in an out of the ordinary way. Believe me, it is my very love of truth which has taught me the beauty of compromise."[12]

If today's smallholders want to achieve significant, positive environmental change, they also must seek to live a sane and lasting life, which offers a model that will attract other people to increase food production, whilst reducing their environmental impact. The attraction of new smallholders will rely on that model balancing the needs of the environment with the needs of the individual.

Finding such a balance involves a continuous process of compromise, and the balance will change according to both internal and external factors. Internal factors include the development of skills and fitness, which enable people to work longer and more efficiently and perhaps reduce their reliance on machinery. Another internal factor is changing age or role in life, which affects the amount of time or physical effort it is possible to devote to land-based activities. External factors include the changing cultural, economic and technological context. During the past decade there has been a rapid rise in the popularity of local and organic food, as more people have become conscious of environmental and health issues. As the price of oil rises, locally produced, organic food is likely to become more commercially competitive compared with imported, non-organic food. The urgency with which we need to address climate change has provided an enormous spur to the development of cleaner, greener technologies, including agricultural equipment, changing the technological context in which smallholders operate. As Gandhi points out, compromise need not represent a failure to achieve the absolute, but a pragmatic step in the general direction of positive change. If compromises are made consciously, then as external and internal factors change they can be modified.

When the human energy equation (see Table 2.1, p.29) is successfully balanced, the result is a quality of life that is the envy of all. In his account of rural life in the Dordogne region of France in the 1930s, Philip Oyler said that,

"French townspeople do not pity the peasant. Far from it, some show resentment at his having such luxury, others envy him and an enormous number are saving as much and as fast as they can in order to buy a little property of their own."[13]

The situation is not so different in the UK today. Large numbers of people would love to have the opportunity to live simply on a piece of land and produce more of their own food. Furthermore, multiple environmental benefits would arise from a larger proportion of the population becoming involved in the efficient management of the land to meet the basic needs of themselves and their communities. Smallholders of the future will be attracted by models that combine efficient, environmentally sound, economically viable farm management, with a high-quality, low-impact lifestyle and the joy and satisfaction of knowing and working with a piece of land. To sustain the growing movement of people who want to live and work on the land, today's smallholders need to demonstrate that they are not merely surviving, but thriving.

Interview questions

A. Personal Questions
1. Why did you decide to live and work like this?
2. What are the main pleasures you gain from living like this?
3. What are the main worries you have about your life here?
4. How often do you feel too tired or overworked to enjoy your life here?
   Often / Occasionally / Seldom / Never
5. How much time do you spend each week on:
   Survival activities
   Livelihood-based activities
   With family/children
   With friends
   Doing other things you enjoy
   Paperwork
6. Are you satisfied with this balance of activities? If not, why not?
7. How is your health compared to before you were living on the land?
8. How long do you think you will live like this?
9. What would you say are the main advantages of living in a (family/ community/ clustered) set-up compared with the others?
10. What are the main problems you experience in day-to-day life?
11. Would you recommend your set-up to others just setting up a land-based project and what changes would you suggest?
12. How do you and your project relate with mainstream culture?

B. Questions about Projects (i.e. smallholdings, farms or communities)
1. What are the aims of your project?
2. What scale is the project? (How many acres? How many people involved? What animals and crops, and how many?)
3. What is the (brief) history of the project?
4. What are the main income-generating enterprises?
5. What are the main subsistence elements in the project?
6. What fossil-fuel-based technologies (including oil-based products such as black plastic, polytunnel plastic) do you use in managing the farm?
7. What non-fossil-fuel-based technologies do you use (e.g. hand tools, horse-drawn tools)?
8. What energy sources do you use domestically?
9. Which activities are done communally and which independently?
10. What plans do you have for the future of this project?

Resources

Training and Advice

Aprovecho Research Centre
80574 Hazelton Road, Cottage Grove, Oregon 97424, USA
(001) 541-942-8198 www.aprovecho.net
Stove Lab, Aprovecho Research Center, PO Box 156, Creswell, Oregon 97426
www.aprovecho.org
This non-profit research and education organisation focuses on appropriate sustainable technology and land-use practices. They publish books and manuals on how to design many different types of stove for cooking, heating homes and water, including the fuel-efficient 'rocket stove' described in Chapter Seven. They also host a 10-week-long internship programme in sustainable living skills, focusing on sustainable forestry, organic gardening, permaculture, and appropriate technology.

Centre for Alternative Technology
Machynlleth, Powys SY20 9AZ
01654 705950 www.cat.org.uk
Since 1973, the Centre for Alternative Technology has been researching and demonstrating ways to live more sustainably. It disseminates this information via practical displays of renewable energy and organic gardening at its visitor centre, its own publications, a range of weekend and MSc courses and a consultancy service.

Chapter 7
The Potato Store, Flaxdrayton Farm, South Petherton, Somerset TA13 5LR
01460 249204 chapter7@tlio.org.uk
Chapter 7 provides free planning advice on the telephone for smallholders, caravan dwellers and other low-impact and low-income people with planning problems. They have an extensive library of planning documents, and publish a number of useful planning guidance publications of their own. They also publish, *The Land*, a journal addressing land access and planning issues.

Low Impact Living Initiative (LILI)
Redfield Community, Winslow, Bucks, MK18 3LZ
01296 714184 lili@lowimpact.org www.lowimpact.org
LILI offer a range of practical courses for smallholders covering subjects ranging from 'How to set up a low-impact smallholding' to straw-bale building, and heating with wood. They also sell a range of books and equipment, such as solar hot-water kits, natural insulation and eco-paints.

Permaculture Association
BCM Permaculture Association, London WC1N 3XX
0845 4581805 (10am-4pm Monday to Thursday)
office@permaculture.org.uk www.permaculture.org.uk
This is an educational charity which helps people use permaculture in their every-day lives to improve their quality of life and the environment around them. It offers a contact point for a wide variety of permaculture courses, designers and learning materials

Resources for Groups

Catalyst Collective Ltd
Nest Farm, High Street, Ilketshall St Margaret, Bungay, Suffolk NR35 2NA
0845 223 5254 info@catalystcollective.org www.catalystcollective.org
Catalyst Collective is a workers' co-op which offers support and legal advice to other co-operatives. They can help set up and register housing, workers and com-munity co-operatives, and offer legal and financial advice. They can also advise on issuing loan stock as a way to raise finance for co-operative projects.

Community Land Trust Website
Community Finance Solutions, Room 214, Crescent House, The Crescent,
University of Salford M5 4WT
0161 295 4454 www.communitylandtrust.org.uk
This website is a central contact point for all those interested in Community Land Trusts as a solution to affordable housing, amenity and workspace in Britain. It offers a directory of existing CLTs, case studies of how CLTs have been established and open access to legal, financial, business and planning advice for aspiring CLTs.

Radical Routes
16 Sholebroke Avenue, Leeds, West Yorkshire LS7 3HB
0845 330 4510 or 0113 362 9365 www.radicalroutes.org.uk
Radical Routes is a network of co-operatives, seeking to achieve a world based on equality and co-operation. They are working towards taking control over housing, education and work, through setting up housing and worker co-ops and co-operating as a network.

Seeds for Change Network
0845 458 4776   oxford@seedsforchange.org.uk
0845 330 7583   lancaster@seedsforchange.org.uk
This non-profit training co-op helps people organise for action and positive social change, and provides training for grassroots environmental and social justice campaigners.   As well as training people in campaigning skills, Seeds for Change also offers workshops on Consensus Decision-Making, Non-Hierarchical Structures, Facilitation of Meetings and Setting up Co-ops.

Tools and Techniques

British Horse Loggers

Heavy Horses, Hill Farm, Stanley Hill, Bosbury, Ledbury, Herefordshire HR8 1HE
01531 640 236   www.britishhorseloggers.org
British Horse Loggers are an independent group of professional full-time and
part-time contractors who work horses by choice in contemporary forestry.
Membership is also open to enthusiasts and supporters. As well as running a register of professional loggers, they run training and demonstration events.

Cart Horse Machinery

Nant-yr-Hyddod, Cwmduad, Carmarthen SA33 6XB
0044 (0) 1267 281684 www.carthorsemachinery.com
Cart Horse Machinery is the leading specialist manufacturer of modern horse-
drawn equipment in Europe. They manufacture and sell hitch-carts onto which
various cultivation equipment can be connected, including the Pintow Triple
System, which incorporates a 25hp petrol engine, transmission, hydraulic pump
and driver platform. Hence, modern farm machinery, which requires a PTO
input and hydraulic control, such as a baler, can be adapted for use with draught-
horses. They also offer tailor-made courses in how to use the implements and
specialist courses in haymaking, ploughing and logging.

Association PROMMATA

La Gare, 09420 Rimont, France
0033 (0)5 61 96 36 60 www.prommata.org Association.prommata@wanadoo.fr
A small business in south-west France, which makes horse- and donkey-drawn
equipment for use at a variety of scales (market garden, vineyards and field cultivation). They run courses, in French, on how to use the tools they sell.

The Scythe Shop

The Potato Store, Flaxdrayton Farm, South Petherton, Somerset TA13 5LR
01460 249204 www.thescytheshop.co.uk chapter7@tlio.org.uk
A mail-order source of Austrian scythes and other equipment necessary for mowing by hand (sharpening stones, peening equipment). The Scythe Shop also runs
courses in how to use and maintain scythes.

The Scythe Network

The Vido Family, 1636 Kintore Road, Lower Kintore, New Brunswick,
Canada E7H 2L4
(001) 506 273 3010 www.thescytheconnection.com
The Scythe Connection website offers a wealth of information relating to mowing
and haymaking. It contains both technical guidance on choosing, fitting and
maintaining scythes, and articles on haymaking and scythe-related miscellany
from around the world.

Supportive Organisations

Soil Association – Local Food Works
South Plaza, Marlborough Street, Bristol BS1 3NX
0117 314 5000 www.localfoodworks.org
The Soil Association's local food team offer a library of technical guides and
reports, advice on funding for local food producers and community food initiatives, and links to regional local food networks. Their 'Cultivating Communities'
website provides a comprehensive directory of community-supported agriculture
schemes throughout the UK.

Sustain: The Alliance for Better Food and Farming
94 White Lion Street, London N1 9PF. 020 7837 1228 www.sustainweb.org
Sustain publish a variety of reports, run campaigns and initiate projects ranging
from getting local and organic food into schools and hospitals to conserving traditional orchards. They can also advise on funding for local food projects.

WWOOF UK (World Wide Opportunities on Organic Farms)
PO Box 2154, Winslow, Buckinghamshire, MK18 3WS www.wwoof.org
WWOOF is a worldwide exchange network, where bed, board and practical
experience are given in return for work. Stays of varied lengths are possible.
WWOOF provides excellent opportunities for organic training, changing to a
rural life, cultural exchange and being part of the organic movement. Members
of the organisation are provided with a directory of hosts, which range from gardens and smallholdings to larger family farms.

Useful Publications

Diggers and Dreamers: The Guide to Communal Living 2008/2009, edited by
Sarah Bunker, Chris Coates and Jonathan How, Diggers and Dreamers
Publications. *Diggers and Dreamers* is a directory of communities of all
descriptions and also contains articles written by observers of and participants
within the communal living movement.

Permaculture Magazine Permanent Publications, The Sustainability Centre,
East Meon, Hampshire GU32 1HR info@permaculture.co.uk
This quarterly magazine combines pragmatism with inspiration. Subjects covered
range from the practical application of permaculture design to the social and
psychological adjustments necessary to make society more sustainable. It also
contains listings of permaculture courses, Global Ecovillage Network news and
reviews of equipment available through their Green Shopping Catalogue.

Small Farmers Journal SFJ, PO Box 1627 Sisters, Oregon 97759, USA
www.smallfarmersjournal.com
This quarterly journal published in the US is the undisputed source for information about modern horse-drawn tools and farming techniques. It contains long
technical articles and helps promote Horse Progress Days, an annual event held in
the Mid-West to showcase new developments in tools design.

References

Chapter One: The Human Energy Equation

1. Sykes, J.B. (1984). *The Concise Oxford Dictionary*. Seventh Edition. Clarendon Press, Oxford.

2. Jones, M. and Gregory, J. (2001). *Biology 2: Cambridge Advanced Sciences*. Cambridge University Press. p.13.

3. Moore, M. (2000). 'Love and Work in the New Millennium: A vision for personal balance and development'. In *Working towards Balance: Our Society in the New Millennium*. Edited by Harry Bohan and Gerard Kennedy. Veritas.

4. Sustain (2006). *Changing diets, changing minds: How food affects mental health and behaviour*. Sustain: The Alliance for Better Food and Farming, 94 White Lion Street, London, N1 9PF.

5. Whitefield, P. (2004). *The Earthcare Manual: A permaculture handbook for Britain and other temperate countries*. Permanent Publications. p.7.

6. World Wildlife Fund (2004). *Living Planet Report*. p.21.

7. Meadows, D. H., Randers, J. and Meadows, D.I. (2004). *Limits to Growth: The 30-Year Update*. Chelsea Green Publishing.

8. Macy, J. (1991). *World as Lover, World as Self*. Parallax Press. p.220.

9. Ibid. pp.15-28.

Chapter Two: Energy Use through the Ages

1. Tate, W. E. (1967). *The English Village Community and the Enclosure Movements*. Victor Gollancz, London. p.55.

2. Pimentel, D. and Pimentel, M. (1979). *Food, Energy and Society*. Edward Arnold.

3. Ibid.

4. Heinberg R. (2003). *The Party's Over: Oil, war and the fate of Industrial Societies*. Clairview Books.

5. Pimentel, D. and Pimentel, M. (1979). *Food, Energy and Society*. Edward Arnold.

6. Leach, G., (1976). *Energy and Food Production*. IPC Business Press Ltd. p.7.

7. Ibid. p.9.

8. Ibid. p.12.

9. Heinberg, R. (2003). *The Party's Over: Oil, war and the fate of Industrial Societies*. Clairview Books. p.25.

10. Leach, G., (1976). *Energy and Food Production*. IPC Business Press Ltd. p.7.

11. Pimentel, D. and Pimentel, M. (1979). *Food, Energy and Society*. Edward Arnold. p.3.

12. Ibid. p.36.

13. Ibid. p.44.

14. Ibid. p.45.

15. Heinberg, R. (2003). *The Party's Over: Oil, war and the fate of Industrial Societies*. Clairview Books. p.47.

16. Tate, W. E. (1967). *The English Village Community and the Enclosure Movements*. Victor Gollancz, London. p.44

17. Ernle, Lord (1922). *English Farming: Past and Present*. Longmans, Green and Co. p.34.

18. Ibid. p.3.

19. Neeson, J.M. (1993). *Commoners: Common right, enclosure and social change in England, 1700-1820*. Cambridge University Press. p.5.

20. Ibid. p.8.

21. Ernle, Lord (1922). *English Farming: Past and Present*. Longmans, Green and Co. pp.169-172.

22. Jefferies, R. (1892). *Toilers of the Fields*. Longmans, Green and Co. p.51.

23. Ewart Evans, G. (1969). *The Farm and the Village*. Faber and Faber. pp.107-109.

24. Heinberg, R. (2003). *The Party's Over: Oil, war and the fate of Industrial Societies*. Clairview Books. p.51.

25. Pimentel, D. and Pimentel, M. (1979). *Food, Energy and Society*. Edward Arnold.

p.15

26. Leach, G. (1976). *Energy and Food Production*. IPC Business Press Ltd. p.15.

27. Heinberg, R. (2003). *The Party's Over: Oil, war and the fate of Industrial Societies*. Clairview Books. p.55.

28. Heinburg, R. (2003). *The Party's Over: Oil, war and the fate of Industrial Societies*. Clairview Books. pp.57-61.

29. Leach, G. (1976). *Energy and Food Production*. IPC Business Press Ltd. p.18.

30. Smil, V. (2001). *Enriching the Earth: Fritz Haber, Carl Bosch and the Transformation of World Food Production*. MIT Press.

31. Clunies-Ross, T. and Hildyard, N. (1992). *The Politics of Industrial Agriculture*. Earthscan.

32. Pretty, J. (1998). *The Living Land: Agriculture, Food and Community Regeneration in Rural Europe*. Earthscan.

33. Pimentel, D. and Pimentel, M. (1979). *Food, Energy and Society*. Edward Arnold. p.48.

34. Maynard, R. and Green, M. (2006). *Organic Works: Providing more jobs through organic farming and local food supply*. Soil Association, Bristol House, 40-56 Victoria Street, Bristol BS1 6BY. p.22.

35. Heinberg, R. (2003). *The Party's Over: Oil, war and the fate of Industrial Societies*. Clairview Books. p.118.

36. Heinberg R. (2003). *The Party's Over: Oil, war and the fate of Industrial Societies*. Clairview Books. p.171.

37. Maynard, R. (2007). 'One planet farming' in *Living Earth* 229, Spring 2007. p.17.

38. Maynard, R. and Green, M. (2006). *Organic Works: Providing more jobs through organic farming and local food supply*. Soil Association. p.29.

39. Monbiot, G. (2006). *Heat: How we can stop the planet burning*. Penguin Books. p.16.

40. Campbell, C. (2005). 'Understanding Peak Oil' in *Permaculture Magazine* No.46, Winter 2005, pp.3-6.

41. Heinberg, R. (2003). *The Party's Over: Oil, war and the fate of Industrial Societies*. Clairview Books.

42. Pepper (1991). *Communes and the Green Vision: Counterculture, lifestyle and the New Age*. Green Print. p.27.

43. Ibid. p.29.

44. Coates, C. (2007). 'The Chartist Land Colonies' in *The Land*, Spring 2007. pp.30-31.

45. Pepper (1991). *Communes and the Green Vision: Counterculture, lifestyle and the New Age*. Green Print. p.30.

46. Ward, C. (1997). 'Whiteway in the Landscape' in *Diggers and Dreamers 1998/99*, pp.5-19.

47. Bang, J.M. (2005). *Ecovillages: A practical guide to sustainable communities*. Floris Books. pp.16-17.

48. Castelnuovo, R. (2007). 'New York Times Slide Show', 26/08/2007 www.nytimes.com/slideshow.

49. Lanza del Vasto (1974). *Gandhi to Vinoba*. Schocken Books, New York. p.21.

50. Lanza del Vasto (1972). *Return to the Source*. Schocken Books, New York. p.106.

51. Ibid. p.105.

52. Pepper (1991). *Communes and the Green Vision: Counterculture, lifestyle and the New Age*. Green Print. pp.69-70.

53. Gamlin, B. (2000). *The Patchwork History of a Community: Old Hall, East Bergholt*.

54. Jackson, R. (2004). 'The Ecovillage Movement' in *Permaculture Magazine* No.40, Summer 2004. p.25.

55. Bang, J.M. (2005). *Ecovillages: A practical guide to sustainable communities*. Floris Books. p.27.

Chapter Three: The Role of the Modern Smallholder

1. Measures, M. and Azeez, G. (2006). 'Soil Carbon: cause or effect' in *Organic Farming*, Summer 2006. p.24.

2. Ibid. p.25.

3. Pretty, J.N., Ball, A.S., Lang, T. and Morison, J.I.L. (2005). 'Farm Cost and Food Miles: An assessment of the full cost of the UK weekly food basket.' *Food Policy* 30 (1), pp.1-20. p.11.

4. London Food (2006). *Healthy and Sustainable Food for London: The Mayor's Food Strategy*. London Development Agency, 58-60 St Katharine's Way, London EW1 1JX. p.44.

5. Jones, A. (2001). *Eating Oil: Food supply in a changing climate*. Sustain: The Alliance

for better food and farming and Elm Farm Research Centre.

6. Ibid. p.15.

7. Measures, M. and Azeez, G. (2006). 'Soil Carbon: cause or effect' in *Organic Farming*, Summer 2006. p.25.

8. Pretty, J.N., Ball, A.S., Lang, T. and Morison, J.I.L. (2005). 'Farm Cost and Food Miles: An assessment of the full cost of the UK weekly food basket.' *Food Policy* 30 (1), pp.1-20. p.4.

9. Maynard, R. and Green, M. (2006). *Organic Works: Providing more jobs through organic farming and local food supply*. Soil Association. p.28.

10. Ibid. p.31.

11. Lobley, M., Reed, M. and Butler, M. (2005) *The Impact of Organic Farming on the Rural Economy in England. Final Report to DEFRA*. CRR Research Report No.11, Centre for Rural Research, University of Exeter. p.78.

12. Ibid. p.8.

13. Soil Association (2006). 'Growing by 30%' in *Living Earth*, Summer 2006. p.9.

14. Sacks, J. (2002). *The Money Trail: Measuring your impact on the local economy using LM3*. The New Economics Foundation and The Countryside Agency.

15. Rivers, P. (1978). *Living on a Little Land*. Turnstone Books. p.92.

16. DEFRA (2004). *Agriculture in the United Kingdom 2003*. The Stationery Office.

17. Maynard, R. and Green, M. (2006). *Organic Works: Providing more jobs through organic farming and local food supply*. Soil Association. p.23.

18. DEFRA (2004). *Agriculture in the United Kingdom 2003*. The Stationery Office.

19. Lobley, M., Johnson, G. and Reed, M. (2004). *The Rural Stress Review: Final Report*. Centre for Rural Research, Exeter University. p.25.

20. DEFRA (2005). *Agriculture in the United Kingdom 2004*. The Stationery Office.

21. Lobley, M., Johnson, G. and Reed, M. (2004) *The Rural Stress Review: Final Report*. Centre for Rural Research, Exeter University. p.51.

22. Office for National Statistics (2006). *Proportional mortality rates for suicide and undetermined injury in farmers etc. Persons aged 20-75 England and Wales 1993-2004*.

23. DEFRA (2005). *Agriculture in the United Kingdom 2004*. The Stationery Office.

24. Maynard, R. and Green, M. (2006). *Organic Works: Providing more jobs through organic farming and local food supply*. Soil Association. p.51.

25. Lobley, M., Reed, M. and Butler, M. (2005). *The Impact of Organic Farming on the Rural Economy in England. Final Report to DEFRA*. CRR Research Report No.11, Centre for Rural Research, University of Exeter. p.118.

26. Lovelock, J. (2006). *The Revenge of Gaia*. Penguin/Allen Lane. p.133.

27. Pretty, J.N., Ball, A.S., Lang, T. and Morison, J.I.L. (2005). 'Farm Cost and Food Miles: An assessment of the full cost of the UK weekly food basket.' *Food Policy* 30 (1), pp.1-20. p.9.

28. Maynard, R. and Green, M. (2006). *Organic Works: Providing more jobs through organic farming and local food supply*. Soil Association, p.48.

29. Fairlie, S. (2007). 'Can Britain Feed Itself?' in *The Land*, Issue 4, Winter 2007-2008. pp.19-26.

30. Maynard, R. and Green, M. (2006). *Organic Works: Providing more jobs through organic farming and local food supply*. Soil Association. p.25.

31. Liebman, M. (1998). 'Polyculture Cropping Systems' in Altieri, M.A. *Agroecology: The Science of Sustainable Agriculture*. IT Publications. p.206.

32. Maynard, R. and Green, M. (2006). *Organic Works: Providing more jobs through organic farming and local food supply*. Soil Association. p.48.

33. IGD (2006). 'Brits spend £13 billion on posh nosh'. www.igd.com/asp?menuid=9&cirid=2085.

34. Mintel (2006). 'Planet Ark: Green is the New Black in Ethical Britain'. www.planetark.com/dailynewsstory.cfm/new sid/38498/story.htm, October 13th, 2006.

35. DEFRA (2005). *Organic Statistics: United Kingdom*. National Statistics, September 2006. p.2.

36. Ibid. p.4.

37. IGD (2006). 'Brits spend £13 billion on posh nosh'. www.igd.com/asp?menuid=9&cirid=2085.

38. Soil Association (2006c). *Organic Market Report*. Soil Association.

39. Institute of Science in Society (2004). 'Corporate Hijack of Sustainable Agriculture'. ISIS press release, November 16th 2004.

40. www.journeytoforever.org/farm.html.

41. *New Scientist*, 12th July 2007. 'Organic farming could feed the world'. Environment Page.

42. Institute of Science in Society. Press Release, November 16th 2004. Editors note, 'Corporate hi-jack of sustainable agriculture'.

43. Rosset, P. (1999). 'The multiple functions and benefits of small farm agriculture: in the context of Global Trade Negotiations'. Policy Brief No.4, Food First, The Institute for Food and Development Policy, Oakland, California, USA. p.7.

44. Rosset, P. (1999). Ibid. p.11.

45. Dawson, J. (2007). 'The Path to Surviving Peak Oil: The Power of Community'. *Permaculture Magazine* No.54, pp.42-45.

46. Lovelock, J. (2006) *The Revenge of Gaia*. Penguin/Allen Lane. p.133.

Chapter Five: Energy-efficient Design

1. Mollison, B. (1988). *Permaculture: A designer's manual*. Tagari Publications, Tyalgum, Australia. p.ix.

2. Whitefield, P. (2004). *The Earthcare Manual: A permaculture handbook for Britain and other temperate countries*. Permanent Publications. p.375.

3. Ibid. p.27.

4. Open University Systems Group (1981). Systems Behaviour. Third Edition. Harper and Row.

5. Spedding, C. (1994). 'Farming Systems Research/Extension in the European Context' in *Rural and farming systems analysis: European perspectives*, Dent, J.B. and McGregor, M.J. (Eds). CAB International.

6. Reijntjes, C., Haverkort, B. and Waters-

Bayer, A. (1992). *Farming for the Future: An introduction to low external input agriculture*. Macmillan. p.4.

7. Lampkin, N. (1990). *Organic Farming*. Farming Press. p.5.

8. Whitefield, P. (2004). *The Earthcare Manual: A permaculture handbook for Britain and other temperate countries*. Permanent Publications. p.13.

9. Mollison, B. (1988). *Permaculture: A designer's manual*. Tagari Publications, Tyalgum, Australia.

10. Whitefield, P. (2004). *The Earthcare Manual: A permaculture handbook for Britain and other temperate countries*. Permanent Publications. p.32.

11. Ibid. p.56.

12. Mollison, B. (1988) *Permaculture: A designer's manual*. Tagari Publications, Tyalgum, Australia. p.90.

13. Clements, B. and Donaldson, G. (1997). 'Clover and Cereals: Low Input Bi-Cropping' in *Farming and Conservation*, Vol. 3, No. 4.

14. Whitefield, P. (2004). *The Earthcare Manual: A permaculture handbook for Britain and other temperate countries*. Permanent Publications. p.268.

15. Fukuoka, Masanobu (1978). *The One Straw Revolution*. Rodale.

16. Whitefield, P. (2004). *The Earthcare Manual: A permaculture handbook for Britain and other temperate countries*. Permanent Publications. pp.272-273.

17. Piper, Jon K. (1993). 'A Grain Agriculture Fashioned in Nature's Image: The Work of the Land Institute' in *Great Plains Research*, 3 (August 1993). Available from Land Institute, 2440E.Water Well Road, Salina, KS 67401, USA.

Chapter Six: Wise Choice of Tools

1. Coleman, E. (1995). *The New Organic Grower: A master's manual of tools and techniques for the home and market gardener*. Chelsea Green Publishing. p.159.

2. Ibid. p.167.

3. Vido, P. (2001) 'The Scythe Must Dance: An addendum on the practical use of the scythe' in *The Scythe Book* by David Tresemer. Alan C. Hood and Co., Inc. p.124.

4. Ibid. p.174.

5. Tresemer, D. (2001). *The Scythe Book: Mowing hay, cutting weeds and harvesting small grains with hand tools*. Alan C. Hood and Company, Inc, Pennsylvannia. pp.20-24.

6. Ibid. p.32.

7. Vido, P. (2001). 'The Scythe Must Dance: An addendum on the practical use of the scythe' in *The Scythe Book* by David Tresemer. Alan C. Hood and Company, Inc. p.162.

8. Tresemer, D. (2001). *The Scythe Book: Mowing hay, cutting weeds and harvesting small grains with hand tools*. Alan C. Hood and Company, Inc, Pennsylvannia. p.46.

9. Bowden, C. (2002). *The Last Horsemen: A year at Sillywrea, Britain's only horse-powered farm*. Granada Media.

10. Castle, W. (2006). 'Horses and machines: Getting the job done'. *Heavy Horse World*, Autumn 2006, pp.52-56.

11. Personal communication with Doug Joiner, Chair of British Horse Loggers, Heavy Horses, Hill Farm, Stanley Hill, Bosbury, Ledbury, Herefordshire HR8 1HE (www.britishhorseloggers.org).

12. Johnstone, J. (2006). 'Horselogging: Learning lessons from abroad' in *Reforesting Scotland Journal – Rethinking Energy*, Issue 35 Autumn/Winter 2006. pp.37-38.

13. Oyler, P. (1950). *The Generous Earth*. Hodder and Stoughton. p.154.

14. Lanza del Vasto (1972). *Return to the Source*. Schocken Books, New York. p.111.

15. Pimentel, D. and Pimentel, M. (1979). *Food, Energy and Society*. Edward Arnold. p.13.

16. Lanza del Vasto (1974). *Gandhi to Vinoba*. Schocken Books, New York. p.40.

17. Lanza del Vasto (1972). *Return to the Source*. Schocken Books, New York. pp.107-108.

18. Ibid. p.111.

19. Parel, A.J. (1997). *Hind Swaraj and other writings*. Cambridge University Press. p.173.

20. Armstrong, P. and Feldman, S. (2006). *A Midwife's Story*. Pinter and Martin Ltd.

21. Pattison, S. (2006). Letter to *Heavy Horse World Magazine*, Winter 2006, p.60.

22. Castle, W. (2006). 'Horses and machines: Getting the job done'. Article No. 8 – Charlie Pinney at Nant-yr-Hyddod, Carmarthen. *Heavy Horse World*, Summer 2006, pp.22-27. p.26.

23. Armstrong, P. and Feldman, S. (2006). *A Midwife's Story*. Pinter and Martin Ltd. p.114.

24. Ibid. p.171.

25. Monbiot, G. (2006). *Heat: How to stop the planet burning*. Penguin/Allen Lane. p.158.

26. Fairlie, S. (2006). 'Biofuel, Horsepower and Hectares' in *The Land*, Summer 2006. The Potato Store, Flaxdrayton Farm, South Petherton, Somerset TA13 5LR. p.13.

27. Monbiot, G. (2006). *Heat: How to stop the planet burning*. Penguin/Allen Lane. p.159.

28. Elsayed, M. A. et al. (2003). *Carbon and Energy Balances for a Range of Biofuel Options*. Sheffield Hallam, for DTI Sustainable Energy Programme.

29. Fairlie, S. (2006) 'Biofuel, Horsepower and Hectares' in *The Land*, Summer 2006. The Potato Store, Flaxdrayton Farm, South Petherton, Somerset TA13 5LR. p.14.

30. Ibid.

Chapter Seven: Domestic Energy

1. Wrench, T. (2001). *Building a Low Impact Roundhouse*. Permanent Publications. Or see Tony Wrench's website at www.thatroundhouse.info.

2. Whitefield, P. (2004). *The Earthcare Manual: A permaculture handbook for Britain and other temperate countries*. Permanent Publications. p.148.

3. Ibid. p.152.

4. Ibid. p.304.

5. Roth, J. (2006). 'Yes it is Rocket Science' in *Permaculture Magazine* No.47, Spring 2006, pp.41-42.

6. www.aprovecho.net.

7. www.greenpowerindia.org/biomass.

8. www.practicalaction.org/ ?id=biogas_christmas.

9. Seymour, J. (1981). *The Complete Book of Self-Sufficiency*. Corgi Books. p.218.

10. Blackaby, A. (2008) 'Power from the People: Why Germany leads the way in

Microgeneration' in *Permaculture Magazine* No. 55, Spring 2008. pp.37-40.

Chapter Eight: Livelihood Strategies

1. Rivers, P. (1978). *Living on a Little Land*. Turnstone Books. p.34
2. National Statistics (2007). *Households spend on average £443 per week: Family spending – The results of the expenditure and food survey 2005/06*, January 18th 2007. www.statistics.gov.uk/pdfdir/efs0107.pdf.
3. Armstrong, P. and Feldman, S. (2006). *A Midwife's Story*. Pinter and Martin Ltd. p.171.
4. Oyler, P. (1950). *The Generous Earth*. Hodder and Stoughton. pp.157-158.
5. Catalyst Collective (2007). 'Loan stock for housing co-ops'. www.catalystcollective.org.
6. Conaty, P., Birchall, J., Bendle, S. and Foggitt, R. (2003). *Common Ground: for Mutual Home Ownership*. New Economics Foundation and CDS Co-operatives. p.16.
7. Kunstler, J. (1993). *The Geography of Nowhere*. Simon and Schuster. pp.268-272.
8. See www.communitylandtrust.org.uk.
9. Conaty, P., Birchall, J., Bendle, S. and Foggitt, R. (2003). *Common Ground: for Mutual Home Ownership*. New Economics Foundation and CDS Co-operatives. p.17.

Chapter Nine: Living and Working Together

1. La Borie Noble (2007). Leaflet about the Community of the Ark at La Borie Noble.
2. Seymour, J. and Sutherland, W. (2003). *The New Complete Book of Self-Sufficiency*. Dorling Kindersley, London. p.289.
3. Pembrokeshire County Council (2006). Supplementary Planning Guidance: Low impact development making a positive contribution. Joint Unitary Development Plan for Pembrokeshire, Policy 52. Adopted by Pembrokeshire Coast National Park Authority (May 24th 2006) and Pembrokeshire County Council (June 26th 2006).
4. Pilley, G. (2000). *A Share in the Harvest: A feasibility study for community-supported agriculture*. Soil Association. p.6.

Chapter Ten: Together or Alone?

1. Lobley, M., Johnson, G., Reed, M., Winter, M. and Little, J. (2004). *Rural Stress Review: Final Report*. Centre for Rural Research, University of Exeter, p.16.
2. Gamlin, B. (2000). *The Patchwork History of a Community Growing Up: Old Hall, East Bergholt, Suffolk*. Privately published. p.41-46.
3. Hrdy, S. B. (2006). 'Meet the Alloparents' in *New Scientist*. 8th April 2006, pp.50-51.
4. Jackson, H. (2007). 'Children and Housing: The birth of an international movement' in *Permaculture Magazine* No. 52, pp.27-29.
5. Pretty, J. (1998). *The Living Land: Agriculture, food and community regeneration in Rural Europe*. Earthscan. p.8.
6. Pepper, D. (1991). *Communes and the Green Vision: Counterculture, lifestyle and the New Age*. Green Print. p.142.
7. Macy, J. (1991). *World as Lover, World as Self*. Parallax Press. p.12.
8. Gamlin, B. (2000). *The Patchwork History of a Community Growing Up: Old Hall, East Bergholt, Suffolk*. Privately published. p.94.
9. Leafe Christian, D. (2003). *Creating a Life Together: Practical tools to grow ecovillages and communities*. New Society Publishers. p.201.
10. Rosenburg, M. B. (2003). *Nonviolent Communication: A language of life*. Puddledancer Press, California.
11. Scott Peck, M. (1990). *A Different Drum: The creation of true community – the first step to world peace*. Rider. p.257.
12. Ibid. pp.86-106.
13. Ibid. p.103.
14. Ibid. p.234.
15. Wood, A. (1997). 'Pecking at the Group Process' in *Diggers and Dreamers: The guide to communal living 1998/99*. D&D Publications. pp.86-92.
16. Leafe Christian, D. (2003). *Creating a Life Together: Practical tools to grow ecovillages and communities*. New Society Publishers. Chapter 17.
17. Scott Peck, M. (1990). *A Different Drum: The creation of true community – the first step to world peace*. Rider. p.220.

Chapter Eleven: The Seven Ages of Men and Women

1. Lobley, M., Reed, M., Butler, M.;Courtney, P. and Warren, M. (2005). *The Impact of Organic Farming on the Rural Economy in England*. CRR Research Report No.11, Centre for Rural Research, University of Exeter. p.34.

2. Maynard, R. and Green, M. (2006). *Organic Works: Providing more jobs through organic farming and food supply*. The Soil Association. pp.51-52.

3. Office of the Deputy Prime Minister. *Planning Policy Statement 7: Sustainable Development in Rural Areas. Annex A: Agricultural, forestry and other occupational dwellings.*

4. Hrdy, S. B. (2006). 'Meet the Alloparents' in *New Scientist*, 8th April 2006, pp.50-51.

5. Lobley, M., Reed, M., Butler, M., Courtney, P. and Warren, M. (2005). *The Impact of Organic Farming on the Rural Economy in England*. CRR Research Report No.11, Centre for Rural Research, University of Exeter. p.47.

6. Jefferies, R. (1892). *Toilers of the Fields*. Longmans, Green and Co. p.31.

7. Lobley, M., Reed, M., Butler, M., Courtney, P. and Warren, M. (2005). *The Impact of Organic Farming on the Rural Economy in England*. CRR Research Report No.11, Centre for Rural Research, University of Exeter. p.46.

8. Lobley, M., Johnson, G., Reed, M., Winter, M. and Little, J. (2004). *Rural Stress Review – Final Report*. Centre for Rural Research, University of Exeter. pp.34-35.

9. Padel, S. (2001). 'Conversion to Organic Farming: A typical example of the diffusion of an innovation' in *Sociologia Ruralis* 41(1), pp.40-62.

10. Lobley, M., Reed, M., Butler, M., Courtney, P. and Warren, M. (2005). *The Impact of Organic Farming on the Rural Economy in England*. CRR Research Report No.11, Centre for Rural Research, University of Exeter. p.46.

Chapter Twelve: Siestas and Fiestas

1. O'Donohue, J. (1997). *Anam Cara: Spiritual wisdom from the Celtic world*. Bantam Books.

2. Lanza del Vasto (1943). *Return to the Source*. Denoel, Paris. pp.108-109.

3. Jones, T. (2007). *Utopian Dreams: In search of a good life*. Faber and Faber. p.66.

4. Louf, D.A. (1983). *The Cistercian Alternative*. Gill and Macmillan, Dublin.

5. Jones, T. (2007). *Utopian Dreams: In search of a good life*. Faber and Faber. p.150.

6. O'Donohue, J. (1997). *Anam Cara: Spiritual wisdom from the Celtic world*. Bantam Books. p.194.

7. Rivers, P. (1978). *Living on a Little Land*. Turnstone Books, London. p.78.

8. Rosenburg, M.B. (2003). *Nonviolent Communication: A language of life*. Puddledancer Press, California.

9. Kindred, G. (1993). *The Earth's Cycle of Celebration*. Distributed by Counter Culture BCM Inspire, London, WC1 3XX.

10. Rivers, P. (1978). *Living on a Little Land*. Turnstone Books, London. p.19.

11. Rosenburg, M.B. (2003). *Nonviolent Communication: A language of life*. Puddledancer Press, California. pp.135-136.

12. Rivers, P. (1978). *Living on a Little Land*. Turnstone Books, London. p.79.

13. Oyler, P. (1950). *The Generous Earth*. Hodder and Stoughton. p.115.

14. Johnstone, C. (2006). *Find Your Power*. Nicholas Brealey Publishing. p.268.

15. Portman, A. and E. (2001). 'Gardening the Self: The heart of permaculture' in *Permaculture Magazine* No. 29, Autumn 2001. pp.46-49.

Chapter Thirteen: Surviving or Thriving?

1. Sykes, J.B. (1984). *The Concise Oxford Dictionary*. Clarendon Press. p.1075.

2. 4th World Ecological Design (2008). *Ecological Footprint Report for Residents of Steward Wood*. June 2008. 4th World Ecological Design, Keveral Farm, St. Martins, Looe, Cornwall PL3 1PA.

3. Howse, M. (2007). *Steward Community Woodland: Carbon Audit*. www.stewardwood.org.

4. Office of the Deputy Prime Minister. *Planning Policy Statement 7: Sustainable*

Development in Rural Areas. Annex A: Agricultural, forestry and other occupational dwellings.

5. Catalyst Collective (2007). 'Loan stock for housing co-ops'. www.catalystcollective.org.

6. Office of the Deputy Prime Minister. *Planning Policy Statement 7: Sustainable Development in Rural Areas.* p.1.

7. Original 'Fifteen Criteria for Sustainable Development' in The Rural Planning Group of Land is Ours (1999), *Defining Rural Sustainability*. Published by TLIO, but now out of print. A shorter version can be found in *Sustainable Homes and Livelihoods in the Countryside* by the PPG7 Reform Group (1999), published by Chapter 7, The Potato Store, Flaxdrayton Farm, South Petherton, Somerset TA13 5LR.

8. Fairlie, S. (2008). 'The Nature of Manual Skill' in *The Land*, Issue 5, Summer 2008. pp.39-41. The Potato Store, Flaxdrayton Farm, South Petherton, Somerset TA13 5LR.

9. Whitefield, P. (2004). 'Of Minimalism and Human Kind' in *Permaculture Magazine*, No.42, p.29.

10. Rose, J. (2008). 'Horsepower, peasants and politics in Poland' in *The Land*, Issue 5, Summer 2008, pp.47-49. The Potato Store, Flaxdrayton Farm, South Petherton, Somerset TA13 5LR.

11. Bunker, S., Coates, C. and How, J. (2008). *Diggers and Dreamers: The guide to communal living*. Diggers and Dreamers Publications.

12. Lanza del Vasto (1974). *Gandhi to Vinoba: The New Pilgrmage*. Schocken Books, New York. p.63.

13. Oyler, P. (1950). *The Generous Earth*. Hodder and Stoughton.

Index

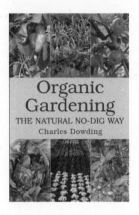
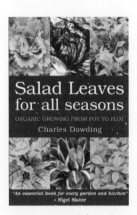